SEXUAL ORIENTATION AND
PSYCHODYNAMIC PSYCHOTHERAPY

SEXUAL ORIENTATION AND PSYCHODYNAMIC PSYCHOTHERAPY

Sexual Science and Clinical Practice

Richard C. Friedman

Jennifer I. Downey

COLUMBIA UNIVERSITY PRESS

NEW YORK

COLUMBIA UNIVERSITY PRESS

Publishers Since 1893

New York   Chichester, West Sussex

Copyright © 2002 Columbia University Press

Library of Congress Cataloging-in-Publication Data
Friedman, Richard C.
   Sexual orientation and psychodynamic psychotherapy :
sexual science and clinical practice / Richard C.
Friedman, Jennifer I. Downey.
         p.   cm.
Includes bibliographical references and index.
   ISBN 978-0-231-12056-2 (cloth : alk. paper)
   ISBN 978-0-231-12057-9 (pbk. : alk. paper)
   1. Psychoanalysis—Practice.   2. Sexual orientation.
I. Downey, Jenifer I.   II. Title.
   RC506
   616.89'17—dc21
                              2002022512

Columbia University Press books are printed on
permanent and durable acid-free paper.
Printed in the United States of America

c 10 9 8 7 6 5 4 3 2 1
p 10 9 8 7 6 5 4 3 2 1

To our patients

Contents

Preface to the Paperback Edition

This book was originally written to further understanding and psychotherapeutic treatment of nonheterosexual individuals. Psychological problems and mental disorders common in the general population are even more prevalent among gay and lesbian persons, a problem of major concern. (Cochran, Mays, and Sullivan, 2003). One reason for this is minority stress, but another equally important reason is internalized homophobia. Adverse experiences of nonheterosexual children with authority figures, family members, and peers may have longstanding painful effects that are conscious and unconscious. When this occurs, self-esteem and security suffer even when the person finds his or her way to positive environments later in life. The long-standing unconscious effects of internalized homophobia may cause chronic anxiety, depression, and impairment in the capacity to work and love (Friedman and Downey, 2007).

The psychological developmental pathways of men and women differ, and in the first part of this book we explain why this difference is crucial for understanding the clinical issues we discuss later. Although some of these issues are similar for gay men and lesbians, some are not. The asymmetrical development of boys and girls, men and women, helps explain these differences.

We have made an effort throughout the book to base our conclusions on sexual science. Since the first edition of this book was published in 2002, additional animal research further supports evidence of the influence of the hypothalamus on sexual orientation (Roselli et al., 2004). Although definitive proof of this in humans is still lacking, it now seems even more likely than before that prenatal neuroendocrine influences shape sexual orientation in some people (LeVay and Valente, 2006).

The title of the original book was changed to emphasize the fact that the therapeutic applications of the psychodynamic principles we discuss are most widely used in psychotherapy rather than psychoanalysis. Throughout the book we note where psychodynamic or psychoanalytic theories need to change in order to align with contemporary scientific knowledge of the brain and sexual behavior.

References

Cochran, S. D., Mays, V. M., and J. G. Sullivan. 2003. Prevalence of mental disorders, psychological distress, and mental health services use among lesbian, gay, and bisexual adults in the United States. *Journal of Consulting Clinical Psycholology* 71(1):53–61.

Friedman, R. C., and J. I. Downey. 2007. Sexual orientation: Neuroendocrine and psychodynamic influences. *Psychiatric Times* 24(9):47–52.

LeVay, S., and S. M. Valente. 2006. *Human Sexuality.* 2d ed. Sunderland, MA: Sinauer.

Roselli, C. E., K. Larkin, J. A. Resko, J. N. Stellfrug, and F. Stormshak. 2004. The volume of a sexually dimorphic nucleus in the ovine medial preoptic area/anterior hypothalamus varies with sexual partner preference. *Endocrinology* 145:478–483.

Acknowledgments

In doing this work we found meetings of the International Academy of Sex Research as well as of the American Psychoanalytic Association, American Academy of Psychoanalysis, and the American College of Psychoanalysts thought provoking and informative. Drs. Kenneth Zucker, Stefan Stein, and Zira DeFries read the manuscript in early stages and provided many helpful suggestions. The book was read in later stages by Drs. Otto Kernberg, Michael Stone, John Oldham, Stuart Yudofsky, and Harold Lief, and their input, both then and through the years when we were developing our ideas, has been invaluable. We are thankful for Drs. Joseph and Judith Schachter's helpful responses to our work as well. The many psychiatric residents, psychoanalytic candidates, and graduate students in psychology we have taught have been a constant source of stimulation and professional enjoyment.

It would not have been possible to carry out this project without the vital assistance of David Lane and Luis Minaya of the Library at the New York State Psychiatric Institute and Columbia University. Our manuscript assistant, Harriet Ayers, has been a crucial member of our team from beginning to end. We are most grateful to Susan Pensak and John Michel, our editors at Columbia University Press.

Finally, throughout years of scholarly effort, our families have provided unending support, for which we are especially grateful.

The following articles were either reprinted or quoted generously, with permission.

Friedman, R. C. and A. A. Lilling. 1996. An empirical study of the beliefs of psychoanalysts about scientific and clinical dimensions of homosexuality. *Journal of Homosexuality* 32:79–89.

Friedman, R. C. and J. Downey, 1993. Neurobiology and sexual orientation: Current relationships. *Journal of Neuropsychiatry and Clinical Neurosciences* 5:131–153.

Friedman, R. C. and J. Downey, 1994. Special Article: Homosexuality. *New England Journal of Medicine* 331:923–930.

Friedman, R. C. and J. Downey, 1995a. Biology and the Oedipus complex. *Psychoanalytic Quarterly* LXIV:234–264.

Downey, J. Counseling homophobic parents of gay and lesbian young adults. *Academy Forum* 40(3):12–15, 1996.

Friedman, R. C. and J. Downey, 1993. Constitutional bisexuality reconsidered. *Academy Forum* 34(4):9–12.

Friedman, R. C. and J. I. Downey, 1998. Psychoanalysis and the model of homosexuality as psychopathology: An historical overview. *American Journal of Psychoanalysis* 58(3):249–270.

Friedman, R. C. 1998. Internalized homophobia, pathological grief, and high-risk sexual behavior in a gay man with multiple psychiatric disorders. *Journal of Sex Education and Therapy* 23(2):115–120.

Friedman, R. C. and J. I. Downey, 1999. Internalized homophobia and gender-valued self-esteem in the psychoanalysis of gay patients. *Psychoanalytic Review* 86:325–347.

Friedman, R. C. and J. I. Downey, 2000. The psychobiology of late childhood: Significance for psychoanalytic developmental theory and clinical practice. *Journal of the American Academy of Psychoanalysis* 28(3):431–448.

Downey, J. I. and R. C. Friedman. 1995. Internalized homophobia in lesbian relationships. *Journal of the American Academy of Psychoanalysis* 23:435–447.

Friedman, R. C. and J. I. Downey, 1995. Internalized homophobia and the negative therapeutic reaction in homosexual men. *Journal of the American Academy of Psychoanalysis* 23:99–113.

We are also grateful to have obtained permission from Lippincott, Williams and Wilkins, and Virginia Johnson to reprint figures on pages 10 and 11 illustrating the male and female sexual response cycle.

SEXUAL ORIENTATION AND
PSYCHODYNAMIC PSYCHOTHERAPY

Part One

Theoretical / Developmental

Introduction to Part 1

This book, written for psychoanalytically oriented psychotherapists, is divided into two parts, scientific/theoretical and clinical. The sections may be read independently or in reverse order. Clinicians working with gay patients who wish to focus on the treatment of internalized homophobia, for example, may wish to get directly to the clinical part of the book and return to the more scientific/theoretical section at leisure. The authors are psychiatrist-psychoanalysts, graduates of the Center for Psychoanalytic Studies of Columbia University, and engaged in the practice of psychoanalysis and psychoanalytically oriented psychotherapy in New York City.

Many traditionally trained psychodynamically oriented clinicians have remained wedded to concepts we now know require revision in light of a knowledge explosion in extra-analytic fields. Our goal in writing the first part of this book was to build bridges between psychoanalysis and these other disciplines. We could not be all inclusive and while respecting the importance of anthropological and sociological research, we focused on other areas. We attempted to integrate selected aspects of extrapsychoanalytic research in genetics and psychoendocrinology, psychological development, and sexology with psychoanalytic theory. Consideration of research from these disciplines, in addition to psychoanalytic observations, results in rich, complex, and empirically supported paradigms of female and male development.

Although Freud's insights about sexual functioning were at the center of psychoanalysis at its inception, the field seems to have moved further and further away from discussion of human sexuality. Much of our emphasis in the first part of this volume is on distinguishing Freud's observations and speculations that remain useful today from those that have not stood the test of time. We particularly emphasize his theory of the Oedipus complex in that regard.

Among the most important revisions in psychoanalytic, developmental, and clinical theories in recent years are those pertaining to homosexual orientation. Discussion of psychoanalytic psychology and homosexuality, because of political controversy, has sometimes been difficult. Throughout this book we stress the need for healthy scholarly inquiry into controversial areas that are often plagued by heated ideological and political debates.

Psychoanalytically oriented psychotherapists are faced with the same challenges as everyone else in adapting to a rapidly changing world in which new networks of information organization and transfer emerge day by day. On the one hand, the analytic couch, both symbolically and as a practical therapeutic modality, seems to us to remain as vital as, for example, Shakespeare's plays. On the other hand, modern developments seem to support the wisdom of those analysts who presciently argued for the usefulness of a systems approach to the understanding of human behavior, at a time when it was not entirely fashionable to do so (Engel 1977). In that respect, recent observations by Thomas Friedman, a social and political critic, seem particularly apt:

> When dealing with any non-linear system, especially a complex one, you can't just think in terms of parts or aspects and just add things up and say that the behavior of this and behavior of that added together makes the whole thing. With a complex non-linear system you have to break it up into pieces and then study each aspect and then study the very strong interaction between them all. Only this way can you describe the whole system. *(Friedman 1999:28)*

The material we discuss in the following chapters is best viewed from the perspective of a complex systems approach, with interactions occurring at many levels of organization from single cells to large social groups.

1

Sexual Fantasies in Men and Women

A major theme of this volume is that males and females develop along different pathways. There are many reasons for thinking this, including the psychoanalytic treatment and study of gay men and lesbians. The brains of men and women are differentially influenced in utero by sex steroid hormones. This difference influences psychological development in many ways. The minds of boys and girls, men and women, develop differently; and important aspects of sexual experience and activity are unique to each sex and not shared by the other. Sexual orientation of any type—homosexual, heterosexual, or bisexual—is best conceptualized as part of the psychology of men or the psychology of women. Sadly, both lesbians and gay men are often discriminated against because of their homosexual orientation. The reasons for and manifestations of this, however, differ by gender. Sex differences in the causes and consequences of homophobia are discussed throughout this book.

We focus on sexual fantasy in this chapter because of its central role in sexual orientation, motivation, and psychoanalytic psychology. It is helpful as a point of departure to be aware of psychoanalytic observations about general aspects of fantasy.

Characteristics of Fantasy

Freud suggested that daydreams—or fantasies—were a continuation of childhood play: "The growing child when he stops playing, gives up nothing but the link with real objects; instead of playing he now phantasizes. He builds castles in the air and creates what are called day dreams" (1907, cited in Gay 1989:439). Person has pointed out that fantasies are a type of imaginative thought that serves many different functions (Person 1995). As Freud observed, they may represent wishes evoked in response to frustration in order to convert negative feelings into pleasureful ones. Fantasies may also soothe, enhance security, and bolster self-esteem or repair a sense of having been abandoned or rejected. Fantasies may (temporarily) repair more profound damage to the sense of self that occurs as a result of severe trauma. They also frequently serve role rehearsal functions, as occurs, for example, in little girls who consider dolls to be their "babies" and play "house" as preparation for becoming adult homemakers. Organized as images, metaphors, and dramatic action, fantasies in the form of artistic productions and mythology have been part of the human heritage probably for the entire life of our species. Freud provided a new framework for understanding these universal forms of human expression by noting that they could be critically analyzed like all other products of the mind.

The Meanings of Fantasy: Conscious and Unconscious

The story line of a fantasy, meaningful in itself, also symbolically expresses additional hidden meanings. Underneath one narrative is another, and under that yet another, arranged in layers as is the mind itself. A fundamental discovery of Freud's and one that remains valid today (unlike many of his ideas about human sexuality) is that some aspects of mental functioning are not subject to conscious recall and that even when unconscious, they may influence motivation. Connections between conscious and unconscious thoughts, feelings, memories occur in the form of "associations." Just as neural networks exist in the brain, so do psychic networks in the mind, although the precise correspondences between the two has not been clarified (Freud 1900, 1915–1916, 1916–1917; Olds 1994). Freud termed his unique method of exploring the pathways of these connections psychoanalysis. His initial explorations in his self-analysis carried out at the end of the nineteenth century led to the recognition that the closer one comes to mental processes that are out of awareness, the more the rules governing mental organization appear to change. Whereas the thinking processes of our ordinary daily life are more or less "logical," unconscious mentation seems to be organized more like dreams. In dreams many ideas, memories, and feelings may be represented by a single image. For example, a grandfather clock may represent the passage of time, one's grandfather, a special occasion upon which the grandfather clock was purchased, a meaningful past residence that had a grandfather clock, and so on. The narrative line of a dream consists of strings of such symbols and emotions that may or may not be ordinarily connected with the images as usually experienced during waking life, all arranged without regard to ordinary time/space rules of the physical universe. For example, someone may dream that a long dead parent was riding a horse and experience in the dream an unaccountable feeling of terror. Or that he was playing in a tennis match even though he had never learned tennis. In dreams anyone can be anyone—man, woman, or child, or even nonhuman—and all is possible. Anything that the mind can imagine can occur in a dream. Freud termed the organization of the unconscious part of the mind the primary process and contrasted it with the secondary process—the system of organization of ordinary, everyday thinking (Freud 1900). A perspective about fantasy unique to psychoanalytic psychology is that beneath the immediately coherent narrative line of waking fantasy are disguised stories that carry hidden meanings. These latent narratives consist of memories of real and imagined events linked in the imagination of the present. Since single symbols can represent multiple meanings, the amount of information carried by sequences of symbols is obviously vast. Beneath the apparently clear meaning of a specific fantasy, therefore, are networks of other meanings.

Another core psychoanalytic idea is that one reason that some story lines are unconscious is that they contain wishes that are unacceptable to the conscience. The mind has the capacity to erase from its awareness certain unpleasant ideas but not the power to completely eliminate their motivational force. For example, a patient dined with a disliked business competitor. Early in their talk he thought: "This guy is such a pain in the neck I wish he would drop dead"—and later "I need this conversation like a hole in the head." That night he dreamt he was riding in a stagecoach with a masked stranger. Pulled by huge black horses, the coach entered a dense forest. Suddenly the stranger pulled off his mask. It was Dracula! The patient pulled a long pencil from the inner pocket of his jacket and stabbed the vampire in the head. His associations led to monster movies, childhood competition with rivals, and, finally, to the hated colleague whom he had wished would die.

Raised by the paradigms presented thus far are important questions: How are symbols and stories selected by individuals and endowed with the dramatic meanings that characterize life narratives? When are they selected?

What are the factors influencing the selection process? How changeable are consciously experienced fantasies? Are the links between conscious and unconscious fantasies fixed and irreversible, or are they potentially modifiable? We discuss some of these questions in this chapter, but they remain important throughout this book. We return to consider them in the clinical sections later on as well.

Definition of Sexual Fantasy

Psychoanalysis is a depth psychology that originally emerged from the study of sexual fantasy. A problem present in the field from its inception, however, has been lack of a definition of erotic fantasy, or even a general sense of agreement about its specific attributes. One reason for this may be that Freud blurred the distinction between the sexual and that which nonpsychoanalytically oriented clinicians might consider nonsexual. In his last published work, *Outline of Psychoanalysis* (1940), he commented:

> It is necessary to distinguish sharply between the concepts of "sexual" and "genital." The former is the wider concept and includes many activities that have nothing to do with the genitals. Sexual life comprises the function of obtaining pleasure from zones of the body—a function which is subsequently brought into the service of that of reproduction. (Freud 1940:23)

Freud hypothesized that "erotogenic zones" under the influence of a sexual instinct invested certain areas of the body with intense pleasure during specific phases of development—oral, anal, and phallic. We agree with psychoanalytic scholars who have argued that Freud's libido theory has not withstood the test of time (Kardiner, Karush, and Ovesey 1959; Person 1980). The psychoanalytic literature contains countless articles, nominally about sexuality, discussing bodily zones invested with so-called libidinal energy. We consider the libido theory, which placed sexual "energy" at the center of all human motivation and all psychopathology, to be of historical interest only, although this position puts us at odds with beliefs that are popular among many psychoanalysts, particularly in Europe and Latin America. Libido theory is not accepted by modern neuroscientists or psychologists (Kandel 1999), and it is important to integrate psychoanalytic theory and practice as much as possible with modern nonpsychoanalytic knowledge. Thus, when we refer to "sexual" or "erotic" fantasies in this article, our meaning is closer to Freud's narrower one (pertaining to the "genitals"), although influenced by research that took place during the decades following his death.

The topic of sexual fantasy is more complex in women than men, and we reserve consideration of its meaning(s) in women until later in this chapter. The first part of the chapter therefore is about sexual fantasy in men.

In this book we define sexual fantasy as mental imagery associated with consciously experienced feeling that is explicitly erotic or lustful. Sexual lust is a specific type of affect. The imagery is nearly always organized in some type of narrative format. Since this volume is directed at readers who are interested in psychoanalytic thought and psychodynamic therapy and are familiar with the concept of unconscious fantasy, we emphasize here that imagery, story line, and erotic feelings of the sexual fantasies we refer to are generally reportable, not unconscious. We discuss situations in the clinical section of this book in which individuals may find it difficult to describe their sexual fantasies. Nevertheless, they tend to be aware of them.

The narrative line of a sexual fantasy tells a more or less elaborated story of objects and situations associated with erotic arousal. Sexual emotion (lust) is associated with physiological changes throughout the body including the central nervous system. Sexual fantasy often occurs during masturbation and during sexual activity. It may be stimulated by pornography (in males more frequently than females) and/or romance fiction (in females more frequently than males) and is often experienced spontaneously (Leitenberg and Henning 1995).

Masters and Johnson and Kaplan

In thinking about sexual fantasy, we find Masters and Johnson's famous depiction of the sexual response cycle and Kaplan's revision of it helpful (Masters and Johnson 1966). According to the Masters and Johnson model, sexual response begins with the subjective feeling of sexual excitement and its attendant physiological changes (vasocongestion of the genital organs, increases in heart and respiratory rate, etc.). The excitement phase builds until orgasm takes place. For a certain amount of time thereafter, the individual, if male, will be in a refractory or "recovery" period during which orgasm is not possible. The male model is diagrammed in figure 1 below. Masters and Johnson pointed out that women's sexual response is more variable. As can be seen from their model of the female sexual response cycle (figure 2), some women, though sexually excited, will not reach orgasm but will rather experience what Masters and Johnson called a plateau of sexual arousal before resolution. Others will experience a single orgasm similar to the male model. Still others are capable of multiple orgasms before they go into the refractory period when no orgasm is possible. During the so-called refractory period, sexual fantasy diminishes, only to surge again with the return of sexual desire and sexual excitement.

Kaplan, a psychoanalyst and sex therapist, observed on the basis of the patients whom she saw that many sexual difficulties seemed to begin before the sexual response cycle as described by Masters and Johnson. She termed this preliminary phase sexual desire. Many of the patients referred to Kaplan complained that they experienced no sexual interest. Kaplan made a distinction between sexual desire and sexual excitement, noting, "Sexual desire is an appetite or drive which is produced by the activation of a specific neural system in the brain, while the excitement and orgasm phases involve the genital organs" (Kaplan 1979:9). She asserted that sexual desire is experienced as specific sensations that motivate the individual to "seek out or become receptive to sexual experience" (10) Kaplan proposed therefore an early phase of the sex-

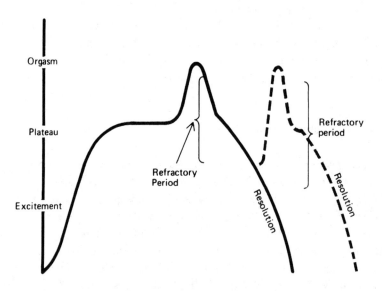

FIGURE 1.1. The male sexual response cycle. From Masters and Johnson, *Human Sexual Response*, p. 5 (Boston: Little, Brown, 1966). Reprinted with permission from Lippincott, Williams and Wilkins, 2001.

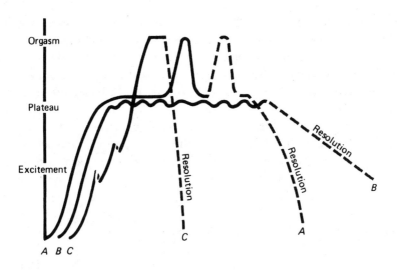

FIGURE 1.2 The female sexual response cycle. From Masters and Johnson, *Human Sexual Response,* p. 5 (Boston: Little, Brown, 1966). Reprinted with permission from Lippincott, Williams and Wilkins, 2001.

ual response cycle when central nervous system changes theoretically occurred and preceded genital changes. In men, however, at least in laboratories studying sexual function, erotic feelings are associated with increased penile blood flow, that is, some degree of erection (Freund, Langevin, and Barlow 1974).

Freud believed that fantasies were the product of wishes that compensated for "unsatisfying reality." Empirical studies of sexual fantasy do not support this, however. Sexual fantasies occur most frequently in people with high rates of sexual activity and little sexual dissatisfaction. Of course, clinically, many patients experience impulsive/compulsive driven sexuality. These individuals are different from relatively healthy people, however, who happen to be highly sexual (Leitenberg and Henning 1995).)

The Components of Sexual Fantasy

Erotic fantasy, as we have discussed above, consists of a few specific components, including a sexual object—usually a human being—either male or female or both. A story line is often present in which the sexual object is involved in a specific situation, such as embracing, engaging in oral sex or intercourse, or undressing. What makes a fantasy erotic, however, is its invariant association with sexual feeling. We do not consider fantasies to be sexual unless the erotic feeling component is present. Erotic fantasy may motivate erotic activity with others or masturbation. It does not always do so, however, and may be experienced privately in the theater of the fantasist's mind.

In both sexes sexual feelings depend on adequate blood levels of androgen. Pharmacological blockage of the effects of androgen eliminates erotic feelings and therefore erotic fantasy and the motivation to participate in sexual activity (Sherwin 1991; McConaghy 1993; Bradford and Greenberg 1996).

Unique Attributes of Male Sexual Fantasy

The reason that male sexual fantasy is different from other types of fantasies is that, in physiologically normal men, it is usually not capable of being repressed for long periods of time, only briefly and transitorily.

A dramatic illustration of this form of everyday life comes form the psychology of teenage boys. Is it possible to eliminate sexual fantasies from their awareness? One can get a laugh from any junior high school teacher by asking that. "Is that a trick question??? Is there anything else up there but sex??? Tell me how to do this so I can get them to learn algebra." Teachers, as well as the world's wisest philosophers, St. Augustine, for example (Oates 1948), know that the answer is no. It has been fashionable at various times in history to maintain that it is possible, and even desirable, for men to eliminate sexual fantasy from consciousness by willpower. "Just think no!" As far as we can determine, there has never been a single instance in which this idea has been successfully implemented as social policy.

Once sexual fantasy is experienced, it may or may not motivate sexual activity, including masturbation and interpersonal sexual activity. Sexual activity in males, however, tends to be preceded by sexual fantasy, and, frequently, sexual fantasy leads directly and immediately to sexual activity.

Development of Erotic Fantasy

In most boys and some girls erotic fantasies occur during childhood. Unlike girls and women, in whom erotic fantasies usually first appear in the context of meaningful involvements with others, in boys the onset of erotic fantasies tends to be independent of romantic, affection, and close relationships (Gold and Gold 1991). In most countries in which sex research is carried out, political constraints are such that it is extremely difficult to investigate the sexual development of children. The data base on which to make inferences about the development of sexuality in normal children is therefore quite limited. Retrospective accounts of adults, both patients and nonpatients, and anecdotal reports or studies of special groups of children, indicate that an age range exists during which sexual fantasy emerges (Gardner 1969; Money and Ehrhardt 1972; Langfelt 1981; Galenson and Roiphe 1981; Friedman 1988; Baldwin and Baldwin 1997; Herdt and McClintock 2000). Many men date the onset of sexual fantasy to their earliest memories—age three to four or so. Most, however, place its onset at about age eight. Some as late as puberty and a few even later. Thus, one can imagine a bell-shaped curve for the onset of male erotic fantasy—with the lower tail beginning at age three to four, the peak at about eight to nine, and the upper tail at about age thirteen. It is apparent that a certain level of cognitive development is necessary for the onset of meaningful sexual fantasy. This distinguishes sexual fantasy from another core component of human psychosexual development: gender identity. Gender identity develops during the first three years of life. During these years, not only is cognitive development at a much more primitive level, but the development of memory systems is as well. Declarative memory—for people, places, and things—is poorly developed during the years that gender identity differentiates, and its time line of development overlaps the very earliest phases of that of sexual fantasy (Kandel 1999). In pointing out that sexual fantasy, as we conceptualize it, seems to begin for some people in toddlerhood, and for others in mid to late childhood, we are not suggesting that very young infants do not experience erotic arousal. Behavioral evidence of sexual arousal and even orgasm has been observed in infants of both sexes. Although this may occur in some children, however, there is no evidence that such events occur in most. In any case, the phenomena that we call erotic fantasy are internal psychological events as well and hence require a certain degree of psychological development.

Most males experience such fantasy passively, as mental events that happen to them. Their first sexual activities tend to be self-masturbation, and the only difference between homo- and heterosexual groups regarding the onset of sexual desire is in the gender of the desired object (Friedman 1988). By adolescence the necessity to cope with intense, specifically erotic fantasies—impulses, desires—is part of the adaptational requirement of boys. Girls are much more diverse, as we discuss later in this chapter (Baumeister 2000).

The erotic fantasies of gay and heterosexual men are similar in important ways, except for the gender of the erotic object. For example, one study found that the most common fantasies experienced by heterosexual men included receiving oral sex, performing oral sex, imaging sexual activity with a current partner, having sex with more than one partner at a time, and being with someone other than a current sexual partner. The comparably frequent fantasies among gay men were of participating in sexual activity with another man, receiving oral sex, performing oral sex, participating in anal sex, and having sexual activity with a new partner (Price, Allensworth, and Hillman 1985). Of course, there are many differences as well, particularly among subgroups of men. For example, men who become sexually aroused when they dress in women's undergarments (e.g., transvestitism) tend to be mostly heterosexual. Men who are involved in such activities fantasize about them. Among gay men various activities associated with anal sexual activity are probably more common. This notwithstanding, the similarities of commonly experienced fantasies are notable.

Lovemaps, Sexprints

After erotic fantasies have formed in most but not all men, they tend to rigidly consolidate, analogous to crystalline structures or pictures within a frame. Once the frame separating erotic and nonerotic fantasy is constructed, that which is outside the frame is not responded to erotically. Men act as if there were a limit on the construction of new types of erotic fantasy and a constraint against the elimination of old fantasy constructed during childhood. Ethel Person coined the term *sexprint* (Person 1980), and John Money *lovemap* (Money 1988) to describe this phenomenon. There is room for some diversity within each person's sexual script, and various types of sexual activities, such as voyeurism, having sex with multiple partners, incorporating force into sexual activity to some degree and in various ways, and other activities may or may not be part of a person's sexual fantasy profile (Person et al. 1989). Whatever diversity exists, however, is programmed in a way such that it is contained within a particular person's frame.

Evidence supporting the idea that sexual fantasy programming tends to be rigid rather than plastic in most men comes from diverse sources. Retrospective accounts of sexual fantasy as described by gay and heterosexual men commonly describe this pattern (Isay 1989; Friedman 1988; Herdt and Mc-Clintock 2000). Since the 1980s the clinical literature contains many examples of gay men treated with psychoanalysis or dynamic psychotherapy whose sexual orientation did not change during treatment, despite attempts to bring this about (Duberman 1991; Isay 1989). Studies of men who have attempted to convert their sexual orientation indicate that this is usually not possible (Gonsiorek and Weinrich 1991; McConaghy 1999).

Studies of men in psychophysiological laboratories provide another source of data. Here, measurements of penile volume and circumference are carried out in response to erotic imagery. In men the correlation between the subjective sense of arousal and blood flow into the penis is substantial. The profile of an individual male, as a general rule, is distinctive. Men aroused by stimuli in category "A" are not aroused by stimuli in category "B," and so on (McConaghy 1999).

Another source of data comes from treatment of men with paraphilias. No matter what therapeutic interactions are used, recidivism is high, and the only certain treatment is to eliminate sexual arousal capacity with potent antiandrogen drugs. Paraphiliac patients are generally male, and tend to first experience arousal to paraphiliac stimuli during childhood (Abel et al. 1992; Bradford 1995; McConaghy 1993, 1999). These patterns have been observed regardless of the sexual orientation of the person.

Juvenile Phase of Development: A Critical Period of Sensitivity for Sexual Fantasy in Males

That the sexual orientation of men often seems fixed from late childhood throughout life raises the question whether it is appropriate to consider the juvenile phase of male psychosexual development a so-called sensitive period with respect to the effects of sexual fantasy. Investigators in animal and human development have described this phenomenon, which consists of a limited window of time when diverse biological and behavioral systems become exquisitely sensitive to the effects of specific stimuli. As a result, they may be irreversibly altered. In an inclusive review of the topic, Bornstein commented:

> Scientists who study structure or function from all but an entirely static perspective inevitably confront the truism that dynamic animate phenomena are shaped by endogenous and exogenous forces interacting

through time. Those forces do not exercise equal effects at all times, however, indeed it is now common to speak of unique phases in the ontogeny of many different structures and functions when evolving transactions among life forces profoundly influence development. These phases are unique in that during select times in the life cycle many structures and functions become especially susceptible to specific experiences (or to the absence of these experiences) . . . during such sensitive periods in development specific experiences may exert a marked influence over future history.   *(Bornstein 1989:179)*

Bornstein went on to point out that although the sensitive period phenomenon was originally described in experimental embryology and ethology, it has been observed in diverse biological, psychological, and social systems and in interactions between combinations of these and in diverse species. Although sensitive periods have been primarily investigated during infancy in birds and mammals, they may arise later in development, and dating their onset and offset has sometimes been possible with great precision and sometimes not so.

There are many examples of sensitive periods in which systems reach full sensitivity gradually, over a time interval that varies between systems and between species. The same is true of the offset of the period of sensitivity. In some instances the offset is prolonged and gradual. In others, however, the period of sensitivity is sharply delineated and relatively brief. For example, in rats, castration of males on postnatal days 1–6 diminishes their capacity for prototypically aggressive male play, but castration after postnatal day 10 does not (Beatty et al. 1981). The neonatal period in rats is equivalent to the prenatal period in many mammals, including primates, with regard to the development of the central nervous system. Interestingly, it has been shown that there is a prenatal critical period of extreme sensitivity to the effects of androgens on the structure and functional organization of the brain in many mammalian species including humans (Gorski 1991; Breedlove 1994). Some of the behavioral consequences of this effect have already been elucidated and many await further investigation.

Critical Periods of Sensitivity and Psychoanalysis

To further complicate this developmental phenomenon, the dependent variables influenced by the input during the sensitive period may not be expressed until after much time has passed. For example, monkeys deprived of contact, comfort, and social interaction during infancy manifest disordered sexual behavior years later, after puberty (Harlow 1986).

This latter phenomenon is compatible with ideas about critical periods of sensitivity commonly accepted by psychoanalysis. Many psychoanalysts believe that the phase of childhood from birth till the postoedipal phase—more or less age six—is a critical period of sensitivity with regard to important dimensions of human motivation. During these years, according to influential theories, templates are hypothetically created that shape future interpersonal interactions. The way in which attachment bonds are formed, and the meaning that they have is influenced, if not determined, by these templates, which are largely unconscious (Atkinson and Zucker 1997). In psychoanalytic treatment the conformity of the patient's relationship with the analyst to the unconscious template is termed transference (Stone 1995). The therapeutic dimension of psychoanalysis is based on the notion that aspects of the unconscious templates may be modified. In structural terms, the components of the templates that are influenced by unconscious conflict may subsequently be altered.

The notion that there is a critical period of sensitivity for the establishment of templates that are in conscious awareness and that influence motivation in a way that is generally more rigid and even more determining than those in the unconscious has not been part of the main body of psychoanalytic thought. Some recent attention has been devoted to this phenomenon by Person, in an extensive discussion of daydreaming (Person 1995). Person has also observed that people have a tendency to form sexual scripts—more or less enduring sexual fantasies—that are found to be uniquely arousing. However, she has not considered the significance of this observation from the perspective of a critical-period-of-sensitivity model, nor has she discussed these phenomena in terms of the role of hormonal influence.

We suggest that in males *there is a late childhood critical period of brain/ mind sensitivity to fantasized images that are associated with erotic arousal.*

This way of viewing male sexual fantasy requires something of a leap, but much less so than one might think at first, in light of the diverse stimuli and responses that have been described in the literature on critical periods.

We conjecture that as the biopsychological processes associated with adrenarche and puberty begin, they are associated with brain sensitivities leading to the encoding of erotic fantasies in the mind as if they were etchings. The gender of the sexual object is encoded, leading to heterosexual, homosexual, or bisexual orientation.

Sexual Plasticity in Individual Men

Although the tendency toward sexprinting exists in most men, in others it seems much less pronounced. Populations or subgroups of men exist that seem to have much more capacity for sexual plasticity than in the statistical norm. For example, Kurt Freund, the investigator who pioneered laboratory investigation of male sexual response using penile plethysmography, found that some homosexual men, without ever having received treatment to become heterosexual, could voluntarily alter their penile responses to respond to heterosexual stimuli (Freund 1963, 1971). This highlights the need for clinicians to use behavioral observations such as these as *guidelines* rather than predictors in assessing change in any aspect of a man's sexual fantasy profile, including sexual orientation change during psychoanalytic/psychotherapeutic treatment. For example, a particular man's sexual orientation may indeed change if he happened to be one of the minority who appears to retain the capacity for sexual plasticity rather than rigid crystallization of sexual fantasies.

It would be erroneous to generalize from a clinical example (analysis of a case or a series of cases of patients with this attribute) that, as a general rule, male sexual orientation is malleable. It would be equally erroneous to exclude the possibility that such cases occur, by extending an observation that is true of the majority of men to include every single case. We discuss this topic more comprehensively in part 2.

Conscious Bisexual Fantasy

The innate capacity to experience bisexual fantasy increases the complexity of the topic of discussion even further. Laumann et al. carried out a population-based study of sexual behavior of a representative sample of Americans (1994). The investigators found that 6.3 percent of men reported current homosexual attraction. Of these only 2.4 percent were exclusively attracted to men and an additional 0.7 percent mostly so. Similar data have been collected from studies in France and the United Kingdom (Sell, Wells, and Wypij 1995; Johnson et al. 1994). Leitenberg and Henning report that, across studies, about 7 percent of heterosexual men have experienced homosexual fantasies (Leitenberg and Henning 1995). Most societies, including our own in the United States, have no bisexual social niche. Most men with bisexual fantasies consider themselves to be heterosexual, but some consider themselves to be gay. This is more or less what might be expected, given widespread social attitudes condoning heterosexuality much more than homosexuality.

Sex Differences in Sexual Fantasy

The following section of this chapter deals with female sexual fantasy. Because men and women are not symmetrical with respect to erotic experience/behavior, it is helpful to consider some sex differences here as well. Men, as a group, seem to be more erotically motivated than women. At every age in which comparisons have been made, they masturbate more frequently and have had more sexual partners (Leitenberg, Detzer, and Srebnik 1993; Oliver and Hyde 1993). Although the tendency to experience sexual fantasy declines during adulthood in both sexes, men fantasize more frequently than women do both during masturbation and also routinely, in daily life. For example, Laumann and colleagues (1994) found that 54 percent of men compared to 19 percent of women had sexual thoughts at least every day. Men also have more diverse sexual fantasies than women (Person et al. 1989). These differences, in addition to those discussed below, are helpful to keep in mind in thinking about the psychology of gay men versus lesbians.

Female Sexual Fantasy

Whereas male erotic fantasy functions as a limit defining the realm of that which is erotically possible, the situation with respect to sexual excitement in women is more variable. In men sexual arousal is generally equated with an awareness of a specific affect (e.g., lust), erection, and intense desire to achieve orgasm. Although this occurs among some women, it is not typical. There is far more variability in the multiple behavioral dimensions constituting sexual experience among women than men.

In discussing sex differences in erotic experience, it is important to note that psychoanalysts and sex researchers tend to assess behavior by different standards. Most sex differences in behavior consist of specific experiences and activities that, when measured, can be described quantitatively. The means for men and women differ statistically, but there is considerable overlap between individuals. For example, men tend to be better at spatial relations than women, but some women perform as well as any man (Collaer and Hines

19

1995). The sculptor Louise Bourgeois, architect Laurinda Spears, and sculptor and architect Maya Lin come to mind here. Similarly women tend to be better at verbal activities than men, but authors John Updike, Saul Bellow, and Philip Roth would hardly be considered verbally challenged. From a sex researcher's perspective it is perfectly understandable that some women experience sexual fantasy similarly to most men.

Psychoanalysts, on the other hand, tend to think of behavioral norms in terms of optimal developmental pathways. This type of conceptualization is more prone to reductionism as a result of stereotyping than is the statistical approach. However, psychoanalysts tend to acquire in-depth knowledge of a few individuals over time. Thus, they have unique access to the meanings that individual people attribute to their sexual experience.

With these caveats in mind, let us consider female sexuality.

Somatic and Subjectively Experienced Aspects of Female Sexual Response

In laboratory situations there is good correlation between a man's awareness of sexual excitement/arousal and objective measurements of erection. This is not so for women. The hemodynamics associated with a woman's genital vasocongestion can be measured utilizing an instrument called a vaginal photoplethysmograph. A number of independent investigators have confirmed that the relationship between what has been termed genital arousal (more or less the equivalent of male erection) and the subjective sense of feeling sexually aroused, is inconstant at best. In fact, at least in experimental situations, women may report little or no sexual arousal even when objective signs of "genital arousal" are unmistakable (Heiman 1980; Laan and Everaerd 1995).

Moreover, unlike men, only a minority of women consider orgasm the most important source of sexual satisfaction with a partner. DeBrulin reported that only 20 percent of women judged orgasm to be the most important source of sexual satisfaction in a sexual interaction with a partner (1982), a percentage that gibes with the findings of other investigators (Bell and Bell 1972; Hite 1976). In addition, whereas erection is necessary for men to achieve intromission, women can participate in heterosexual intercourse without sexual arousal. Common sense, clinical experience, and research data indicate that they frequently do so. Whereas most men who achieve intromission during intercourse experience sexual orgasm, substantial numbers of women do not (for example, Laan notes that over 50 percent of women with masturbatory experience do not orgasm during coitus [Everaerd and Laan 1994]). These data indicate that women tend to participate in sexual activity, including intercourse, for many reasons, only some of which would be considered "erotic" by standards applied by men to their own behavior (DeBrulin 1982; Hatfield and Rapson 1993; Laan and Everaerd 1995).

Laan and Everaerd (1995), Rosen and Beck (1988), and others have suggested that women's sexual arousal may be helpfully conceptualized according to cognitive-emotion theory as proposed by Schacter and Singer (1962). Laan and Everaerd (1995) have discussed this as follows:

> A given situation will not be experienced as sexual despite the presence of genital arousal, without the occurrence of the appropriate emotional attribution. Thus, a situation (a stimulus) is not intrinsically sexual, it becomes sexual by its transformation. *(44)*

> Sexual arousal is best construed as an integrated multimodality processing system consisting of subjective, physiological and behavioral components. These components may be at least partially independent. We assume that this information processing system includes parallel cognitive processing of both situational dimensions and bodily changes. *(45)*

Whereas men tend to experience sexual arousal in a simple unitary way, women experience it more contextually in terms of combinations of emotions. Nuances of feelings, meanings, and attitudes toward real and imagined experience are more characteristic of the consciously experienced female than the male experience. For instance, Dekker reported that subjective reports of sexual arousal of men were almost exclusively limited to sexual excitement, whereas women reported many other positive and negative emotions concurrent with sexual excitement (Dekker and Everaerd 1988). Numerous authors have reported this sex difference for nonsexual situations as well.

A woman presented with a stimulus that a man might find immediately erotic (a picture of the nude member of the opposite sex) may or may not experience it as sexually arousing. After all, what is traditionally considered "pornography" is largely consumed by men. On the other hand, men do not consume romance novels in any great numbers. From a male perspective, endless attention is devoted in these novels to a certain type of context and setting in which sexual arousal may possibly be mobilized. The stories that pique the interest of so many women bore men (Stoller 1975a). It seems evident that the characteristics and meanings of "erotic fantasy" differ between the sexes (although, of course, some overlap does exist). Laan has pointed out that women do respond with excitement around pornography that is "woman made" and focuses on the excitement of the female actor (Everaerd and Laan 1994).

At the beginning of this chapter we put forth a definition of sexual fantasy for men. The question naturally arises: Is it possible to put forth a definition for women as well? Perhaps the most important sex difference that bears on the question of definition concerns the onset of the feeling of sexual arousal, which women report much more variably. Should the sexual situation for women be defined very broadly in a way that includes experiences that provide a context within which erotic desire is likely to emerge? How does one deal with the problem that genital changes consistent with sexual arousal are often present without concurrent subjective arousal, an observation of women made by a number of sex researchers (Heiman 1977, 1980)?

The second question is easier to deal with. Although it is true that genital arousal might occur without subjective arousal, there is no evidence that the converse commonly occurs (although this area has been sparsely investigated). In any case, we take the position that sexual arousal in women should be defined subjectively—that is, subjective reports of arousal are necessary for sexual fantasy to be so labeled. With regard to the question of experiences conducive to the development of sexual arousal, we take the narrow view that the term *erotic fantasy* should be restricted to fantasy that is associated with the actual sense of being aroused. When circumstances that lead to sexual excitement are discussed—romantic fantasies, for example—they should be so labeled.

The notion that female sexual fantasy depends more on relational context than male sexual fantasy is also compatible with evolutionary psychology. It is adaptive for women to seek partners who can provide resources and protect them and their offspring. Men, on the other hand, should (according to an evolutionary model) seek sexual encounters with as many different partners as possible (Buss and Schmitt 1993).

Sexual Fantasy and the Menstrual Cycle

In an article discussing female sexual arousal, Laan and Everaerd commented:

> Feminists have long criticized the notion that the behavior and abilities of women are uniquely determined by their biology. This criticism led to

an almost total rejection of the role of biology in the construction of gender (Birke and Vines 1987). It also contributed, unfortunately, to an
image of female sexuality devoid of the body.   *(Laan and Everaerd 1995:34)*

In a society of gender inequity, is it possible to consider biological influences
on the behavior of the gender discriminated against, or does that foster prejudice? We believe that discrimination should be challenged at the sociopolitical level, but that it is not only possible but desirable to consider biological as well as psychological and social factors that influence behavior, even
among groups of people who have been prejudicially treated. It is our view
that most behavior is neither determined by biological factors nor social
ones, but rather by interactions between biological, psychological, and social
levels of organization in individuals and groups (Friedman and Downey
1993a, b; Engel 1962). This is certainly the case for behavior and the menstrual cycle.

Rather than look at phenomena as purely biologically determined or
purely culturally determined, we feel it is more helpful to consider experiences
and behaviors during the menstrual cycle as resulting from interactions between biological, psychological, and social factors.

In the late 1930s a psychoanalyst, Benedek, and a gynecologist, Rubenstein, began an astonishingly original research project on the relationship between the hormonal fluctuations of the menstrual cycle and verbalized sexual
fantasy during the psychoanalytic process (Benedek 1973). This investigation
opened an entirely new vista onto human sexual fantasy. The psychoanalyst
Karen Horney had earlier criticized Freud's view of female sexual development
and held Freud to task for masculine bias, but she had not carried out systematic research (Horney 1924, 1926). Benedek noted that Freud "did not investigate the function of procreative sexuality as a psychobiologic process"
(1973:409). She observed that the male's "reproductive function depends upon
a single act, the motivation of which is experienced as a compelling desire for
orgiastic discharge." The woman's more complex and phasic psychosexuality
was organized differently.

The investigators began their work with the prospective investigation of
a single woman in analysis with Benedek. The patient was instructed to take
daily vaginal swabs and rectal temperatures. These data were analyzed blind
by Rubenstein, who used them to date the physiological events of the cycle.
After ten cycle phases had been completed, Benedek reviewed detailed notes
that she made of each analytic session (the references to actual menstruation
having been edited out) and accurately predicted, on the basis of the patient's

verbalized sexual fantasies and associations, the precise date of ovulation during every cycle. The investigators went on to study fifteen patients, for variable lengths of time, in whom Benedek accurately and blindly predicted cycle phase. She wrote:

> We became blatantly aware of the obvious. . . . Sexual impulses, wishes, drives in adults are normally accessible to consciousness. Even if hidden in fantasies and dreams, they precipitate moods and feelings which are experienced and for the most part understood by the person even if not admitted. Psychoanalysts are so accustomed to searching for repressed sexual tendencies that we often forget that we arrive at them from currently experienced or experienceable phenomena such as dreams, fantasies and from behavior. *(Benedek 1973:134)*

Benedek and Rubenstein described phasic alteration in the fantasies of their patients (Benedek and Rubenstein 1942). Early in the first part of the cycle self-esteem was high and erotic interest was primarily motivated by the desire for sexual stimulation. As ovulation approached the patients tended to experience increased sexual tension and conflicts associated with this. Immediately following ovulation, there was a sense of relaxation. After this, during the luteal phase, there was a pronounced change in the quality of sexual fantasies. The women tended now to focus on procreational aspects of sexuality. Needs to be nurtured and protected were more pronounced; imagery of babies and mothers was more plentiful. This was followed by a brief phase prior to menstruation when ego defenses appeared to weaken. Negative affects increased, as did the patients' level of regression.

Benedek and Rubenstein were aware that the phenomenon of estrus characteristic of lower animals did not regulate human sexual activity. They speculated, however, that despite the freedom from regulation of sexual activity by the hormones of the cycle, woman might experience an equivalent of estrus in fantasy.

The investigation undertaken by Benedek and Rubenstein, although achieving instant acclaim, has been mostly ignored in subsequent psychoanalytic thought about sexual fantasy. No attempt to replicate it has ever been carried out at a psychoanalytic institute. Components of Benedek's observations have been validated in many nonpsychoanalytic studies (Hedricks 1994; Severino and Moline 1989; Friedman et al. 1980). Others still remain to be investigated.

A compressed way of summarizing a large interdisciplinary body of work in this area would be as follows. There is substantial variability between women regarding the timing of physiological events of the cycle and the experience and meaning of psychological events. Diverse subgroups exist, and more extreme and repetitive fluctuations occur among some than others. For example, premenstrual "regression" as described by Benedek may have been a function of the neuroticism of her patients and not of women in general. The sequential progression of fantasies from stimulatory to procreational may characterize a subgroup of women rather than women as a whole. It is evident from menstrual cycle research that many subgroups exist with regard to virtually all psychobiological parameters of the female reproductive cycle and that substantial variability exists not only between women but also within individual women (Hedricks 1994). Across studies, and in many different societies, however, there is little question that the inner mental experience of women is cyclic in many ways and that this is true of the intensity and quality of sexual fantasies as well as other aspects of their cognitive and emotional life (Persky et al. 1978, 1982). The notion of cyclicity does not suggest that any dimension of experience or behavior is not influenced by psychosocial events or that any dimension of experience or behavior is somehow intrinsically more problematical (e.g., negatively valued) than among men, nor does it suggest that women are under "biological influence" to a greater degree than are men.

Benedek's research indicated that the quality of sexual fantasies in women and their many meanings may change phasically. Psychoanalysis as a whole treats sexual fantasy as if it is either trait-related or a result of reactions to specific life events and traumata. The notion of innately influenced cyclicity imposes a requirement on clinicians to utilize more complex behavioral paradigms. For example, cyclicity by no means implies the notion of biopsychological events occurring in a vacuum without social context. In fact, the meanings attributed to psychological events during the cycle, including sexual fantasies, may be greatly influenced by interpersonal experience, including sexual experience, and may also influence the way such experience is psychologically processed by the woman. It might well be that the transference relationship with the analyst, a crucial aspect of psychoanalytic treatment, is influenced by the menstrual cycle. Whether or not this is the case, however, remains to be explored by empirical research. With regard to the significance of cyclicity, we particularly emphasize the following:

1. The cyclic fluctuations of hormones during the menstrual cycle have no parallel in male physiology.
2. Many mental events associated with the menstrual cycle have no parallel in male psychology. This is true of certain dimensions of sexual fantasy.
3. The conflicts associated with cyclicity are also experienced cyclically. This means that at conscious and unconscious levels the psychological functioning of the sexes differs in crucial ways. This area is not well understood at present and may be illuminated in the future with the use of modern brain imaging techniques.
4. The onset of menstrual cyclicity during the life cycle creates a discontinuity in female development that has no parallel among males. This applies to menopause as well.

Cyclicity apart, however, Benedek's point that procreative fantasies are a crucial dimension of the sexual experience of women is central. We suspect that erotic fantasy is much more tightly linked to procreative fantasies in women than men. These may include the wish to become pregnant, to deliver, to raise children, or any component of this sequence.

Sexual Fantasies in Women and Other Life Cycle Issues

We have written in our earlier work about a phenomenon much more common in women than men, the need to be "kindled" by an intimate relationship before sexual excitement can emerge. The original "kindling hypothesis" comes from animal electrophysiologic models and has been adopted by researchers in other areas such as depression (Kendler, Thornton, and Gardner 2000). As we use it, we refer to the phenomenon of initial experience (in this case, of a relationship that acquires a sexually exciting quality), which makes patterns of processing that can be activated in the future by less and less substantial cues. Havelock Ellis wrote that

> in women . . . sexual excitement also tends to occur spontaneously, but by no means so frequently as in men. In a very large number of women the sexual impulse remains latent until aroused by a lover's caresses. The youth spontaneously becomes a man; but "the maiden—as it has been said—must be kissed into a woman."
> (1942:2:241)

Once the girl or woman is awakened to these sexually exciting feelings, she is much more sensitive to situations in the future that may elicit them. In those situations the girls or women involved may not have entertained fantasies that are explicitly sexual originally; their fantasies may have been purely romantic. Once sexual awakening has taken place, purely sexual fantasies may (though they may not) take their place beside the romantic ones.

A related phenomenon has to do with kindling of new sexual feelings in adulthood, an event that seems to occur more often in women than in men and that has led us to suggest that women may have more capacity for sexual plasticity than men (Baumeister 2000; Downey and Friedman 1998). Thus it is not uncommon for women whose behavior has been exclusively heterosexual and their fantasies primarily heterosexual to experience the kindling of passionate sexual feelings and fantasies toward a woman with whom they have developed a close and intimate friendship.

The content of women's sexual and romantic fantasies differs considerably from that of men's. For instance, Person et al. (1989) reported about a study of gender differences in sexual fantasy that women significantly exceeded men on just a few items, of which the most common fantasy was "being rescued from danger by one who will become my lover." The men endorsed more often fantasies of sex with a variety of partners and initiatory behavior. Many authors have pointed out women's tendency to imagine scenes of seduction by a powerful man, scenes of being forcibly required to engage in sexual acts, as well as scenes of being so sexually attractive that the partner is overcome with passion and/or willing to change his life forever, and scenes of being preferred to the partner's current or previous lover. We are struck by the features of power, transgression, and danger in these fantasies as well as the relief of guilt that attends a fantasy in which the woman is required to engage in sex and the oedipal triumph that comes from superseding the partner's lover. Such fantasies, as Person points out, replay and remediate childhood traumas and exclusions, among which is the very common one of being excluded from the parents' relationship. Throughout all these fantasies the woman as fantasist retains control of the events and thus can modulate any fearful aspects. Further, she does not have to act out the fantasies or even share them with her lover but can simply enjoy them privately in whatever way she wishes.

A recent movie, *The Tango Lesson*, by Sally Potter, seems to us to illustrate many of the aspects of an extended female sexual fantasy. The protagonist, played by Ms. Potter, is a successful middle-aged screenwriter stuck on a script when she attends a tango performance, is entranced by the young male partner of the performing couple, and approaches him for tango lessons. In the course of their relationship, she becomes a skilled tango dancer herself and performs with him on stage. The physicality of his dramatic dance sequences done for her at a time when he lacks the words to communicate, and the awe in which he is held by other dancers, thrill her. The appearance of his young and beautiful partner and other instances when his interest in her seems to flag become sources of conflict. She resolves this difficulty by deciding to make a movie out of her relationship with her partner, Pablo, and tango. The film ends with an extended sequence in which she takes Pablo to Buenos Aires, dances expertly with two other men as well as Pablo (no other women are present), excites his jealousy, and in every way exerts total control over the events because she is, in fact, literally writing the script.

Oedipal Themes in Female Sexual Fantasy

Just as with men, oedipal and preoedipal themes are regularly revealed in the sexual fantasies of women during the psychoanalytic/therapeutic process. It is helpful in thinking about the meaning of such material from a theoretical/developmental perspective to briefly review aspects of classical psychoanalytic thinking about the female Oedipus complex.

Freud conceptualized the early maternal-child relationship as a love relationship that fundamentally structured the development of erotic life for both sexes. In the boy the pathway from preoedipal to oedipal love was straightforward. The girl is faced with a developmental task—shifting her love object from mother to father and shifting the organ of sexual stimulation/arousal from clitoris to vagina. The girl also responds to awareness of the genital difference between the sexes with anxiety, anger, and depression. She feels that she once had a penis and has been deprived of it by her mother, whom she blames for this "castration." During the oedipal phase, as well, she experiences hostility toward her mother whom she regards as a rival for father's attention and love. Just prior to the oedipal developmental phase, both sexes were hypothesized to experience heightened sexual/erotic responses involving the genitalia.

In classical psychoanalytic theory the concept of a phallic/oedipal developmental phase is used to connote the stage when object-related erotic fantasies occur and become elaborated. Freud believed that, in the girl, castration anxiety ushers in the Oedipus complex. The girl realizes that she lacks a penis and develops a reparative wish—to have a baby. The competition with her mother for her father's love is associated with an incestuous desire; that he impregnate her. The hostile/matricidal components of the "complex" and the incestuous wish then become repressed during the next developmental phase, as occurs in male development. This is associated with maternal identification and enhanced feelings of femininity.

Freud and subsequent psychoanalysts have emphasized that these developmental phenomena coexist with complex positive feelings about both parents that occur during development. The result is ambivalent attitudes about parents and subsequent sexual objects (Freud 1931; Moore and Fine 1990, 1995). In classical psychoanalytic theory different components of this complex developmental pathway are retained in a condensed and otherwise disguised way in the erotic fantasies of women.

We disagree with most parts of this model and believe that they have not stood the test of time. In keeping with many modern psychoanalysts, we reject the notion that psychobiology dictates that girls are inherently determined to begin life with awareness of a body/self defect. We also reject the notion that the girl's desire for a baby, during normal childhood development, is predicated upon an incestuous wish. Such wishes are, of course, often (although not universally) expressed either directly or indirectly by adult women during psychoanalysis. The commonly expressed procreational component of women's sexual fantasies, however (in contrast to men's), and their greater interest in involvement with infants and procreative matters generally has a different explanation than any Freud proposed, in our view.

Maternalism

In discussing the development of maternalism in girls and women, it is important to begin with a qualification. A biologically influenced predisposition that affects the behavior of most individuals in a group should not be equated with a developmental norm, necessary for psychological health. We emphasize this distinction throughout this book. There is no implication from psychobiological or developmental data that women "have to feel maternal" in order to be psychologically healthy. The issues concern feelings and wishes that most girls and women are likely to experience. In developmental psychobiology there is no unitary construct analogous to the early psychoanalytic idea of the prototypical girl.

Just as almost all female mammals have innately determined patterns of behavior that lead them to show interest in and care for their young, so—we suggest—do human females. There is little question that this interest is present in young girls, much more than young boys, long before pubertal development, and remains so later in life. An important reason for this has to do with prenatal psychoneuroendocrine functioning. It is likely that innate maternal interest in neonates and very young infants is diminished in males as a consequence of prenatal sex steroid influences on the embryonic brain. The behavioral evidence for this is substantial for many nonhuman animals and in humans, although indirect, is also compelling. Little girls are far more interested in maternal doll play and in babies, from toddlerhood on (Maccoby 1990, 1998; Leaper 1994). In girls who are exposed to excessive androgen prenatally as a result of genetically determined adrenal steroid metabolic disorders, or for other reasons, maternal interest tends to be diminished. In childhood they show less interest in maternal doll play than normal children. The theme of interest in maternal doll play and in infant care is built on and elaborated during middle childhood and again is a feature of the development of girls and not boys. Still later, after puberty occurs, procreative themes expressed in fantasy and dreams take on a more adult quality and may occur cyclically in some women, as observed by Benedek and Rubenstein.

During childhood, as cognitive development occurs and mental archives of social experience grow larger and larger, oedipal themes appear in the fantasies of girls. These involve competition and hostility toward the mother and desire for attention and love from the father. These themes sometimes do involve fantasies of having the baby of the father or a father figure. We stress the following critical points, however: 1. Little girls have maternal interest for psychobiological reasons and not because they seek to have their fathers' baby. In fact, the younger the child, the more likely it is that interest in dolls and babies do not involve pregnancy fantasies. Children differ as to the age when they understand the meaning of pregnancy. Their understanding of the relationship between pregnancy and sexual intercourse tends to occur after the beginnings of gender identity differentiation and after the earliest interest in maternal doll play. Aspects of oedipal material that involve triangular and ambivalent relationships with the parents take place as a result of narrative constructions that are superimposed on a stratum of fantasy that occurs in children as a result of the way their brains differentiate and, in a more general sense, as a consequence of evolutionary influences. 2. When psychoanalysts consider oedipal issues in girls, the themes tend to be conceptualized in terms of romance or romantic competition but rarely erotic arousal in the narrow sense that we have discussed it in this chapter. In that regard an observation of Leitenberg and Henning is relevant. They summarized research on

> stories of 150 children 5 to 10 years old. . . . The authors did not specifically try to elicit psychosexual imagery or any other specific content. Each child told two stories to the investigators over the course of a year. Twenty-four children told tales with reference to either sexual or romantic behavior. Of these, 9 boys told psychosexual stories and 4 boys told romantic stories, whereas no girls told psychosexual stories and 11 told romantic stories. *(1995:475).*

As a general rule, the spontaneous stories told by younger children (under the age of five) contain content expressing aggression, loss, insecurity, morality, bodily hurt, but not erotic fantasy and extremely rarely material about reproduction (Ames 1966; Pitcher and Prelinger 1963).

Parenting and Erotic Fantasy

Among common fantasies in women is the desire for a high-status and desirable mate to coparent offspring with them. Their fantasies of the ideal mate may be influenced by those they have entertained about the kind of child or children they desire: handsome or beautiful, highly intelligent, sharing some maternal trait such as height or hair color or having the opposite, etcetera. Indeed, the idea of conceiving a child is sexually highly arousing to many women (and some men as well). For instance, a young single woman involved in an affair with a socially prominent married older man entertained as her main sexual fantasy the prospect that he would impregnate her in one of their episodes of passionate lovemaking. She imagined that when she shyly confided the pregnancy to him, he would realize how much he loved her, leave his wife, and marry her. This is a sexual fantasy embedded in a romantic one. The part she used to arouse herself was that his powerful semen would cause her to conceive, no matter what precautions they took, and she would be rewarded with a tiny version of her lover.

Clinicians who treat patients suffering from infertility observe that many such couples report a loss of sexual interest and excitement. Although this is commonly attributed to the rigors of infertility evaluation and treatment, we think that this is not the whole story. Rather, couples struggling to conceive without success lose contact with powerful, sexually arousing fantasies of conception. Mental images of failure and barrenness inflict narcissistic injury on the infertile couple as well. It is our impression that women are more likely to be adversely affected by the loss of the sexually exciting fantasy of conceiving a child, whereas both men and women may experience intense pain from the narcissistic injury of inability to conceive. Individual differences are to be expected, however. Clinicians who do psychoanalytic work realize that fantasies are endlessly variable and cannot be predicted on the basis of demographic features alone, even such powerful ones as gender.

Procreational Fantasies in Lesbians

Today lesbian couples frequently have children together, using a variety of new reproductive technologies. While there are numerous differences between these couples and heterosexual ones, many of the fantasies of the women in these partnerships are similar. Fantasies of impregnation are powerfully exciting, however that impregnation may be accomplished: via sperm bank and turkey baster, mutual recruitment of an attractive sperm donor, or a sexual encounter with a male lover.

We are not aware of data about frequencies of sexually exciting, procreative fantasies in men and women. In general, however, it is our impression that reproductive fantasies fuel erotic desire more frequently in women, regardless of sexual orientation, than in men. Since women who conceive children in lesbian partnerships also often report arousing fantasies of conception, we conclude that this fantasy is linked to maternal and nesting desires rather than penetrative sex with a male partner.

Idealization of the Partner

Women's fantasies about their romantic/sexual partners and coparents of their children also have unique attributes. We have been struck by the great importance women put on their *admiration* of the potential partner. The need to maintain admiration in the face of sometimes glaring deficiencies of the partner leads to dramatic instances of denial that become the province of the psychodynamic clinician. Indeed, the degree to which the idealized picture of the potential mate gibes with the real person may serve as an index of how much psychopathology suffuses the relationship. Denial is used to preserve admiration so as to enhance sexual excitement. Such admiration is multidetermined: the high status of the partner obviously enlarges the woman's own self-esteem. The fact that the mate is powerful and capable is security enhancing—such a partner can more ably provide care for the woman. The desire for such a partner derives developmentally from early childhood when the child looks up to and unquestioningly loves the parent. The admired partner may obviously partake of the ego ideal as well as aspects of the "imaginary playmate," depending on what childhood predeterminants of object choice exist in the individual's personal biography. Although men may also idealize their partners, our clinical experience suggests that among women admiration of the partner is far more frequently a requirement for sexual relationships than among men. Obviously, the fantasy requirement for the woman's partner need not include male gender. The gender of the preferred object depends on many determining factors of sexual orientation, which we discuss further in section 1 of this volume.

Dominance/Submissions/Oedipus

During childhood it is certainly common for girls to idealize their fathers in a romantic way and to resent attentiveness to their mothers. It is also common for girls to fear retaliation because of their jealous impulses, usually in the form of disapproval and loss of love from their mothers, although themes of bodily damage are also commonly experienced. These wishes and fears are usually kept secret. It is easy to trace their elaboration and displacement into fantasies in which the father figure is symbolically represented by a powerful older man who seduces the woman, overcoming her protestations, forcing her to succumb to his will, even raping her. This type of fantasy certainly is the bedrock of women's romance novels, so-called bodice rippers. It is probably experienced by many women under diverse conditions and provides one type of imagined setting in which erotic excitement can develop (Stoller 1979).

In almost all societies the rules regulating male and female sexual experience differ, with male experience being valued much more positively. Abuse of women by men is common, and overt physical abuse, including systematic rape, bodily mutilation, and sexual slavery are still prevalent in many nations. This difference in power and status interacts with the biological influences to lead to a final common pathway with respect to many behavioral sex differences including sexual fantasy. For example, the theme of being overwhelmed by a powerful male who stimulates but also protects need not refer exclusively to the father, but, understandably, probably emerges commonly in response to the differential treatment of the sexes throughout entire societies. This observation is more or less in keeping with a psychoanalytic perspective first expressed by Karen Horney (1924, 1926). In any case, the oedipal fantasies of both sexes express themes of power and dependency.

Limitations of space do not permit us to review the manner in which modern ideas about the development of gender identity led to alteration of Freud's developmental model for girls. This topic has been discussed extensively by others, however, and interested readers are referred to Zucker and Bradley (1995), Tyson (1982, 1994), Tyson and Tyson (1990), and Downey and Friedman (1998).

Reflections of Sexual Fantasy and Passionate Desire in Men and Women

In the history of psychoanalytic thought, the frameworks necessary to inform discussion of sexual fantasy include object relations theory (Kernberg 1976, 1980), self, ego, and relational psychology (Sullivan 1953; Hartmann 1964; Kohut 1971, 1977), in addition to a body of thought that we loosely term Freudian, by which we mean all of Freud's original theories and speculations.

Human beings are social animals. Therefore, it is no surprise to recognize that a major purpose of sexual arousal is to motivate interpersonal contact—not only to experience physical pleasure via stimulation of the body. The vast majority of sexual fantasies are interpersonal; hence sexuality is part of the repertoire of communications signifying what people want and need from each other. In adults sexual passion and sexual fantasy must be conceptualized in an interpersonal framework.

Psychoanalytic psychology views social behavior from a number of unique perspectives. As we have pointed out earlier, one of its assumptions is that observable behavior and conscious experience always contain unconscious messages and motives within it. Another is that the meaningful past is always included in mental depictions of the present. The attribution of meaning to specific situations is therefore influenced by the person's life history in ways that may or may not be immediately apparent. Psychoanalysts recognize that different people experience different subjective realities although they may be in the same or similar social situations. To a psychoanalyst, as to a cognitive neuroscientist, the term *reality* refers to subjective representations. These not only involve representations of the self and of others but of self and others engaged in meaningful action and interaction. Via the mechanisms of condensation and symbolization, representations of the self during different points of development and of others over vast periods of time are often fused experientially with images of present relationships.

One of Freud's particularly important insights is that human relationships are inherently ambivalent. Crystals of antipathy are always contained within the pattern of our meaningful affections. Unambivalent friendliness, exuberance, expansive playfulness, and joy are certainly part of our repertoire, but these feelings are never unalloyed for long in ongoing meaningful interpersonal experience. As have virtually all major psychoanalytic theorists, Freud recognized that feelings of fear and anxiety and rage and hostility are inevitably mobilized in ongoing relationships, although they may be experienced in ways that are repressed or denied.

Thoughtful psychoanalytic scholars have realized that the concept of ambivalence is, in a condensed and often disguised way, an integral component of sexual passion. Thus, during sexual arousal human beings tend to experience more than a unitary sense of "lust." Men as well as women experience feelings of anger and anxiety that are usually associated with a sense of danger. Mixtures of these feelings influence the attributions given to erotic fantasy. To put this in less formal language: when we become sexually aroused we feel lustful, but also fearful and often angry, and we process mixtures of these feelings with our characteristic defenses. As part of our mental processing activities we create dramatic narratives to which we (later) return in the form of memories. As we become more sexually excited, the fantasy, with its different components, is experienced more and more vividly. These fantasies provide the stimuli for masturbatory activities and also endow specific, actually occurring sexual situations with meaning. During intense interpersonal sexual activity, the fantasy constructs of people appear to come to life and feel as if they are shared. Both aspects of the actual activity—the enactment in external reality of subjective wishes and narratives and the sharing of such experience, with its evoked mutual identifications—are experienced as thrilling.

The psychoanalytic and sexological scholar Robert Stoller has emphasized the hostile component of sexual excitement, but the anxious component is also embedded in the concept of childhood "traumas." He wrote:

In the absence of special physiological factors (such as a sudden androgen increase in either sex) and putting aside the obvious effects that result from direct stimulation of erotic body parts, it is hostility—the desire overt or hidden, to harm another person—that generates and enhances sexual excitement. The absence of hostility leads to sexual indifference and boredom. The hostility of eroticism is an attempt, repeated over and over, to undo childhood traumas and frustrations that threatened the development of one's masculinity or femininity. The same dynamics, though in different mixes and degrees are found in almost everyone, those labeled perverse and those not so labeled.   *(1979:6).*

Sexual fantasy is rooted in bodily experience—one's own and that of others. The first relationship in which one's body is more or less completely explored by another is with the mother or mothering person. Hence psychoanalysts have noted that representations of the maternal-child relationship and of the mother's body are symbolically included in manifest sexual fantasy experienced during adulthood by both sexes (Chasseguet-Smirgel 1986).

Kernberg advanced Stoller's thinking, putting sexual emphasis on the polymorphous perverse aspects present in all interpersonal sexual activity.

The fantasied early polymorphous perverse relations to the parental objects are condensed with the admiring and invasive relation to the lover's body parts. Erotic desire is rooted in the pleasure of unconsciously enacting polymorphous perverse fantasies and activities, including symbolic activation of the earliest object relations of the infant with mother and of the small child with both parents. All this is expressed in the perverse components of intercourse and sexual play—in fellatio, cunnilingus and anal penetration and in exhibitionistic, voyeuristic and sadistic sexual play. Here the links between the early relationship with mother of both genders and the enjoyment of the interpenetrating of body surfaces, protuberances and cavities is central.   *(1995:26)*

Both Kernberg and Stoller stressed that sexual passion is associated with a sense of risk and defiance of convention. Kernberg drew attention to the importance of the sexual couple's dynamics, especially the excitement of fantasied shared transgression against societal restrictions (Kernberg 1995).

Sexual passion brings the self to the boundary in the experience of pleasure associated with emotional intensity. At the outer boundary of the self, there is always a feeling of danger of dissolution, and then a feeling of relief, relaxation, and of being soothed when the intensity passes and the self inhabits its customary, familiar, surroundings. When sexual passion is shared with another person, the loss of self-boundary is associated not only with what is usually termed communication in conventional usage but also with the sense that the inchoate matter of one's interior and the other's interior are mixed. This type of experience, whether actually occurring and encoded in memory or only wished for but nonetheless psychologically represented in some form, endows sexual fantasy with the power of mysterious enchantment.

It is difficult to capture the subjective qualities of sexual fantasy in laboratory research settings or via questionnaire studies. On the other hand, research using psychoanalytic techniques is time-consuming and extremely difficult to implement. Moreover, many aspects of sexual fantasy and sexual arousal were unnoticed by psychoanalytic psychology and could never have been discovered via psychoanalytic exploration. It was only because of the physiological investigations of Masters and Johnson that psychoanalysis revised its erroneous model of female development and psychosexual functioning, with its emphasis on the vaginal orgasm and devaluation of the clitoral orgasm (Masters and Johnson 1966). The pioneering work of gender identity researchers led to similarly far-reaching revisions of psychoanalytic models of the mind (Stoller 1968; Kohlberg and Ullian 1974; Money and Ehrhardt 1972). Psychoanalytic exploration alone could never have described the crucial distinction in women between genital and subjective arousal.

In its earliest phases psychoanalysis resisted accepting the findings of nonpsychoanalytic researchers about psychological development and functioning. Fortunately, this is much less true today. The field has moved away from its original interest in sexuality, however. Psychoanalysts are unique in having access to the uncensored expressions of fantasy. Moreover, they get to know individual patients in depth and are able to observe how these fantasies are elaborated and changed over time. Many questions about the somatic, psychological, and social determinants and consequences of sexual fantasy and activity remain to be illuminated. Hopefully, collaborative efforts between behavioral scientists and psychoanalysts will allow us to better understand human sexuality in the future.

2

Genetic Influences on Sexual Orientation

In chapter 1 we suggested that one consequence of the extensive recent attention that psychoanalysis has devoted to homosexuality has been its increasing sophistication about sex differences in erotic experience and behavior. Psychoanalytic and psychotherapeutic experience with gay men and lesbians contributes to an understanding of male and female psychology as well as that of sexual orientation. We now turn out attention to homosexual orientation beginning in this chapter with discussion of genetic influences.

Extrapsychoanalytic research in the areas of genetics and psychoneuroendocrinology is often invoked in many clinical and nonclinical discussions about sexual orientation. Research in these areas is relevant to psychoanalytic understanding not only of lesbian/gay people but also of psychological development generally. Psychoanalytically oriented psychotherapists use developmental models in their clinical formulations. The research we review in the following chapters is relevant for the validity of these models.

We begin by discussing how psychoanalytically informed research on twin children separated at birth and raised by different families, illustrates the need to distinguish between psychodynamics and etiology. We then consider extrapsychoanalytic research carried out on twins studied during adulthood who had also been separated at birth and raised in different environments. Intelligence, psychopathology, and many areas of personality functioning are influenced by genetic factors to a much greater degree than generally appreciated in psychoanalytic theory.

This discussion allows us to place questions about the possible role of genetic influences on homosexual orientation into perspective. After considering ethical issues, we discuss the literature on genetic influences on homosexuality, and the relevance of such genetic studies for psychoanalysis.

Is Homosexuality Genetic?

At clinical conferences one often hears discussants commenting that "homosexuality is genetic" and, therefore, that homosexual orientation is fixed and unmodifiable. Neither assertion is true. These ideas were sometimes put forth in the 1980s in a debate that has long since ended about change in homosexual orientation during psychoanalysis. It was once believed that only after sexual orientation changed to heterosexual could the psychoanalysis of a gay person be deemed successful. Persistence of homosexual desire was viewed as evidence that oedipal and/or more primitive preoedipal conflicts persisted and that the psychoanalysis had failed. Even though we now know this to be erroneous, the reason that homosexual orientation does not change during analysis is not simply that "homosexuality is genetic." Homosexual orientation results from interaction of many factors, including genetic influences in varying degrees across individuals. Genetic origin of a behavior or other attribute does not necessarily mean that the attribute is fixed and unmodifiable, however. The assertion that homosexuality is genetic is so reductionistic that it must be dismissed out of hand as a general principle of psychology.

Psychoanalysis and Genetics: Psychodynamics Versus Etiology

How is the topic of genetics relevant to psychoanalysis? The answer to this is perhaps best illustrated in a case discussion.

Clinical Vignette

Amy, a ten year old who had been adopted shortly after birth, was shy, had psychosomatic symptoms and somatic worries without organic cause, severe anxiety, gender identity/role confusion, and was believed by mental health professionals to be pathologically immature. She was prone to nightmares, had episodes of enuresis, and had been a tense and demanding baby.

Amy's behavior was studied as part of a research project by a team that attributed her difficulties primarily to parental rejection. As his wife did, Amy's father favored her seven-year-old brother, who was handsome and academically successful. It was hypothesized that Amy was alienated in her family setting, insecure as a result of maternal inadequacies during her preoedipal phase of development, and unable to adequately resolve oedipal phase conflicts because of defective input from both parents. This type of reasoning seems credible enough, and we have been at many psychoanalytic case conferences in which elaborate formulations of character development and symptom formation would be presented on the basis of the above data.

Interestingly, the research project of which Amy and her adoptive family were part was of identical twins, separated at birth and raised in different families. Identical twins result from the division of a single zygote, or fertilized egg, during the first two weeks after conception. Since they come from one zygote, they are often referred to as monozygotic twins, in contrast to fraternal or dizygotic (DZ) twins—essentially brothers or sisters who happen to be born at the same time. Monozygotic (MZ) twins who are separated at birth (as a result of life's vicissitudes) and raised by different families provide unusual opportunities to study nature/nurture influences on development.

In the case of Amy—if the clinical teams' speculation about the etiology of her symptoms was correct—then Beth, her twin, raised in a different setting, should have had a different developmental course.

Whereas Amy's family was lower class, Beth's was financially well-to-do. Amy's mother had low self-esteem and was threatened by Amy's attractiveness. Beth's mother was described by the research team as "pleasant, chic, poised, self-confident, dynamic, and cheerful" and she consistently discussed Beth in a loving, accepting, positive way. Beth's father was more available, nurturant, and supportive to Beth than Amy's. Beth also had a brother. Unlike Amy's, however, Beth's brother suffered from learning disabilities and behavioral difficulties of various types. Clearly, Beth's brother was not preferred by their parents and Beth was not seen as an outsider by the other family members. Beth did not experience the type of maternal deprivation that Amy experienced. Lawrence Wright summarized Beth's developmental course as follows:

> In nearly every respect, however, Beth's personality followed in lockstep with Amy's dismal development. Thumb-sucking, nail-biting, blanket-clenching, and bedwetting characterized her infancy and early childhood. She became a hypochondriac and, like Amy, was afraid of the dark and

of being left alone. She, too, became lost in role playing and the artificial nature of her personality was more pronounced than that of Amy's. She had similar problems in school and with her peers. On the surface, she had a far closer relationship with her mother than Amy did with hers, but on psychological tests she gave vent to a longing for maternal affection that was eerily the same as her identical sister's. . . . The differences between the girls seemed merely stylistic; despite the difference in their environments their pathology was fundamentally the same.   *(Wright 1997:5)*

This is a clinical vignette of unusual power because it emerged from a longitudinal investigation directed by a child psychoanalyst, Dr. Peter Neubauer (Neubauer and Neubauer 1990). Not only were the children studied over time but their parents and familial interactions were as well. The example illustrates the distinction between psychodynamics and etiology. The term *etiology* refers to causation—the factors necessary and sufficient to produce a specified behavior. The term *psychodynamics,* on the other hand, has a much more delimited meaning. We use it to refer to aspects of unconscious function that have been warded off from conscious awareness, or repressed, and that exert an influence on motivation, experience, and/or activity. For example, when Amy's mother physically left her, she was prone to separation anxiety. Perhaps she unconsciously experienced her mother as abandoning her. To speculate further, this fantasy might have been a response to feelings of anger she harbored toward her mother for any number of reasons. Perhaps Amy believed, in an unconscious and irrational fashion, "My mother is punishing me by abandoning me because I was angry at her. Mother has gone away and will not return. I am all alone." (We did not actually examine Amy and are alluding to her situation for the purpose of making a point about the distinction between psychodynamics and etiology.) These unconscious phenomena were not etiological, however. In fact, the whole fantasy sequences may have resulted from genetic influences in the first place. That does not mean that clinicians who treat patients such as Amy should ignore their fantasies, of course. The traditional methods of psychotherapy can often be quite helpful to patients such as Amy (or Beth, for that matter). Such clinicians, however, must be careful not to accept a narrative line that they create—and that seems plausible and reasonable—as a necessary and sufficient explanation of their patient's symptoms and/or personality functioning. One clinical consequence of what has now been learned, not only from the study of twins but from behavioral genetics generally, is that family history should be part of the initial assessment of all patients treated by mental health clinicians, including psychoanalysts and psychoanalytically oriented psychotherapists.

Patients, too, invent theories that explain the origins of their behaviors. For example, Neubauer discusses a different twin set: men in their thirties, separated early in life and raised by families in different countries. Each was neat and orderly. One attributed the reason for this to having been raised by a mother who was highly organized, punctual, tidy, and insistent that he be the same way. The other, however, decided that his penchant for cleanliness and order emerged as a reaction against a mother whom he described as a "slob" (Neubauer and Neubauer 1990).

The Minnesota Twin Studies

Neubauer only reported on a handful of cases. As interesting as his findings are, their small number necessitates caution in generalizing from the results. A research group at the University of Minnesota (independently) capitalized on the type of experiment in nature reported above, in which monozygotic twins were separated at birth, raised in different families, and studied during adulthood. Meticulous behavioral and physical studies of a series of such individuals, whose genetic material is identical, provided a solid basis for inferences about the role of genetic influences on behavior. The findings were compatible with those of Neubauer. Genetic influences on behavior are far more significant than psychoanalysts had realized. The project was directed by Dr. Thomas J. Bouchard Jr., and the first of a series of articles discussing the results of its pioneering work was published in the journal *Science* in 1990. Thus, the last decade of the twentieth century was ushered in by empirical investigation whose results challenged many assumptions about the relationship between etiology and psychodynamics of psychoanalytic therapists and theoreticians throughout the world. We note that, with regard to one central theme of this volume, homosexuality and psychoanalytic psychology, this research was published after the major critiques by Isay (1989), Lewes (1988), and Friedman (1988), which were so influential in leading to the demise of the pathological model of homosexuality in psychoanalysis. Psychoanalysts and dynamic psychotherapists need to be conversant with research demonstrating genetic influences on many aspects of behavior in order to place research on genetic influences on homosexuality in perspective.

Bouchard read of MZ twins separated at birth and reunited at age thirty-nine in a local newspaper. The article noted uncanny psychological similarities between the two including a love of carpentry and mechanical drawing and a taste for Miller light beer. Each chain-smoked Salem cigarettes. The twins accepted an invitation to be investigated at the University of Minnesota, and the project began. They were tested and interviewed independently, and further similarities in their life course emerged. They each followed stock car racing and had an aversion to baseball. They pursued their passion for carpentry in elaborate workshops that each had installed in his home basement. Both had worked part-time as sheriffs. Their similar health histories included hypertension, headaches, strabismus, migraine headaches present from teenage years, hemorrhoids, and a history of a ten-pound weight gain occurring at the same age in each man. Each bit his fingernails, and each had had a vasectomy. Each wrote love notes to his wife, which he left scattered about the house. Psychological tests, administered independently, revealed results so similar for measures of intelligence and personality functioning that they could have been tests of the same person on two different occasions.

There is no *psychoanalytic* model or way of looking at behavior that accounts for these astonishing empirical findings, given that these men were reared in two completely different families. Studies of other twin pairs yielded equally unexpected results that were so far from generally accepted ideas about psychology they seemed almost weird. For example, a set of MZ women, also separated at birth and reunited at age thirty-nine, met for the first time in 1980.

Each appeared wearing a beige dress and a brown velvet jacket. They greeted each other by holding up their identical crooked little fingers—a small defect that had kept each of them from ever learning to type or play the piano. They discovered that they were both frugal, liked the same books, had been girl guides, hated math in school, chose blue as their favorite color. . . . Both had the eccentric habit of pushing up their noses, which they each called 'squidging.' They liked their coffee black and cold. Both had fallen down the stairs at the age of 15 and claimed to have weak ankles as a result. . . . Although both loved to talk, Bouchard was interested in the fact that each fell silent whenever the conversation turned to more provocative subjects such as politics. In fact, neither had ever voted, except once when they were both employed as polling clerks.

(Wright 1997:53)

Similar behaviors have been described in many other early separated twin pairs (Segal 1999). We now turn our attention to a more detailed consideration of the Minnesota Twin Study findings, discussed in light of additional research as well.

Intelligence

Of behavioral traits intelligence has been studied most extensively by research scientists and is highly "heritable." We discuss it here because it illustrates important issues we shall return to when we consider genetic influences on homosexuality. Heritability means the proportion of variation in a trait present in a population that is attributable to genetic differences among its members. Comparison of MZ twins to DZ twins or siblings is a good way of assessing heritability. The reason for this is that DZ twins and siblings share half their genes but MZ twins share all of them. If, for example, one of a pair of MZ twins happens to become ill with tuberculosis, the chance of his twin also having the same illness is about two and a half times as great as would be the case if the twin was DZ. This means that there is a heritable tendency for a person to get tuberculosis. The tuberculosis example illustrates the way in which genetic influences are usually multifactorial in leading to a final result. Thus, the twins in this example would both have to be exposed to the same pathogen—the bacillus responsible for tuberculosis—to fall ill. Once that occurred, their immune systems would either be able to fight off the invader or not. In this instance genetic influences interact with other factors—including exposure to a pathogen—to result in an illness. We note this in order to emphasize that final results are usually the result of systemic interactions, not simply "effect follows cause." Let us now return to the topic of genetic influences on intelligence.

The term *intelligence* is generally used to describe a set of cognitive abilities that may be measured in various ways. The most commonly used measure is the "IQ" test, and correlations between individuals express the degree to which they are alike. As might be expected, the highest correlations are between MZ twins. Although the correlations are slightly higher for MZ twins reared together (.86) than apart (.75), these differences are small and may be artifacts of the fact that different groups were assessed at different ages. The heritability of intelligence increases with age, being less during childhood than adulthood. For example, in a large study of Swedish twin pairs, older MZ twins, despite living in different environments, were more similar in IQ than younger pairs. Older fraternal twins were somewhat less similar. These and other data indicate that MZ twins become more and more alike in cognitive abilities *over time*—even if they live in different environments (McClearn, Johansson, and Burg 1997). When reared together or apart, MZ twins are much more alike in intelligence than DZ twins, siblings, parents and children, half-siblings, or cousins (Segal 1999). In fact, comparisons of the IQ test scores between MZ twins often yield the same pattern as test-retest scores of the same person. The similarity in IQ of MZ twins is an empirical fact resting on a solid data base, having been established by many research groups (Bouchard 1998).

In thinking about the significance of these results, it is important to note that the high correlation does not apply to every twin pair tested. Considerable IQ differences among individual twin pairs studied have been reported. The reasons for this are thought probably to be the influences of *non-shared environments*. These environments may include the prenatal physiological environment—even MZ twins can have somewhat different intrauterine environments as a result of differences in placental circulation, for example, Postnatally, the *shared environment* includes environmental influences experienced by all family members. One person, however, can experience a unique injury, illness, or event that results in a different subsequent psychosocial adaptation. As people age and leave their family settings, the influence of the *non-shared* environment increases.

This does not mean that parental input early in life is unimportant, however. With regard to the attribute of intelligence—as well as a number of others—the role of parents may well be to provide an adequate enough interpersonal environment for the child's abilities not *to be permanently impaired*. This is to say that dysfunctional families possess a great deal of destructive potential. A different point concerns the possible beneficent effects of good parenting on psychological sequelae of trauma, such as occurs from illness, accidents, or as a result of many other causes. Absent adequate parenting, many children become derailed.

Personality Traits and Psychopathology

Once again the empirical findings are at variance with what might be expected from a conventional psychoanalytic developmental view that emphasizes the importance of identification. The role of identification in child development might well be important, pervasive, subtle, and even in individual instances determinative of many forms of experience, fantasy, and behavior. However, with regard to personality traits that have been investigated, the evidence indicates that similarities are much more likely to be explained by shared genes than environmental influences. For psychoanalysts this raises the intriguing possibility that the psychological mechanisms involved in making identifications are themselves often likely to be determined by genetic influences.

Researchers have extensively studied five major personality dimensions: extraversion-introversion, agreeableness–lack of agreeableness, conscientiousness–lack of consciousness, emotional stability–emotional instability, openness to experience–resistance to experience. Genetic influences are substantial for all five major personality traits, although less so than for IQ. Interestingly, as was the case with IQ, reared-apart twin studies indicate that shared environment—that is, the familial environment of rearing—has little or no influence on the emergence of many core personality traits. Segal described it as follows:

> Identical twins reared apart and together are about as similar as identical twins reared together in personality traits such as Well Being, Stress Reaction, and Aggression. In contrast, Social Closeness (affiliation) was more susceptible to the shared environment than the other traits. A surprise was the Traditionalism, the endorsement of traditional family and moral values, did not show common family effects. In other words living with someone does not lead to agreement on standards of conduct. . . . The last decades has witnessed a run of twin studies that have generally confirmed these findings.
> (Segal 1999:76)

To the best of our knowledge, in no study has the frequency of a specified personality trait (or other behavior for that matter) been greater in DZ twins or in siblings than in MZ twins, whether reared apart or together (McGue and Bouchard 1998).

Segal suggests that genes directly influence 20–50 percent of variation in personality, shared environment very little, and non-shared environment the lion's share of the rest. From the psychoanalytic perspective the term *non-shared environment* is not restricted to psychosocial phenomena (different experiences happening to a person) but must include different internal worlds. Suppose, for example, that one twin becomes depressed and the other does not—for any of a number of possible reasons. The depressed twin is more likely to evaluate interpersonal experiences in a bleak, pessimistic way. The nondepressed twin may place a more optimistic spin on interpreting events that seem similar to the outside observer. The twins thus may have non-shared psychological environments, despite the similarity in the appearance of observable activities.

There are a number of other ways of assessing genetic influences on behavior. For example, one can assess a behavior in family members across generations—the family pedigree method. The more closely people are related, the more genetic material they share. Siblings share more genes than cousins, for example. The proportion of people expressing a particular trait should be similar to their degree of closeness—siblings more frequent than cousins—if that trait is directly influenced genetically. With regard to the nature versus nurture question, one can compare frequencies between blood relatives and people adopted into families. The latter can also be studied in relation to their own blood relatives. One can also estimate whether a trait is likely to be sex-linked by studying the family pedigree. For example, males have XY sex chromosomes, the "Y" coming from the father and the "X" from the mother. If a trait is sex-linked and transmitted on the X chromosome, it is likely to be expressed more frequently on the maternal side than the paternal side of the family pedigree. This is by no means an inclusive discussion of methodology. There are other more biologically sophisticated ways of studying behavioral genetics, of course. Based on these traditional methods, as well as others not discussed here, a large list of behavioral syndromes, traits, symptoms, and disorders has been found to be at least modestly heritable. We refer readers interested in further discussion of this to the following references: Berkovic et al. 1998; Gatz et al. 1997; Heath et al. 1997; Holden 1997; Kaprio, Koskenvuo, and Rose 1990; Kendler et al. 1991; Kendler et al. 1993; Losoya et al. 1997; Lykken et al. 1993; Lyons et al. 1995; McConigle et al. 1993; Plomin and Daniels 1987; Price et al. 1985; Reiss et al. 1995; Robinson et al. 1992; Roy et al. 1991; Roy, Rylander, Sarchiapone 1997; Saudino and Plomin 1996; Segal et al. 1990; Sherman, McGue, and Iacono 1997; Swan, Carmelli, and Cardon 1997; and Waller et al. 1990.

Sources of Complexity

Behavioral effects may be due to single genes, such as occur in Huntington's chorea, a neurodegenerative illness with behavioral symptoms. A more common situation, however, is one in which the effects are polygenic: many genes interact with each other, such as occurs in schizophrenia and in the determination of IQ. Furthermore, environmental stressors may trigger genetic vulnerabilities that then shape various types of behaviors. Interestingly, the question whether genetic influences of any type influence *the capacity to respond positively to* psychoanalysis or psychoanalytically oriented psychotherapy is an open one. Even a single study comparing the psychoanalysis of MZ versus DZ twins would yield important results. Certain genetic influences may not be expressed until mid or later life, having no discernible effect during childhood (Plomin and Daniels 1987). Finally, the types of coincidences in tastes, abilities, and eccentricities observed in the lives of MZ twins reared separately are probably due to extremely unusual sequences of gene combinations (termed emergenesis) (Lykken 1992; McGue and Bouchard 1998). These combinations produce shared traits that would be impossible to occur conjointly in any pair that did not share all their genes.

Other qualifications and complexities concern the topic of homosexuality itself. No matter how the terms *homosexuality* or *homosexual orientation* are defined, they cannot be considered unitary entities. Moreover, the time line during the life cycle for the emergence of erotic imagery, the psychosocial experiences that precede such emergence, and the consequences of such imagery, are quite different for men and women. In men erotic imagery emerges by late childhood, is not a function of intimate, loving experiences, and limits future sexual options. In women erotic imagery emerges in conscious awareness over much a much lengthier time line. Unlike men, women may not experience full erotic arousal until adulthood—sometimes mid adulthood or even later. Although most women do experience erotic imagery, some never do. The comparable experience in men—never to be aroused by erotic imagery—occurs so rarely in male development as to be virtually unknown. These women who have not experienced erotic imagery still have a gender identity as female and usually experience themselves as having a sexual orientation as well (e.g., "Even though I have never felt sexual arousal, I am heterosexual—or lesbian," etc., etc.). We suggest that sexual orientation, no matter how defined, be understand as a behavioral dimension that is organized by gender. Male sexual orientation, homo, hetero, or bi (however the terms are defined), is fundamentally different from female sexual orientation. Of course, just as men and women share certain attributes, such as symmetrical body design, for example, with one head and torso and two legs and arms, so there are some common features to their sexual orientations. Be that as it may, the differences are dramatic and certainly as important for understanding sexual orientation as the similarities.

Finally, let us turn our attention to the empirical literature dealing with genetic influences on homosexuality. Although the results of these studies vary, no modern investigations that have been replicated suggest that homosexuality is as heritable as IQ or that it *is not* influenced by environmental factors, although there remains some uncertainty about the precise nature of these factors.

Ethics of Research on Genetic Influences on Homosexuality

We begin by addressing an ethical issue. Some scholars have questioned the ethics of studying genetic (or other biological) influences on homosexuality, since knowledge resulting from such investigation could be used to discriminate against gay people. If the genetic "causes" of homosexuality are known, might not antihomosexual parents, for example, seek medical assistance to prevent their offspring from becoming gay? The question has particular salience in light of the discoveries that led to sequencing of the human genome just as this volume was being completed (*Science* 2001).

We believe that it is ethical to investigate genetic influences on homosexuality (or other controversial areas such as intelligence, for example) with appropriate ethical-scientific guidelines in place. These are routinely guaranteed by institutional research review boards—and include informed consent and other precautions against violations of ethics. We note that the concept of *gender identity* was established at a time when discrimination against women by men was even more extreme than exists today (Money and Ehrhardt 1972). Were investigation of the intermediate psychobiological mechanisms leading to the establishment of a female and feminine sense of self interdicted on the grounds that results might be used to discriminate against women, this whole line of research could have never been carried out. There is no question that the social consequences of this new knowledge were advantageous for both men and women. Even the most well-intentioned social policy makers slide down a slippery slope when advocating censorship of scientific investigation. Critics who believed they were on the moral high road were opposed to Masters and Johnson's research, for example. Psychoanalysis has been indebted, however, to this nonpsychoanalytic research, which led to revision of psychoanalytic models of female psychosexual development and functioning.

Erroneous ideas that gay people were sociopathic led to discriminatory policies in the 1950s and sixties that influenced immigration and naturalization, child custody, occupational choice, and many other areas (Gonsiorek and Weinrich 1991). The incorrect basis for these political decisions was illuminated only because of empirical research comparing homosexual and heterosexual people. Had this research not been carried out, we doubt that high-minded argument, in itself, would have influenced the political process. The more information that can be acquired about the origins of homosexual orientation, the more will be learned about bisexuality and heterosexuality.

Studies of Genetic Influences on Homosexuality

Kallman (1952a, b) reported on a consecutive series of eighty-five homosexual males, all of whom had twin brothers. When the twin pair was MZ (forty pairs), the concordance for homosexuality was 100 percent, far greater than among the DZ pairs. Concordance of 100 percent for a behavioral trait would be extremely unlikely in a sample representative of the population as a whole, however, and it was not long before many reports of MZ twins discordant for homosexuality orientation were published (Friedman 1988). Sanders (1934) had earlier reported five of six MZ twin pairs concordant for homosexuality, however. Habel had described no concordance in five DZ twin pairs but concordance in three of five MZ pairs (Habel 1950).

Eckert and colleagues (1986) studied two sets of MZ male twins, separated at birth and raised in different families. Sexual histories were obtained during adulthood. One pair was concordant for homosexuality, and each twin had experienced "feelings of femaleness" before age nine (Friedman 1988). One twin in the other pair had been exclusively homosexual after age nineteen. The other was married and considered himself to be heterosexual. He had, however, been involved in a homosexual relationship between ages fifteen and eighteen). None of four sets of MZ females was concordant for homosexuality (Eckert et al. 1986).

Whitam, Diamond, and Martin (1993) reported on two additional sets of MZ twins. One was discordant for homosexuality, the other concordant. Reared independently in different cities, they each experienced early puberty at age nine, and "at 10 years of age, each experienced full and pleasurable sexual relations with an adult man" (201).

Evidence supporting genetic influence on homosexuality was substantially strengthened by the research of Bailey and Pillard (1991). Sexual orientation was investigated among MZ ad DZ twins of homosexual probands and also adoptive brothers. Fifty-six homosexuals had an MZ co-twin; of these co-twins, 52 percent were also homosexual. This was in contrast to the fifty-four homosexual subjects with DZ twins for whom sexual orientation could be determined; only 22 percent of these were homosexual. Of 57 adoptive brothers of homosexual probands, only 11 percent were homosexual. The investigators concluded that there is substantial heritability of homosexuality. These same investigators (1993) later presented preliminary data suggesting a genetic component in female homosexuality as well. Of the relatives of lesbian probands whose sexual orientation could be rated, 48 percent (34/71) of MZ co-twins, 1.8 percent (6/337) of DZ co-twins, and 5.3 percent (23/435) of adoptive sisters were homosexual (1993). In addition, two studies have reported that the frequency of homosexuality or bisexuality in sisters of homosexual female probands was elevated in comparison to heterosexual probands (Bailey et al. 1993; Bailey and Benishay 1993).

Whitam, Diamond, and Martin (1993) reported similar findings. In addition to the small sample of MZ twins reared in different environments, they discussed a more traditional sample comparing MZ and DZ twins reared together. Of thirty-four MZ pairs 64.7 percent were concordant for homosexuality. Among these were cases whose sexual histories so resembled each other that they were reminiscent of the observations of the Minnesota investigators.

> Another pair of homosexual MZ twins, aged 35, both accountants, reported that they did not reveal their sexual orientation to each other until fairly late. After mutual revelation, they discovered that both, completely independently and unknown to each other, simultaneously for a period of about a year while living in different cities, had photographed shirtless construction workers over the age of 40, and later at home, masturbated to the photographs.   (Whitam, Diamond, and Martin 1993:195)

Findings for DZ twins were markedly different: of fourteen DZ twin pairs, only 28.6 percent were concordant for homosexuality.

Whitam, Diamond, and Martin (1993) also discussed three sets of triplets. One set consisted of MZ men, concordant for homosexuality, and a heterosexual woman. A second set consisted of MZ lesbians with a DZ heterosexual sister. A third set consisted of three MZ homosexual males. Each had married, fathered a single child, divorced at about age forty, and self-defined as gay.

The data summarized above, taken in conjunction with the evidence for familial aggregation of homosexuality, support the notion that homosexuality seems to be heritable.

The situation in that regard is somewhat more complex than it seems in light of an ambitious, meticulously designed study recently reported by Bailey, Dunne, and Martin (2000).

The investigators observed that all previous studies of heritability of homosexuality used volunteers recruited from homophile organizations or word of mouth and were therefore subject to the criticism of volunteer bias. To overcome this limitation they utilized a large representative sample of Australian twins who were recruited to participate in a study of sexuality, but not explicitly of homosexuality. Questionnaires were completed by 4,901 twins. Sexual orientation was assessed in terms of subjective phenomena, not sexual activity with others, since individuals may be responsive to homosexual stimuli yet not involved in interpersonal sexual activity. Thus the nature of sexual fantasy and sexual attraction provided the relevant measures.

The results indicated that among 1,683 men and 2,704 women, 90 percent were rated exclusively heterosexual. The distribution of nonheterosexual scores was quite different for men and women, however. Whereas women were more likely than men to have slight to moderate homosexual feelings, men were much more likely to be predominantly or exclusively homosexual in fantasy and desire. This empirical observation is but one of many suggesting that male and female sexual orientations are dissimilar in numerous ways. It was true for both men and women, however, that they more often reported only a slight amount of sexual attraction/fantasy for members of the same sex rather than predominant or exclusive attraction. In women the difference was dramatic, and in men, slight but measurable.

Interestingly and in contrast to previous reports, the MZ concordance rates for men were only 20 percent and for women 24 percent, significantly lower than concordance rates in most previous studies. The investigators speculated that participants in previous studies might have decided to participate in light of what they knew about the sexual orientation of their co-twin. They qualified their conclusions about women, since only seven pairs of female MZ twins were predominantly or exclusively homosexual.

Because of the design of this research, the observations above would have made important contributions to the literature even without other findings.

The investigators went beyond simply studying homosexual orientation, however. They also utilized standard measures to assess childhood gender nonconformity. Not only did they find that childhood gender nonconformity was far greater among homosexual than heterosexual subjects, they also observed that the degree of gender nonconformity was related to the degree of adult homosexual orientation. Men and women who were predominantly or exclusively homosexual reported more than those who were only slightly so. The later group reported more childhood gender nonconformity than subjects who were totally heterosexual, however.

Whereas this study did not demonstrate that homosexuality is heritable, it did in fact show that *childhood gender nonconformity was heritable for both men and women.* Childhood gender nonconformity was strongly associated with adult homosexual orientation for males in this study, and somewhat less so for females. In discussing their results the authors observed that childhood gender nonconformity has been associated with adult homosexual orientation in many independent studies. In fact, this is one of the most robust associations in the behavioral sciences (Bailey and Zucker 1995).

Kendler and colleagues (2000) carried out a questionnaire study in a U.S. national sample of twin and nontwin sibling pairs. The investigators asked a single question about sexual orientation: "How would you describe your sexual orientation? Would you say you are heterosexual (sexually attracted only to the opposite sex), homosexual (sexually attracted only to your own sex), or bisexual (sexually attracted to men and women)?" They rated subjects as either heterosexual or nonheterosexual. Among 2,907 individuals, 3.1 percent of men and 2.5 percent of women reported nonheterosexual orientation. The concordance rate for nonheterosexual orientation in the MZ twins was 31.6 percent. Pair resemblance for nonheterosexual orientation was greater in MZ twins and DZ twins or siblings. Because of the small number of cases in this investigation, data for nonheterosexual males and females were pooled. The investigators concluded that familial factors, at least partially genetic, influence sexual orientation.

An additional area of research about genetic influences on homosexuality concerns the question whether male homosexuality is a sex-linked trait, transmitted on the X chromosome. In July 1993 Hamer and colleagues reported the results of a pedigree and genetic linkage study. They carried out an analysis that revealed increased frequency of homosexuality in the mother's brothers, and in sons of the mothers' sisters, but not on the father's side of the pedigree. This is precisely what one would expect to find with sex-linked transmission if the gene for the trait was carried on the mother's X chromosome.

Hamer and colleagues reasoned that if homosexuality were heritable via the mother's X chromosome, modern genetic linkage techniques should be able to demonstrate this. If one studied brothers, each of whom was predominantly or exclusively homosexual, one should be able to demonstrate that they shared a group of polymorphic genetic markers at a site on the X chromosome that came from the same genetic territory that carried the homosexuality gene. Such marker concordance was in fact demonstrated in thirty-three of forty sibling pairs—each of whom was homosexual.

On face inspection it would appear that the study provides strong support for the genetic hypothesis. This conclusion must be qualified, however. First, let us look more critically at the design of the study itself. The forty homosexual brothers were highly selected, both with regard to sexual orientation—none was bisexual—and also for pedigree—all came from families selected for transmission of homosexuality on the mother's side. Other investigators have looked at family pedigrees of homosexual subjects and have not found that they contain an excess of male homosexual members on the mother's side (Bailey et al. 1999). This suggests that families containing such an excess on the mother's side are unusual—and not representative of families containing a homosexual subject in the general population. Looking back at Hamer et al.'s study, seven sets of siblings, each of whom was homosexual, were discordant for markers. This immediately implicates additional types of transmission of homosexuality, including the possibility that homosexuality was not at all related to genetic transmission in this subgroup of subjects. Furthermore, predominant/exclusive homosexuality sometimes occurs in families in which father and son are homosexual, further suggesting additional mechanisms of transmission.

A much more important issue indicating that the findings of Hamer and colleagues require cautious interpretation concerns *replication*. Before scientific results are accepted as valid, they must be replicated by independent researchers. Hu and colleagues (1995) did report a replication study for men in which subjects who came from families where there appeared to be *nonmaternal* transmission for homosexuality were excluded. The investigators also studied homosexual women and found no such effect. These researchers, however, came from the same laboratory that reported the original sex-linked finding.

Rice et al. (1995) carried out an independent investigation with negative results. These investigators studied four markers in fifty-two pairs of gay brothers and found that the brothers were no more likely to share the X chromosome markers than would be expected by chance. In an additional independent investigation, Sanders (1998) found only a statistically insignificant trend of an X linkage among fifty-four gay brother pairs.

The research team of Rice et al. has argued that if there is an X-linkage effect, it is a weak one, accounting for so little variance of homosexuality in the population as to be unimportant (Rice 1999). Hamer (1999) and Rice (1999) have debated the significance of their studies, but as of the time of writing of this volume, the conclusion that male homosexuality is even sometimes determined as a result of X-linked transmission cannot be accepted as valid. This is not to say that it has been definitively disproven, but rather that, as is true so frequently in science, more information must be accumulated before the X-linked transmission hypothesis can conclusively be accepted or rejected.

Genetics, Homosexuality, and Evolutionary Psychology

The studies of genetics inevitably raise a question from the perspective of evolutionary psychology. If the purpose of evolution is to foster reproductive fitness, how could homosexual orientation facilitate that aim? The question really involves male behavior to a much greater degree than female behavior (since women of all sexual orientations may become pregnant), and only pertains to predominant or exclusive homosexual activity. The answer to the question of the evolutionary advantage of homosexuality is not known, but a common theory involves the concept of kin selection and kin altruism. This proposes that the infertile gay person assists family members who share some of his genes in their adaptive tasks. This increases the likelihood that these genes will be passed on to the next generation (Ruse 1981). This is but a speculation, however, and the empirical observation that there seem to have been homosexual people throughout history and in most or all societies is perhaps best accepted as a simple fact. Although some degree of homosexual attraction is more common, about 3 percent of the male population and 1.5 percent of the female population consider themselves to be homosexual (Michaels 1996). Although the percentages are low, they still account for millions of people through the world, however, and many patients seen by psychotherapists.

The scientific questions raised by possible genetic influences on homosexuality are formidable. Psychoanalysts are indebted to the scientific community for immense efforts that have resulted in the steady accumulation of data. Despite this, important questions remain. The most important points to draw from the complex material outlined above are as follows.

1. There are far more data available about males than females. Evidence for genetic transmission of homosexual orientation in females therefore rests on a less solid database than in males.

2. The distribution of nonheterosexual orientation is different for women and men. Predominant or exclusive homosexual orientation is more common among men. Even so, most men who have experienced homosexual feelings do not become predominantly or exclusively homosexual in orientation (McConaghey 1999). Gay men constitute a subgroup of men who have ever experienced homosexual desire. One way of looking at this is to invoke the concept of categorical versus dimensional thinking about sexual orientation. For many men homo , hetero desire/feelings/fantasies are best described dimensionally. Those who are truly gay, however, seem to be categorically different from the rest in the sense that the many nonsexual attributes of being gay coalesce in the self with the imagery of sexual desire to form a unique psychological entity.

3. It is common for MZ twins to be *either* concordant or discordant for homosexuality. Although in the latest large study discordant twins occurred more frequently than in previous investigations, it is possible that a large enough sample in a similarly designed investigation will demonstrate that homosexuality is heritable to some degree. This remains to be seen. The best available evidence to date indicates that male homosexuality is familial (Bailey et al. 1999). Among special subgroups (as opposed to variance in the population at large), there seems little doubt that genetic influences on homosexual orientation are present. Even though familial clustering does not prove genetic influence (native language runs in families, for example, but is not genetically determined), these studies, taken in conjunction with the twin research, are certainly highly suggestive. The ways in which the sexual histories of some twins are similar, for example, are not explicable by an environmental hypothesis. The degree to which genetic factors directly influence the variance of homosexuality in the general population, however, remains to be determined. What this indicates is that there is no *general* theory explaining the *balance* between genetic effects

and other influences on the origins of homosexual orientation at this time. The more information about sexual development that can be obtained by scientific research, the more likely such a theory will emerge in the future.

4. The relationship between childhood gender nonconformity and adult homosexual orientation has been demonstrated beyond doubt in numerous investigations (Bailey and Zucker 1995). One recent investigation, discussed above, has found that childhood gender nonconformity is heritable (Bailey, Dunne, and Martin 2000). A number of scholars have argued that there is a causal relationship between these two behavioral dimensions, although the intermediate mechanisms remain to be ascertained (Bem 1996, 2000; Friedman 1988). Even this association, however, is not interpretable in a simple way. Although the vast majority of gay men and most lesbians have experienced more childhood gender nonconformity than heterosexuals, many gender nonconforming children do not become gay or lesbian. It seems apparent that there is no "one-to-one" relationship in which "A" precedes and causes "B." It is noteworthy that in every instance in which childhood gender nonconformity has been assessed in MZ twins discordant for homosexuality, it has always been present/greater in the homosexual than the heterosexual twin (Segal 1999). As we discuss in the next section of this book, the most likely influences on childhood gender nonconformity are neuroendocrine. Moreover, much remains to be learned about this area as well.

5. The exact nature of environmental effects on sexual orientation remains to be ascertained. Such effects theoretically include both pre- and perinatal hormonal influences and those of shared and non-shared interpersonal environments.

As we pointed out earlier, the concept of shared versus non-shared environment in MZ twins become more complex when looked at from a psychoanalytic developmental perspective. For example, in boys, sometime during late childhood, erotic fantasies become either heterosexual or nonheterosexual. If the twins are divergent for sexual orientation, they may seem to share their familial environment, but actually the internal psychological environment of each twin is different. This difference may also be associated with differences in internal representation of familial relationships. For example, in an investigation of MZ male twins discordant for homosexuality, both twins in a pair remembered their father's actual behavior in similar fashion but valued it differently and attributed different feelings to him. The heterosexual twin described him as silent and strong, the homosexual twin as detached and withdrawn (Friedman 1988). Our purpose here is not to discuss the role of the father in the psychological development of gay men but rather to simply point out that in this instance the psychological environments of these twins might have seemed—to an external observer—to have been shared, yet their internal psychological environments were quite different.

It seems clear that theory building about the origins of any type of sexual orientation requires a multifactorial model—with biological, psychological, and social factors exerting influences at different times and in different degrees. A suitably complex paradigm certainly allows room for unconscious influences on behavior in diverse ways. It is apparent, however, that data garnered from the psychoanalytic-psychotherapeutic situation cannot be the sole basis for an adequate approach to the substantial theoretical and clinical problems involving sexual orientation that still await clarification.

3

Psychoendocrinology and Sexual Orientation

In this chapter we discuss hormonal influences on homosexual orientation. Our consideration of this area is relatively brief, since we selected only those aspects of the field that we felt it essential for psychoanalytically oriented therapists to be aware of. The reason that this line of research is so important for psychoanalytic developmental theory is that it is about *prenatal* influences on brain and mind. During the years that psychoanalysis was created, these influences had not yet been described. The psychoanalyst Robert Stoller was the first to direct the attention of the psychoanalytic community to the burgeoning new field of gender studies, which included prenatal hormonal effects on brain and mind (Stoller 1968). His contributions greatly influenced psychoanalytic ideas about gender identity/role and the psychological development of males and females. Stoller did not emphasize homosexuality in his writings, however, and his line of thought was different in important ways with that proposed in the following chapters. Since Stoller's death, continuous research has led to the need to revise psychoanalytic thought to an even greater degree than he had proposed.

We begin this chapter with criticism of the concept of biological determinism. Sexual orientation is usually not determined by biological factors alone. Biological influences are significant, however, and the way in which they act in concert with psychological and social influences to shape sexual orientation are crucial for psychoanalysts to be aware of. The psychoanalytic-psychotherapeutic process is, after all, based on hypotheses not only about present psychological functioning but also about psychological development.

In order to understand the psychobiology of human sexual orientation, it is necessary to (briefly) consider hormonal influences on nonhuman sexual behavior. We discuss these in light of recent research on humans suggesting that prenatal hormones might influence key areas of the brain that later affect sexual fantasy and perhaps sexual activity as well.

Reflections on Psychoanalysis and Neurobiology

The idea that homosexuality is biologically determined has been the subject of controversy for more than one hundred years. The nature-versus-nurture debate about the origins of human sexual orientation has waxed and waned, often accompanied by ill will and bitterness. The scientific issues have been framed by antihomosexual attitudes that have been common in many societies. Questions pertaining to sexual behavior have been inextricably bound to issues of stigma and victimization.

The notion that homosexuality is the effect of biological causes has been used to justify antihomosexual views on the one hand and an accepting, tolerant stance toward homosexuality on the other. Some have argued that a biological paradigm for homosexuality may lead to a biomedical perspective and hence to a tendency to pathologize homosexuality and even attempt to prevent or eliminate it (Schmidt 1984). Liberal theorists have used biological ideas about sexual orientation to argue against such tendencies. They have pointed out that homosexuality, being biologically determined, is not voluntarily chosen. It is experienced and expressed by people who are indistinguishable from others in society and is not associated with any type of defect. It is analogous to left-handedness, perhaps, or having red hair; attributes that are innocuous, although not those of the majority (Isay 1988; Robinson 1989).

A few points require summary and emphasis at this time:

- Neither homosexuality nor heterosexuality nor bisexuality is a unitary entity. No matter how these are defined, none is likely to have a unitary cause. At present there is no biological test that distinguishes people on the basis of sexual orientation.
- Any study or article focused on homosexuality will inevitably be about heterosexuality as well. Any study or article focused on heterosexuality will inevitably be about homosexuality as well. It is impossible to consider one without considering the other.
- The problem of antihomosexual bias is serious and continuing in many societies, including that of the United States. Great strides have been made in overcoming this, but much still remains to be done. Responsi-

ble scientific research provides the type of knowledge that must ultimately weaken the ignorance upon which bias and prejudice rest.

In struggling to place the new biological findings about homosexuality in perspective, many consumers of scientific information feel caught between the Scylla of biological determinism and the Charybdis of psychosocial reductionism. The pressure to avoid the complexities and ambiguities with which the field abounds is great because of anxieties evoked by the topic of sexuality generally, and homosexuality in particular, in contemporary culture. Yet it is important that scientists and clinicians not succumb to the temptation to see biology and psychology as antipodal forces vying for dominance in the area of human sexuality.

A recurrent wish expressed with some urgency in nonscientific publications, and even echoed in university settings, has been to find specific unitary answers to the question What causes homosexuality? It is apparent that biological, psychological, and social factors, interacting in complex and various ways, shape human sexual orientation. It is equally apparent that the specific mechanisms that lead to homosexuality, heterosexuality, and bisexuality in individual human beings still remain to be described.

In this and the next few chapters we discuss a different area of science than genetics that is helpful for a modern psychoanalytic understanding of sexual orientation: psychoneuroendocrinology, the science of how hormones influence the brain and behavior. Beginning with a review of empirical research, we move on to consider how these scientific advances necessitate modification of psychoanalytic ideas about the Oedipus complex and the significance of this for theoretical and clinical issues pertaining to sexual orientation.

Much research that has led to basic psychobiological principles has involved the physiology and behavior of nonhuman mammals. Discussion of behavior in other species sometimes evokes anxiety among psychoanalytically oriented therapists whose daily work is based on language and symbolic thinking. Understanding aspects of behavior in other species that parallel behavior in humans, however, does not imply that humans are identical to them.

One important difference between the sexual behavior of primates generally and that of so-called lower animals, such as rodents, is in the relationship between sexual activity and reproduction. In rats, for example, sexual activity is tightly linked to reproductive physiology. The biochemical and physiological systems controlling reproductive physiology also control sexual behavior, which in adult animals may properly be called "mating behavior." This occurs when females are physiologically ready or "in heat." Primates, and especially humans, are more variable in this regard; for example, sexual activity occurs through the menstrual cycle (Friedman et al. 1980). Sexual activity in humans is multidetermined and serves many functions, only one of which is reproduction (Katchadourian and Lunde 1972; Bardwick 1971).

Although sexual activity between same-sexed individuals occurs throughout the animal kingdom, there is no nonhuman mammalian species in which predominant or exclusive homosexuality occurs in the way that it does in humans. For example, among the primates, only humans may form meaningful, lengthy, sexual affectionate relationship between members of the same sex and not seek sexual activity with members of the opposite sex. Moreover, sexual behavior in humans is greatly influenced by gender identity, a psychological construct that influences behavior in a way for which there is no animal model (Ford and Beach 1951; Bell, Weinberg, and Hammersmith 1981).

These facts have been used as fuel for antihomosexual bias on the one hand and rationale for positive attitudes toward homosexuality on the other. The idea that human homosexuality is somehow "unnatural" has long been an argument fostering prejudice, as if human beings have a moral obligation to organize their sexual behavior similarly to that of nonhuman animals. Many types of human behavior, universally considered virtuous, are unique to our species, however. Although it is sometimes anxiety provoking to ponder our similarities and differences with other species, such consideration can also add a useful perspective to inform psychoanalytic theory and practice.

Nonhuman animal studies of sexual behavior involve observation of what subjects do with each other sexually. Human studies may include observation and quantification of interpersonal sexual behaviors and physiological responses to erotic stimuli, but they may also involve assessment of what people feel about each other, sexually and nonsexually. Psychoanalytically oriented psychotherapists are unique among behavioral scientists since their patients reveal otherwise private feelings, wishes, conflicts, and fears. Psychotherapists are therefore able to help understand the diverse meanings of human sexuality and distinguish its similarities to and differences from the sexual behavior of animals.

The Brain and Sexual Arousal

Many parts of the brain and spinal cord are involved in human sexual response, as are the autonomic nervous system and endocrine systems. Trying to conceptualize this can be overwhelming, and some illustrations of how biological regulation of human sexuality actually works may be helpful. A recent investigation, for example, used PET scanning to study the brain's response to sexual arousal of adult, physically healthy (heterosexual) male volunteers. The PET scan is a brain imaging technique that studies the functional activity of the brain via the use of radioactive isotopes. When the subjects became sexually aroused as a result of exposure to erotic films, certain areas of their brains became activated. These included cortical visual association areas, other areas involved in integrating sensory input with emotional states, and yet another area of the cortex ("left anterior cingulate cortex") involved in the higher regulation of the autonomic and endocrine nervous systems. The investigators suggested that different areas of the cerebral cortex were involved in integrating psychological processes including labeling visual stimuli as sexual, assimilating these stimuli with other emotions so that they were experienced as meaningful for motivation, and integrating these with the physiological responses involved in sexual response (Stoleru et al. 1999:17).

Throughout the brain and spinal cord are areas involved in providing different levels of integration of human sexual response. These areas are in two-way communication with each other, utilizing communication systems, analogous to telephone or telegraph wires, and also chemical-hormonal messages that constitute a wireless system. Even the idea of a bidirectional highway linking upper and lower levels of the nervous system is far too elementary to model events as they actually occur in nature. Feedback loops, both positive and negative, parallel influences involving messages carried by nerves and chemicals carried outside of the nervous system, sensitivities of responding systems, and elaborately orchestrated cascades of behavioral responses are all involved in what to the outsider (or participant) might seem to be a smoothly unfolding pattern of sexual behavior.

These feedback loops influence and are influenced by fantasy, conscious and unconscious, in day-to-day psychological functioning (Herbert 1996; Pfaff 1999; Whalen and Schneider 2000; Meston and Frohlich 2000).

The Hypothalamus

The hypothalamus is a small area at the very bottom of the brain, above the pituitary gland, located just above the roof of the mouth. It is an important nodal point and an information processing/generating center in the bidirectional communication pathway between the mind, the higher brain, the spinal cord, the autonomic-endocrine system, and interpersonal sexual activities. It is an area of the brain about which much research has been done. Many investigators have suggested that it may somehow be involved in shaping sexual orientation. One reason for thinking this has to do with studies of male and female sexual behavior in nonhuman animals.

The idea that there may be certain types of sexual behavior characteristic of one gender or the other may be provocative—even offensive—to some readers. This concept, however, provided the rationale for a well-known recent study indicating structural brain differences between heterosexual and homosexual men (LeVay 1991). In his book, *The Sexual Brain* (1993), LeVay commented:

> There are separate centers within the hypothalamus for the generation of male-typical and female-typical sexual behavior and feelings. . . . The foregoing, seemingly innocuous statement, is calculated to raise the hackles of numerous critics. They will say: "How dare you define what is sex-typical behavior, thus branding anything else as pathological or deviant?" "How can you speak of a center for sex when we know that many brain regions are involved?" and "How can you say the hypothalamus has anything to do with feelings, when feelings are conscious and therefore must be produced by the cerebral cortex and the thalamus." . . . I call behavior and feelings, "male-typical or female-typical" when they are more common in one sex than the other. Taking the insertive role in sexual intercourse, for example, is male-typical behavior. Taking the receptive role is, for men, sex-atypical behavior. But in no way do I intend by this to label such behavior as undesirable or pathological. *(71)*

The investigation that LeVay carried out followed upon many years of research on mammals and other species indicating that there are anatomically distinct areas in the hypothalamus that control "male-typical" and "female-typical" sexual responses. One region, termed the medial preoptic area (MPOA), controls male-type copulatory behavior—mounting, insertion of the penis, and pelvic thrusting. An adjacent hypothalamic area, the dorsomedial nucleus, controls ejaculation (Slimp, Hart, and Goy 1978; Perachio, Marr, and Alexander 1979; Gorski et al. 1980; Oomura et al. 1988; Allen et al. 1989).

A neighboring area of the hypothalamus called the ventromedial nucleus (VM) regulates female-typical sexual behavior. As is also true in the case of the male, female-typical sexual behavior actually consists of complex patterns and sequences whose end result consists of the "lordosis response." The animal arches her back in such a way as to accept the mounting male. In non-human primates this is called "presenting." Stimulation-ablation studies (e.g., cells in the nucleus are electrically or chemically stimulated or destroyed) reveal the VM's central role in female-sex typical responses. These responses are also influenced by estrogen and progesterone hormones secreted during the estrous cycles of female animals (Pfaff 1999).

Prenatal Hormonal Influence on Sexual Behavior

Thus far, as we have considered sexual behavior in lower animals, we have framed it as being "male-typical" or "female-typical," in keeping with the convention employed by Simon LeVay and others (LeVay 1993). However, experimental research reveals that male-typical and female-typical sexual behaviors are subject to the organizing influences of sex steroid hormones. What this means is that during a critical period of pre- or (depending on the species) perinatal life, androgen secreted from the fetal testis changes the structure of the hypothalamus. This eliminates the female endocrine reproductive cycle, greatly diminishes female stereotypic behavior (lordosis, sexual receptivity, etc.), and increases male stereotypic behavior. If the embryo is female, no androgen is secreted and the brain develops as female.

In humans the period during which testosterone secretion in the human male fetus first increases is between the eighth and twenty-fourth weeks of pregnancy. During this interval plasma testosterone in the fetal male tends to be eight to nine times that of the fetal female and fourfold greater than that of the mother. Sex differences in the structure and function of the central nervous system (CNS) that derive from the effects of gonadal steroids secreted during a critical period of pre- or perinatal life occur throughout the vertebrate kingdom (Goy and McEwen 1980). Among the manifestations of these CNS effects are certain differences in both sexual and nonsexual behavior.

Of possible relevance with regard to sexual orientation is that the critical periods during which the different mating centers are responsive to hormonal influence are slightly different. Thus it is possible experimentally to create an animal that demonstrates *both* female typical and male typical sexual responses (e.g., lordosis and mounting) (Collaer and Hines 1995; Gorski 1991; Arnold and Gorski 1984).

Prenatal Hormones and Human Sexual Orientation

Some scientists, taking an overview of the different ways that male and female sex-typical sexual behavior could be influenced by prenatal hormones in different species, hypothesize that in humans a prenatal androgen deficit results in male homosexuality and that a prenatal excess results in female homosexuality (Phoenix et al. 1959; Money and Ehrhardt 1972). Since this hypothesis involves prenatal biological events, it is compatible with the fact that neither plasma hormone values nor other endocrine tests distinguish groups with regard to sexual orientation (Gooren, Fliers, and Courtney 1990; Meyer-Bahlburg 1993; Friedman and Downey 1993a).

It is obviously not possible to make inferential leaps from studies of lower animals that lead to conclusions about human sexual behavior. Some psychotherapists might even wonder what the relevance of all this is for understanding their patients. Had Simon LeVay and others, interested in the differences in brain structure and function not only between homosexuals and heterosexuals but also between men and women, never undertook their research, we might question the relevance of animal research on sexuality as well. LeVay carried out research on humans, however, precisely because he was aware that extensive nonhuman animal research (much not discussed here) made it at least credible that homosexual orientation in humans may have biological determinants.

LeVay (1991) performed a neuropathological study of areas in the hypothalamus previously observed to be sex-dimorphic in order to test the idea that these areas might vary with the gender of the sexual object (i.e., sexual orientation) rather than the gender of the subject. LeVay obtained brain tissue at autopsy of forty-one adults, of whom eighteen were homosexual males, one was a bisexual male, sixteen were (presumed) heterosexual males, and six were (presumed) heterosexual females. Following appropriate histological procedures, slides of brain tissue of all subjects were examined and outlines of four hypothalamic nuclei were traced. The volume of each hypothalamic nucleus was compared between the experimental groups: homosexual men, heterosexual men, and heterosexual women.

The neuroanatomic loci for comparison had been selected on the basis of previous work by other researchers who observed that two key hypothalamic nuclei were larger in males than females (Allen et al. 1989). The area of the brain in which these differences between the sexes occurred regulates sexual behavior in mammals. LeVay found that one of these two nuclei was the same size in homosexual men and in women and smaller than in heterosexual men. In criticizing the design of his own research, LeVay pointed out he studied brain structure, not brain function. One could not conclude that, as a result of similarities in the volumes of hypothalamic nuclei, homosexual men were sexually attracted to men similar to the way heterosexual women are. He observed, however, that the size of a similarly located brain nucleus in the rat is dependent on exposure to circulating androgens during a sensitive period of perinatal life. Variability in size of this nucleus (the sexually dimorphic nucleus) among normal males is correlated with the amount of male-typical sexual behavior they express. He speculated that in humans the same type of responsivity to perinatal androgens might occur and that the effects on the brain might influence sexual orientation later in life.

LeVay's research was difficult to carry out and, as is common with exploratory projects, had a number of important limitations in design. For example, hardly any biographical information was known about the subjects, including information about their sexual histories. The study included no (known) homosexual women, and some of the subjects had AIDS. Moreover, although statistically significant differences between experimental and control groups were present, some presumed heterosexual men had small brain nuclei in the critical area, and some presumed homosexual men had nuclei large enough to be within the heterosexual range.

In keeping with pressure to find scientific "answers" to the many social problems that are associated with sexual behavior in American society, LeVay's research attracted great public attention. A recent attempt to replicate that research illustrates how complex the scientific issues actually are (Byne et al. 2000a, b). The investigators obtained autopsy material from the brains of heterosexual men, heterosexual women, and homosexual men. Some of their subjects were HIV+, some HIV-, and they established that the volume of the key brain nucleus discussed by LeVay in his study of homosexual men was not in fact influenced by HIV status. This nucleus, called INAH3, occupied a larger volume and contained more neurons in heterosexual men than women. This in itself was an important result, in keeping with previous reports by Allen et al. (1989) and LeVay (1991). Other brain areas were studied, but no sex differences in brain structure were found. The researchers observed that hypothalamic nucleus INAH3 is therefore the only area of the human brain that has been reported to be structurally different between the sexes by independent laboratories; no laboratories have reported to the contrary. (In contrast, negative as well as positive findings have been reported by different investigators with respect to a number of other brain areas [Fox, Tobet, and Baum 1999].)

Byne and colleagues (2000b) found the size of INAH3 in homosexual males to be greater than females but smaller than heterosexual males. These findings did not reach statistical significance, however. (Researchers refer to such effects as a "trend.") The researchers were able to determine the number of neurons in INAH3 and found no difference between homosexual and heterosexual males, although both had more neurons than females. They speculated that the (possible) difference in size of INAH3 between homo- and heterosexual men, despite no difference in number of neurons, might have been due to some type of laboratory error or perhaps to differences in the density of neuronal cells. Neither the physiological significance of the sexual dimorphism in INAH3 nor any possible differences in neuronal cell density between men of different sexual orientations is known.

The elegant investigation carried out by Byne and coinvestigators provides a sober counterbalance to those who seek to find simple "scientific" solutions to complex social problems. Carefully designed research studies often raise as many questions as they appear to answer. One research project leads to another, and definitive conclusions are few and far between. The investigators put it as follows:

> Considerable speculation has addressed the possible functions of INAH3, particularly regarding a potential role in regulating male-typical sexual behaviors. *(Allen et al. 1989; LeVay 1991)*

> Based on the results of the present study as well as those of LeVay (1991), sexual orientation cannot be reliably predicted on the basis of INAH3 volume alone. *(Byne et al. 2000b:10)*

LeVay had speculated about the prenatal androgen hypothesis of homosexual orientation. Are there other data from studies of humans supporting this hypothesis?

Congenital Adrenal Hyperplasia

The answer to this is affirmative, but although the support clearly exists it is not particularly robust or dramatic. The best illustration of the complex nature of the supporting evidence that prenatal androgen influences adult homosexual orientation comes from studies of women. The hypothesis states that if females are exposed to excess androgen during embryonic life it will influence their brains in such a way as to increase the likelihood that homosexual orientation will develop when they are adults. One way of testing this would be to find so-called experiments of nature—situations in which pregnant women were somehow exposed to increased androgen levels during their pregnancies. The frequency of homosexual orientation in the daughters of such women should theoretically be increased.

Such a group of women does in fact exist, and behavioral studies of their offspring have been carried out. The women were born with a genetically determined metabolic disorder of their adrenal glands termed congenital adrenal hyperplasia (CAH). Because of defects in certain enzymes, the pathway for secretion of cortisol is blocked off and precursors are shunted into a pathway leading to synthesis of adrenal androgens. Thus babies born with this syndrome have two major types of biological difficulties. The first is too little cortisol. This is a dangerous problem requiring early correction, since cortisol is a vitally important hormone necessary for the preservation of life. The second biological difficulty is that these children synthesize too much androgenic hormone. These processes occur during prenatal life, and continue—until medically corrected—after birth. The increased levels of androgen masculinize the appearance of the external genitalia: the clitoris is hypertrophied and the labia may be partially fused. In addition, the increased androgen has an influence on the embryonic brain. Because the disease is diagnosed and treated during infancy, the behavior of the girls who have been exposed to excess androgen may be seen as resulting from prenatal hormonal effects.

With proper medical treatment (including surgical correction of genital abnormalities, if necessary), girls with CAH develop normal secondary sex characteristics, and, although some have delayed puberty, in most instances puberty develops normally. Most have ovulatory menstrual cycles indicating that the degree to which their brains had been androgenized prenatally was not enough to alter the normal feminization pattern of the area of the ventral hypothalamus that controls the secretion of gonadotrophic hormones, the hormones that regulate the menstrual cycle.

With respect to their sexual orientation, most girls grow up to become heterosexual women. Compared to control groups, however, the frequency with which homosexual fantasy occurs in the CAH group is undeniably increased. The women who experience this do not, however, tend to define themselves as lesbians. Although behavioral studies of outcome have been clear in this regard, psychoanalytically informed research has not been carried out on these individuals. Hence, from the perspective of developmental psychodynamics, we have little information comparing object relations or self-representation development between girls who develop homosexual fantasy and those that do not (Ehrhardt, Epstein, and Money 1968; Money and Ehrhardt 1972; Money, Devore, and Norman 1986; Dittmann, Kappes, and Kappes 1992; Money 1994; Zucker et al. 1996).

Administration of Masculinizing Hormones During Pregnancy

Several decades ago progestins, synthetic analogues of naturally occurring progesterone, were administered during pregnancy in an effort to prevent miscarriage. Only later was it realized that these compounds had a masculinizing effect on some fetuses. Affected neonates appeared similar to CAH girls, and similar observations were made on their psychosexual functioning. The same type of pattern of development was observed in these girls as in those with CAH. Most became heterosexual, but more had increased homosexual fantasy/activity than would be expected by chance or that occurred in controls (Ehrhardt and Money 1967; Meyer-Bahlburg, Grisanti, and Ehrhardt 1977; Ehrhardt, Grisanti, and Meyer-Bahlburg 1977; Ehrhardt and Meyer-Bahlburg 1981; Money and Mathews 1982; Ehrhardt et al. 1985; Edelman 1986? 1987?; Meyer-Bahlburg et al. 1988; Ehrhardt et al. 1989; Friedman and Downey 1993a).

Another hormone preparation which, like the progesterone compounds, was used several decades ago in an effort to prevent miscarriage, is diethylstilbestrol (DES), a synthetic estrogen. DES is particularly interesting because in nonhuman animals it has been shown to masculinize and defeminize sexual behavior but not to masculinize play patterns. (In the next chapter we discuss the significance of the fact that prenatal androgens not only influence sexual orientation but also masculinize childhood play.) The findings of an outcome study on behavioral effects of fetal DES exposure on women were consistent with these observations. Childhood play was not masculinized in the DES-exposed women (Ehrhardt et al. 1989), but homosexual orientation in the experimental group was greater (Ehrhardt et al. 1985). However, even though homosexual responsiveness was increased, compared with control women, most of the DES-exposed women were still largely heterosexual (Meyer-Bahlburg et al. 1995).

It is striking that the same type of behavioral results have been obtained regardless of whether prenatal masculinization occurred via an experiment of nature, as in CAH, or as a consequence of medication administered during pregnancy. In both types of individuals—those with CAH and those exposed to exogenous hormones secondary to medical treatment—only limited, incomplete prenatal androgenization occurs. However, under these conditions even a modest effect in the expected direction on dimensions of sexual orientation is meaningful.

Animal research illustrates that sexual behavior is subject to neuroendocrine control. Research on the control of sexual experience activity in humans suggests both similarities and differences between human beings and our mammalian relatives (LeVay 1996). The concept that prenatal hormones could influence human sexual behavior originally derived from animal research. It has found some support in research on sexual orientation in girls who experienced increased androgen prenatally, and in studies showing structural brain differences between heterosexuals and homosexuals. These include LeVay's research as well as reports of increased size of the suprachiasmatic nucleus of the hypothalamus and increased size of the anterior commissure in homosexual men (Swaab and Hofman 1990; LeVay 1991; Allen and Gorski 1992). The studies of masculinizing hormones have been replicated. Those of structural brain differences still require adequate replication before they can be accepted. The line of thought that we have outlined in this chapter must be supplemented by another dealing with a different developmental domain—gender role behavior—in order to place research on homosexuality in appropriately complex perspective.

4

Psychoendocrinology and Gender Role Behavior

In the last chapter we discussed the evidence that prenatal sex steroid hormones may influence the sexual orientation of adults. The idea that something that occurs very early in development can influence adult behavior is a familiar one to psychoanalysts. In traditional psychoanalytic theory the earliest *time of* potential influence on the mind and personality is the oral phase of infancy, and the *type of* influence is interpersonal (e.g., the maternal-child relationship). The prenatal hormonal theory hypothesizes an earlier occurring influence—during prenatal life—and one that involves the brain directly. The two types of theories are not mutually exclusive but rather involve different levels of organization of brain, mind, and personality. Prenatal sex steroid hormones, however, also exert an important influence on childhood gender role behavior. Behavioral studies and clinical experience also indicate that childhood gender role behavior must be understood in order to make sense of the developmental pathways leading to the different types of adult sexual orientation.

In this chapter we discuss inferences about psychosexual development from two very different sources. The study of children with unusual medical conditions that used to be termed hermaphroditism and are today called intersex disorders has provided an important source of data about the respective influences of nature and nurture on childhood gender role behavior and adult sexual orientation. These studies indicate that although prenatal sex steroid hormones appear to influence both domains of behavior, the effect on childhood gender role is robust, and the effect on sexual orientation weaker and more variable.

The life narratives of gay/lesbian people constitute an entirely different data base suggesting that childhood gender role behavior is associated in some fashion with adult sexual orientation. We discuss the relevance of this association for the prenatal hormone hypothesis of sexual orientation.

We conclude the chapter by considering the significance of these lines of nonpsychoanalytic sex research for psychoanalytic theory and practice.

Gender Role Behavior

The term *gender role* was first used by the sexologist John Money (1955) and referred to the public communication of one's gender identity. By this was meant everything someone did or said that communicated to others that she was female, or he was male. More recently, Bailey and Zucker observed that gender role must be understood in historical and social context.

> Compared to Money's original definition the term gender role is now defined more narrowly. Many scholars use the term to refer to behaviors, attitudes and personality traits that a society, in a given culture and historical period, designates as masculine or feminine, that are more "appropriate" or typical for the male or female social role. In young children the measurement of gender role behavior includes several easily observable phenomena, including affiliative preference for same vs. opposite sex peers, interest in rough and tumble play, fantasy roles, toy interests and dress-up play. *(1995:43)*

Sex Stereotypic Behavior in Children with CAH

In the last chapter we discussed the possible influence of prenatal androgens on homosexual orientation in women. Prenatal androgen has, however, a much stronger and earlier occurring influence on child development—it influences gender role behavior. In girls who have early-treated CAH, the components of gender role behavior (and internal experience) that are influenced are quite specific. The CAH girls tend to have less interest than average in maternal doll play and infants, in self-adornment (e.g., jewelry, lipstick, and other makeup), and stereotypically feminine clothing (e.g., lace and frills). They have few daydreams of becoming a wife and mother when they grow up and tend to place more importance on career than marriage. A question that a psychodynamic clinician might ask at this point might be: "Couldn't these fantasies be influenced by the type of parenting the girls received? Perhaps their mothers discouraged a homemaking role, or were themselves primarily career oriented. Couldn't these effects simply be due to maternal identification?" The answer to this is that, as far as can be determined from developmental research, the effects occur in children of homemakers and career women alike. They occur more frequently in children with CAH than control subjects, including their sisters, for example, no matter what their parents' attitudes about appropriate womanly role behavior are. Although there is always need for psychoanalytic inquiry into the lives of children such as these, the best available evidence points to overriding prenatal hormonal effects, rather than rearing influences alone, on childhood fantasy in these children.

Compared with controls, CAH girls have a greater preference for boy playmates, and display higher energy expenditures and participation in more rough-and-tumble activities. A recent study of adolescents with CAH demonstrated that the preference for male stereotypic activities and careers persisted into adolescence and did not dissipate with more years of the same sex-role socialization pressures (Berenbaum 1999). As is true with most behavioral research, this tendency towards cross-gender stereotypical behavior has been found in many but not all girls with CAH (Hines and Kauffman 1994). We suspect that this is because there is a spectrum of sensitivity of the brain with regard to prenatal sex steroid hormonal influences.

In considering the developmental pathways of girls with early corrected CAH, we emphasize the following points.

The influence of prenatal androgen on their childhood gender role behavior is robust, has been demonstrated in many independent studies, and occurs when there is virtually no androgen in the blood.

These behavioral effects are not explicable in psychoanalytic terms. They cannot be explained by psychoanalytic ideas about the role of introjection, identification, and projective identification in development, for example. The effects of prenatal androgen occur among children whose genitalia have been minimally impacted by the disease process as well as those with more substantial genital deformity (e.g., clitoral hypertrophy).

Most girls with CAH are drawn toward male sex stereotypical behavior and away from female sexual stereotypical behavior to some degree. Of those, only a minority experience an increase in homosexual fantasy and most grow up to become heterosexual women. The modest increase in homosexual fantasy that has been reported in this group of patients is substantial enough, however, to support the prenatal androgen hypothesis. An important area for future research is to compare the family and developmental histories and psychodynamics of girls who develop homosexual fantasy with those who become exclusively heterosexual. This type of research might clarify the multifactorial pathways leading to different sexual fantasy patterns during adulthood among girls with similar constitutional predispositions toward male gender role behavior. It would help clarify the way in which the evolving self-representation is related to conscious and unconscious ideas about masculinity and femininity and the development of sexual fantasy.

The influence of androgen on childhood play/activity patterns is precisely what would be expected from research on nonhuman animals. A particularly striking finding from research on monkeys, for example, was that prenatal testosterone administration influenced certain sexually dimorphic nonmating behaviors in female offspring in addition to sexual behavior per se. Pseudohermaphroditic female rhesus monkeys threatened, initiated play, and engaged in rough-and-tumble play more frequently than control females, although somewhat less than males. They also withdrew less often from threats expressed by others. These observations about the effects of prenatal testosterone were made when the animals were between two and five months of age (that is, well before adulthood) and only occurred if testosterone had been administered during a critical prenatal period (Goy and Goldfoot 1974). Similar effects of prenatal androgen on play behavior have been well described in numerous species (Meaney 1989).

Sexual Differentiation

CAH is but one of a group of medical disorders that are characterized by some type of abnormality of physical sex differentiation. It is helpful to have a roadmap of the different physical markers of biological sex to make sense of the developmental principles learned from the study of intersex patients.

Males and females have different sex chromosomes—males are XY and females XX. A sex-determining gene is located on the Y chromosome (Donohoe and Schnitzer 1996). This gene directs the fetal gonad to differentiate as a testis that then secretes testosterone. Target tissues must have normal androgen receptors in order for fetal testosterone to exert its effects. If little to no androgen is produced (as would be the case in normal females with XX chromosomes) or androgen receptors are absent, the external genitalia have a female appearance and testosterone's influence on the brain is not present. A different substance is also secreted prenatally in the event that fetal differentiation is male. This "Mullerian inhibiting substance" causes the uterus, fallopian tubes, and upper vagina to melt away, leaving the anlage that becomes the prostate, vas deference, and seminal vesicles in place (Carr 1998).

Normally the chromosomal sex, prenatal hormones, internal reproductive structures, and external genitalia are congruent. At birth (or, in our age of high technology, before), a baby's sex is identified and announced. As soon as the child is born, everyone in her or his interpersonal network reacts to her or him as girl or boy. Thus the psychosocial messages transmitted from caretakers during the child's infancy remain congruent with the biological messages that were transmitted to and from the embryo in utero (Money and Ehrhardt 1972). In every society boys and girls are treated differently by caretakers throughout their development, however (Friedman, Richard, and Vande Wiele 1974; Maccoby 1998). Such differential treatment shapes behavior, but not exclusively so. Prenatal sex steroid hormones exert effects as well.

Androgen Insensitivity Syndrome

One way of determining the role a substance plays in development is to study the behavior of people who are born without it or whose bodies do not respond to it for some reason. The androgen insensitivity syndrome (AIS; Morris 1953; Morris and Mahesh 1963; Perez-Palacios et al. 1987; Rutgers and Scully 1991; Brown et al. 1993; Griffin 1992; Quigley et al. 1995; Radmayr et al. 1997) is of interest in this regard. In the complete form of this genetically determined disorder, the chromosomal sex of the child is XY—male. The initial part of the sexual differentiation sequence is normal, and a message is transmitted to the fetal gonad for it to differentiate as a testis and not an ovary. The testis then secretes testosterone as it should. Because of a genetically determined malfunction, however, the developing embryo lacks androgen receptors. As a result, testosterone has no influence on any of its target tissues. The external genitalia appear to be female, and there is no malelike effect of male hormones on the brain. As far as the people in the infant's social network are concerned, the newborn infant is a normal little girl, and they treat her accordingly. When she is a toddler she has a typically "girl-like" profile of interests and play. Her gender role behavior is prototypically feminine and remains so for life (Costa et al. 1997; Hampson, Hampson, and Money 1955; Imperato-McGinley et al. 1991; Masica, Money, and Ehrhardt 1971; Slijper et al. 1998; see also Money, Ehrhardt, and Masica 1968; Slob et al. 1993; Meyer-Bahlburg 1999). These girls are often diagnosed as having their unusual disorder during adolescence. Since they lack ovaries and internal female reproductive structures, they do not menstruate and seek medical attention to determine the reason that this is so.

Even though these patients have amenorrhea and some other abnormalities, they have the physical habitus and psychological profile of normal women. Their gender identity is female and their romantic-sexual interests are directed toward men. There is perhaps no medical disorder that better illustrates that chromosomal sex, in itself, does not determine a person's gender identity.

Prenatal Androgen, Gender Identity, and Gender Role Behavior

Babies with intersex disorders are often born with ambiguous genitalia and multiple other abnormalities. These patients are the subjects of ongoing study by interdisciplinary teams of medical-behavioral researchers, and treatment guidelines for their optimal care are continually being revised and updated (Diamond 1997; Meyer-Bahlburg 1998; Kipnis and Diamond 1998).

A general principle that has emerged from investigation of intersex patients is that the more extreme and prolonged the exposure of the prenatal brain has been to androgen and its metabolites, the more likely it will be that the child will experience prototypically *masculine* gender role behavior. These behavioral consequences of the influence of androgens on the prenatal brain occur in children whose parents have diverse attitudes about norms for appropriate childhood sex-role behavior. The masculinizing effects become pronounced in mid to late childhood and influence peer relationships and the development of the child's social persona and his or her internalizations. In the case of children assigned to female gender at birth, the disparity between gender of rearing and progressively intense and persistent male gender role interests and preferences can be quite painful. Patients in this category often have multiple physical abnormalities as well, including ambiguous genitalia at birth. Review of each syndrome is outside the scope of this book, and the interested reader is referred to Zucker's inclusive discussion of this topic (1999). Sometimes the person's gender identity changes in childhood, adolescence, or adulthood from that of rearing to that in keeping with ever more persistent male-stereotypical interests and activities (Imperato-McGinley et al. 1986; Imperato-McGinley et al. 1974; Imperato-McGinley et al. 1979; Imperato-McGinley et al. 1991; Mendez et al. 1995; cf. Perez-Palacios et al. 1984; Mendonca et al. 1996; Al-Attia 1996; Elsayed et al. 1988; Hochberg et al. 1996; Taha 1994; Mendonca et al. 1987; Rosler and Kohn 1983; see also Gross et al. 1986). In other instances individuals who have been born with ambiguous genitalia and incongruities between components of sex gender seem to develop conflicted gender identities whose features are different from those of the two that occur most commonly in nature, male or female. Stoller termed this hermaphroditic gender identity (Stoller 1968).

Thus the degree of male typical gender role behavior during childhood varies with the amount of prenatal androgenization of the brain. To a lesser but perceptible degree, the more the brain is exposed to prenatal androgen, the greater the likelihood that the sex object later in life will be female.

Traumatic Loss of the Penis During Early Childhood

Comparison of two tragic cases in which boys who lost their penises during early childhood as a result of accidents and were raised as girls is instructive, particularly from the perspective of developmental psychology.

A seven-month-old boy, one of a set of MZ twins, had his penis accidentally ablated as a complication of circumcision. In keeping with the principles of gender identity development that were accepted at that time, he was reared female. From the perspective of developmental psychoanalytic clinical theory, it is important to note that for practical reasons this decision was not made until age seventeen months and surgical castration and genital reconstruction were carried out at twenty-one months.

Following the accident, the parents, who were obviously psychologically traumatized, sought consultation about the best way to raise their child. They found their way to a team at Johns Hopkins Medical Center who had carried out the benchmark studies of gender identity differentiation in intersex patients, and were advised to raise the child as unambiguously female. They also did not disclose the accident to the twins. As the affected child grew into mid and late childhood, she felt more and more masculine and more and more abnormal in comparison to her female peers. Despite the fact that girls tend to be much more tolerant of cross-gender behavior than boys are, in this particular child's case the behavior was so pronounced that it did in fact lead to peer rejection and abuse. In keeping with her masculine interests and activities, she began slowly but progressively to develop a self-concept that was male, and she decided that despite sex of rearing, she was truly male. (Her genitalia had been reconstructed as female, but abnormalities persisted, included a hypertrophied clitoris). Against medical advice, she refused female hormones during adolescence and rejected her female gender identity. At that time her parents apprised her of the accident that had befallen her as an infant, and her response was one of relief. The self-concept that she had fashioned now appeared to have an explanation. This person embraced an adult male gender identity role, married at age twenty-five, and adopted his wife's children. Throughout his life the objects of his sexual desire had been female (Money and Ehrhardt 1972; Diamond 1982; Diamond and Sigmundson 1997; Colapinto 2000).

The second case report is that of a boy whose penis sloughed off at age two months following electrocautery circumcision. At age seven months, castration and other surgical intervention was made as well as the decision to raise the child as female. Although this young girl also became a tomboy during mid to late childhood, her movement towards masculine interests/activities and away from feminine activities/interests appeared somewhat less pronounced than in the first case. For example, she preferred female to male playmates, and throughout childhood had a best friend who was a girl. Although she had masculine interests, she experienced herself as female, and never wished to be a male. This patient had vaginoplasties at ages sixteen and twenty-six with the expressed desire of making the vagina suitable for sexual intercourse with men. She experienced sexual desire for males as well as for females and had sexual experiences and durable sexual romantic relationships with both women and with men. She considered her sexual orientation to be bisexual (Bradley et al. 1998).

These contrasting cases provoke much food for thought. An important difference in their biographies concerned the age of the traumatic insult and the age of behavioral interventions. Many other differences existed as well, however. Masculinization of gender role occurred in both instances, but more extremely so in one than in the other. Since the brains of both had been completely masculinized, the reasons for the difference in gender role are unclear. Perhaps innate brain differences in androgen responsivity were present. Core gender identity was affected in one but not the other. More variability in sexual object was present in the second than in the first case as well. Neither was investigated from a child psychoanalytic perspective. Additional cases of penile ablation have been reported, but none investigated with psychoanalytic informed research (Zucker 1999).

Inferences for Psychoanalytic Theory

One major theme that is relevant for psychoanalytic developmental theory is that although prenatal sex steroid hormones influence both the genitalia and the brain, the latter influence is much more important for the development of subsequent gender role behavior than the former. This is an empirical fact, directly opposed to Freud's ideas about psychosexual development (Freud 1905). A second point that we have earlier emphasized is that the highly specific effects of prenatal sex steroids cannot be explained by developmental psychoanalytic theory as it now exists.

In the next section of this chapter we discuss the relationship between childhood gender role behavior and adult sexual orientation.

Childhood Cross-Gender Behavior and Adult Homosexuality

Homosexual women are much more likely than heterosexual women to report having been extreme tomboys as children. Although tomboyishness is quite common in the female population at large, the more extreme and enduring forms of the behavior are less so, as common sense would suggest. Although the studies performed have not been uniform in defining the extent and nature of tomboyism, there is a persistent pattern in the proportion of women reporting a childhood preference for stereotypic boys' activities and boys as companions. In two large population-based studies comparing heterosexual and homosexual adults, the finding were quite similar. Saghir and Robins (1973) reported that 70 percent of homosexual women but only 16 percent of heterosexual women recalled being "boylike" in childhood. Bell, Weinberg, and Hammersmith (1981) found that 71 percent of homosexual women versus 28 percent of heterosexual women enjoyed typical boys activities (e.g., team sports) in childhood "very much."

For men the data are comparable: homosexual men are much more likely to report gender-atypical behavior during childhood than are heterosexual men. Thus Saghir and Robins (1973) found that 67 percent of homosexual men but only 3 percent of heterosexual men recalled being "girl-like" as children. Homosexual men often had no male buddies, avoided boys' games, played predominantly with girls, and were teased and called "sissy" by other boys. Bell, Weinberg, and Hammersmith (1981) reported that 70 percent of heterosexual men but only 11 percent of homosexual men had enjoyed sex-stereotyped boys' activities such as baseball and football in childhood. Conversely, 46 percent of the homosexual men but only 11 percent of the heterosexual men reported enjoying stereotypic girls' activities.

J. Michael Bailey, a behavioral geneticist, and Kenneth J. Zucker, a developmental psychologist, reviewed all studies published in English from 1960 on in which homosexual and heterosexual individuals were queried about their childhood cross-gender-typical interests and activities. Forty-one articles were uncovered, and their comparisons involved 1,583 heterosexual women, 1,539 homosexual women, 3,315 heterosexual men, and 4,966 homosexual men. They observed that in every study, regardless of when it was published, method of sample selection, or specific details of design, childhood gender role was recalled by homosexuals as being more atypical with regard to sex stereotypic behavior than by heterosexuals. Bailey and Zucker computed effect size of sex stereotypic behavior differences across studies by calculating the difference between the means of the homosexual and heterosexual groups and dividing these for the behaviors in question by their pooled standard deviations. Differences were highly significant, but more so for men than women (Bailey and Zucker 1995).

Cross-Cultural Studies of Childhood Behavior of Homosexuals

Whitam and Zent (1984) carried out a study in which they selected four societies that differed with regard to tolerance for and acceptance of homosexuality. They found that in all four—the United States, Guatemala, Brazil, and the Philippines—the same childhood developmental pattern was present among male homosexuals. Homosexuals reported having been more interested during childhood in doll play and sewing and cooking, cross-dressing more frequently, tending to be regarded as sissies, preferring play activities with girls, and preferring the company of adult females to that of adult males. Whitam and Mathy (1991) have reported similar findings for childhood cross-gender behavior in lesbians studied in Brazil, Peru, the Philippines, and the United States. In all four societies, despite radically different prevailing attitudes toward homosexuality, homosexual women were significantly more likely to report that as children they played with boys' toys, had little interest in girls' toys, dressed up in men's clothing, had little in dressing up in women's clothing, and were regarded as tomboys.

Whitam (Whitam and Zent 1984; Whitam and Mathy 1991) has argued that this association is evidence of a strong biological influence on sexual orientation. If this is so, the specific nature of this influence remains to be established. There is reason to suspect, however, that the prenatal androgen environment might substantially contribute to childhood play and activity preference patterns in ways that are relevant to the establishment of later sexual orientation.

Cross-Gender Behavior in Boys and the Prenatal Androgen Hypothesis of Sexual Orientation

Of the many behaviors that are part of a gender nonconformity pattern of boys on gay developmental track, one of the most common is aversion during late childhood to rough-and-tumble play (RTP) and play fighting. Data supporting this observation are substantial and come from diverse sources, including studies of patients and nonpatients alike (Friedman 1988; Bell, Weinberg, and Hammersmith 1981; Saghir and Robins 1973; Zucker and Green 1991; Zucker 1991; Green 1987; Bieber et al. 1962; McConaghy and Blaszczynski 1980).

As is true of sex differences in behavior, differences between homosexuals and heterosexuals in RTP and play fighting (and childhood peer aggressivity generally) refer to behavioral differences between groups, not between individuals. Some boys who become heterosexual men avoid RTP and some boys who become gay men do not. The fact that there are many adult gay athletes including boxers, football players, and others attests that many gay men participate in and enjoy RTP. During late childhood, however, this is much less frequently the case. The differences in childhood history between gay and heterosexual groups are striking. The time period when this difference is marked is roughly between ages six and twelve.

The reasons that males on a gay developmental pathway engage in less rough-and-tumble play during childhood than do heterosexual males is not known. It is credible to hypothesize, however, that this difference may be an expression of differences between the two groups in the way in which androgen influences brain development during a critical prenatal developmental phase. Prenatal androgen influences the childhood expression of RTP. This leads to sex differences in RTP that occur long before puberty, at a time when no differences between the sexes in blood level of androgen are found. This sex difference in behavior is found among many mammalian species and is thought to be the result of the fact that prenatal androgen influences the organizational structure of key areas of the brain (Maccoby and Jacklin 1974; Collaer and Hines 1995; Pellegrini and Smith 1998).

Based on these data, it seems possible that many or even most males on a gay developmental track are not exposed to the prenatal organizational effects of androgen in the same way as those on a heterosexual developmental track. If this were so, it should not, however, be taken to mean that such boys would be somehow "defective." Speculation about "deficits" in androgen might lead some social theorists, particularly those naive about science, to conclude that the group manifesting such deficits, i.e., male homosexuals, are somehow "defective." The concept of normality here is used in a biostatistical and not in a pathological sense. If one group has less androgen than another—and this has not yet been demonstrated to be the case among gay males—this does not mean that the group in question "should" have more androgen. Nature contains no such prescriptions.

In this chapter we discussed the relationship between childhood gender role behavior and adult homosexuality. This chapter followed one in which we discussed the prenatal hormonal theory of homosexuality. We observed that the same prenatal sex hormones that are thought to influence adult homosexual orientation also influence childhood gender role behavior. In order to understand the former set of influences, it is necessary to understand the latter.

At present there is no biological test that discriminates between people on the basis of their sexual orientation. Despite the fact that there is no unitary biological "cause" of any type of sexual orientation, we agree with Isay that it makes sense to consider homosexual orientation to be innate in most gay men and in life-long lesbians (Isay 1989, 1996). One reason for adopting this view is that a meaningful relationships exists between childhood gender-atypical behavior and adult homosexual orientation.

Cross-gender interests during childhood among gay/lesbian individuals occur across cultures that differ with respect to attitudes about gender role behavior. At least one recent study found that childhood gender nonconformity is heritable (Bailey, Dunne, and Martin 2000). (This investigation did not study prenatal hormonal effects, and it is possible that the intermediate mechanisms shaping sexual orientation somehow involved prenatal hormones.) Another intriguing area supporting the relationship between childhood cross-gender behavior and adult homosexual orientation is that of prospective studies of children with gender identity disorder (GID). These children have pronounced cross-gender interests prior to age four. We have elected not to discuss the topic of gender identity disorders in this volume and refer readers interested in childhood GID to Zucker and Bradley (1995) and the *DSM-IV* (American Psychiatric Association 1984). At present there is debate in psychiatric circles over whether these children should be classified as having a specific "psychiatric disorder." We mention them here simply because follow-up studies show that, as time passes, most develop homosexual orientation (Green 1985, 1987; Friedman 1988). On the one hand, most gay men have not experienced childhood GID, and therefore we do not believe generalizations about psychodynamics of sexual orientation can be made from studies of such children. On the other hand, however, the fact that many but not all of these children tend to develop homosexual fantasy/attraction patterns later in life is compatible with the literature on the relationship between atypical childhood gender interests and adult homosexual orientation. Interestingly, no biological "cause" of childhood GID has yet been identified. The condition is rare, and there is no evidence that it runs in families (Coates 1992).

The links between biological influences, gender atypical behavior during childhood, and adult homosexual orientation have not yet been worked out. We find it difficult to imagine any reason for the connections that have been established, other than a strong biological predisposition toward both in subgroups of the general population. Moreover, this should not be taken to mean that strong cross-gender interests during childhood always predict homosexual orientation. They do not. Although most gay/lesbian people have had such interests, there is no solid evidence that most people with such interests become gay or lesbian adults.

The fact that the development of boys and girls is asymmetric with respect to gender nonconformity is crucial in understanding the developmental pathways of gay/lesbian people. Boys are much less tolerant of gender nonconformity in other boys than girls are in either boys or girls. Tomboys are likely to be accepted by boys and girls unless their behavior is extreme. The very term *sissy,* however, is inherently devaluing. There is no word equivalent in meaning to *tomboy* for boys whose gender role behavior does not conform to rather narrow social norms. These norms exist among their peers as well as in the society as a whole. In later chapter we discuss the significance of this for the development of homophobia.

Exotic Becomes Erotic

In 1996 Daryl Bem proposed a general theory of the origins of sexual orientation that was influenced by much of the data about childhood gender nonconformity and adult sexual orientation that we discussed here (Bem 1996). He suggested that biological variables, including genes and prenatal hormones, code for childhood temperaments such as aggression and activity level but not for sexual orientation per se. Childhood temperament, in turn, predisposes to sex-typical versus sex-atypical activity preferences that predispose to same-sexed or opposite-sexed playmates. The most important aspect of Bem's theory is the hypothesis that the awareness of being different from same-sexed peers

> produces heightened physiological arousal. . . . The theory claims that every child—conforming or nonconforming—experiences heightened, nonspecific physiological arousal in the presence of peers from whom he or she feels different. For most children this arousal is neither affective toned nor consciously experienced. *(Bem 2000:533)*

This childhood arousal is subsequently transformed into erotic attraction. Bem pointed out that his theory "is not intended to describe an inevitable, universal path to sexual orientation, but only the modal path followed by most men and women in a gender polarizing culture like ours" (Bem 2000:543).

Our perspective is similar to Bem's in certain respects but different in others. The model he proposes seems helpful for understanding development in many children, but it has limitations. For example, it does not address the issue of "spectrum of sensitivities" with regard to predisposition toward sexual orientation. We conjecture that genes and hormones interact in diverse ways to influence brain functioning in such a way not only to facilitate certain types of sexual orientation in subgroups of individuals but also to limit options for the emergence of other types. For example, we conjecture that there are many children who, because of genetic and/or prenatal hormonal influences, are extremely unlikely to develop homosexual orientation in any type of postnatal psychosocial environment. We speculate that, for similar reasons, some children are extremely unlikely to develop a heterosexual orientation. In between these polar groups we hypothesize that there are considerable numbers of children whose brain-mind responsiveness falls along a spectrum of sensitivity for sexual orientation programming. The development of many such children is probably compatible with the Bem paradigm. Another problem with Bem's model is that it invokes a concept of "childhood" in a somewhat global way. Even if gender nonconformity usually precedes nonheterosexual orientation, for example, there is great need to empirically ascertain how frequently the two occur simultaneously in development, and whether same-sexed desire occurs first in some children.

We also agree with critics of Bem's who have suggested that his paradigm is more applicable to male than female development (Peplau et al. 1998).

With regard to the development of many boys and some girls, Bem's theory is compatible with a psychoanalytic developmental model. The psychological mechanisms that intervene between physiological arousal and erotic desire, for example, probably involve unconscious wishes and fears (Friedman 1988). No matter what the intermediate childhood mechanisms of causation, we suggest that among most gay men, and lifelong lesbians, it is helpful for clinicians to conceptualize homosexual orientation as being innate. It is important for psychotherapists always to keep in mind, however, that general theories might or might not apply to their particular patients.

In this chapter, and the one preceding it, we discussed research that we judged to be of particular interest to psychoanalytically oriented psychotherapists. Our discussion was therefore selective. The areas that we did not discuss include cerebral laterality (Lalumiere, Blanchard, and Zucker 2000; Geschwind and Galaburda 1985a, b; McCormick, Witelson, and Kingstone 1990; Rosenstein and Bigler 1987), cognitive functioning (Kimura 1999; Sanders and Ross-Field 1987; McCormick and Witelson 1991), and sibship order (Blanchard and Bogaert 1996a, b; Blanchard and Sheridan 1992; Blanchard and Zucker 1994; Blanchard et al. 1995; Blanchard et al. 1996). A number of studies, for example, indicate that gay men tend to be born later in groups of siblings than do heterosexual men. The reasons for this remain to be determined.

Although the material discussed in chapters 3 and 4 was primarily descriptive and not psychodynamic, it provides background necessary for understanding the critical discussion of oedipal theory that follows in the next chapter of part 1.

5

Freud, Oedipus, and Homosexuality

Throughout the history of psychoanalysis Freud's ideas about the Oedipus complex have arguably been the single most important influence on the way psychoanalysts think about childhood development. Indeed, this influence remains pervasive to this date, and oedipal theories still provide the structure for much formulation about the psychodynamic functioning of adults (Greenberg 1991; Friedman and Downey 1995). Even though the central role of the preoedipal maternal child relationship in psychological development received full psychoanalytic attention, nonetheless, the emphasis on orality and preoedipal functioning complemented but did not replace or invalidate many of Freud's views. Freud's ideas about the Oedipus complex in turn influenced generations of psychoanalytic thinkers about the factors leading to the development of homosexuality. Indeed, in the 1970s, when there was great debate among psychoanalysts about whether to follow the lead taken by organized psychiatry in depathologizing homosexuality, much opposition came from psychoanalysts who believed that such action would be incompatible with the central role given the Oedipus complex in psychoanalytic theory. This argument has subsided in the United States but is still expressed in many sectors of the international psychoanalytic community.

That being the case, it is important to consider Freud's ideas about the Oedipus complex in the light of scientific advances since his death. We begin with a look back at Freud's ideas about Oedipus Rex. Freud was fascinated with the story of Oedipus long before he ever created psychoanalysis. In this chapter we review the Sophoclean version of Oedipus Rex. In a letter to his dear friend Wilhelm Fleiss written in 1897, Freud expressed his excitement at discovering

the Oedipus complex during his self-analysis. Throughout his lengthy and pro-
lific career, he believed that the Oedipus complex was biologically determined
and universal (Sulloway 1979). Despite the dissent of such influential psychoanalysts as Karen Horney (Horney 1924, 1926; Friedman and Downey 1995),
Freud's theory of the Oedipus complex continued to be influential long after
his death and still remains one of the pillars of the psychoanalytic edifice. Within psychoanalysis Freud's ideas were illustrated (sometimes in modified form)
in countless articles. As an example of this, we critically consider a particularly
influential article by Loewald (1978). We then discuss extrapsychoanalytic research and the contributions of some modern psychoanalysts that raise doubts
about the validity of Freud's oedipal theory. We conclude the chapter by considering the significance of the Oedipus complex in development in light of recently revised psychoanalytic theories about homosexuality.

Freud and Oedipus

There is no question that Freud felt a strong kinship with Oedipus. In a letter written to Arnold Zweig, for example, he referred to himself as Oedipus
and his daughter Anna as Antigone. During his youthful years, when he was
a medical student, Freud wished that one day he would be as famous as the
professors whose sculptured busts were on display. The ambitious student
imagined that his own bust would bear the inscription from *Oedipus Rex:*
"Who divined the famed riddle (of the Sphinx) and was a man most mighty."
Ultimately, Freud's fantasy proved Delphic. Today, alongside the busts of his
great teachers at the University of Vienna, is one of Freud, inscribed exactly
as he had wished (Sulloway 1979:480).

It is noteworthy that Freud selected the Oedipus legend as being of unique
importance in the narrative of his own life many years before he hit upon the
developmental and clinical significance of the "Oedipus complex" as a general
psychological principle. His personal narrative pulled him toward the myth that
subsequently became an organizing image for his psychoanalytic ideas.

The Legend of Oedipus

Freud's observation that the story of Oedipus Rex exerts widespread if not
universal fascination is born out by history. The legend has existed, only min-

imally altered, in many societies and during many periods of civilization. Documentation of the Oedipus legend has been provided for cultures in medieval Europe, the Near East, modern Europe, and those in Africa, Asia and the Slavic countries. Freud appears to have been familiar primarily or exclusively with the Sophoclean version of the story, as revealed in the great tragedian's plays *Oedipus Rex* and *Oedipus at Colonus.*

The story of Oedipus as told in the plays of Sophocles goes like this:

The king of Thebes, Laius, is told by the oracle at Delphi that he is destined to die at the hands of a son yet to be conceived. His wife, Jocasta, becomes pregnant and gives birth to a boy. Laius binds the infant's feet together (in one form of the legend they are pierced) and orders him placed in a mountain wilderness to die. The infant is rescued by a kindhearted shepherd and given to another shepherd. Unaware of his history, this shepherd presents the baby to the king of Corinth, who raises him as his own. The boy is given the name Oedipus ("Swollen Foot").

He grows up in Corinth, and when he is a young adult a drunken companion reveals that he was adopted, and not the true son of the King of Corinth. Oedipus confronts his adoptive parents, who refuse to discuss his past. Feeling an urgent need to discover his origins, Oedipus seeks out the oracle at Delphi. The oracle does not reveal who his parents are and instead makes a horrifying prediction: Oedipus is fated to murder his father and marry his mother.

Resolving to save his parents and himself from an incomprehensibly terrible fate, Oedipus flees the city. This decision is predicated on the belief that his adoptive parents are in fact his biological parents. In fact, neither his adoptive parents nor the oracle at Delphi have confirmed this.

At a place where three roads meet, Oedipus has a violent confrontation with an older man. Each refuses to let the other pass first. They fight and the man is slain.

Having no idea who the stranger was, Oedipus continues his journey. The scene now shifts to the city of Thebes, which is suffering on two counts. Thebes is without a king, and travelers to and from the city are being preyed on by the Sphinx. A female monster, half-lion but with a human face, requires passersby to answer a riddle. What animal walks on two, three, or four feet, yet speaks with one voice? She devours everyone unable to solve the puzzle. Desperate, the king of Thebes offers the kingdom and the hand of Jocasta to whomever answers the riddle correctly. Oedipus, known to be brilliant, responds correctly. "The answer is man." He thus became king of Thebes and husband of Jocasta. The Sphinx then kills herself.

Oedipus and Jocasta have four children, and he reigns contentedly for many years, until a plague falls upon the city. A blind prophet, Teiresias, accuses him of polluting Thebes and causing the affliction. Oedipus, seeking assistance from the oracle, is advised that the murderer of Laius must be driven from the city for the plague to end. Forced to search systematically for the killer, he uncovers his past. Confronted with a horrifying story of which she had previously been unaware, Jocasta hangs herself. Oedipus pokes out his eyes.

Exiled, he wanders from place to place assisted by his loyal daughter, Antigone. He finally reaches Colonus, where he achieves a state of wisdom and exalted grace. At Colonus he disappears into the earth, never to be seen again (Edmunds 1985; Rudnytsky 1987; Sophocles 1947).

Homosexuality and the Oedipus Myth

A final word about the Oedipus story concerns an additional theme that involves Laius. Before conceiving Oedipus, Laius was said to have raped a young boy, Chrysippus. The father of this child cursed Laius. If he ever fathered a son, that son would murder him. The destiny of Oedipus was therefore dictated by the act of homosexual violence carried out by his father. This part of the story has been elaborated on by some psychoanalysts in their explication of the "negative Oedipus complex" in which the son unconsciously identifies with the *mother* (Freud 1923; Wiedeman 1995).

In 1897 Freud carried out his self-analysis, a unique feat in the history of thought. The experience of psychoanalysis is daunting, even with the help of a mentor-guide. Freud simultaneously discovered and experienced the analytic process all alone. Others who have been psychoanalyzed have had good reason to be awed by the unusual combination of traits Freud exhibited when he ventured into such uncharted and foreboding territory.

On October 15 of that year, he wrote to his dear friend Wilhelm Fleiss:

Dear Wilhelm,
My self-analysis is in fact the most essential thing I have at present and promises to become of the greatest value to me if it reaches its end. . . .

If the analysis fulfills what I expect of it, I shall work on it systematically and then put it before you. So far I have found nothing completely new, just all the complications to which I have become accustomed. It is by no means easy. Being totally honest with oneself is a good exercise.

A single idea of general value dawned on me. I have found, in my own case too, the phenomenon of being in love with my mother and jealous of my father, and I now consider it a universal event in early childhood, even if not so early as in children who have been made hysterical. . . . If this is so, we can understand the gripping power of Oedipus Rex, in spite of all the objections that reason raises against the presupposition of fate; and we can understand why the latter "drama of fate" was bound to fail so miserably. . . . The Greek legend seizes upon a compulsion which everyone recognizes because he senses its existence within himself. Everyone in the audience was once a budding Oedipus in fantasy and each recoils in horror from the dream fulfillment here transplanted into reality, with the full quantity of repression which separates his infantile state from his present one. *(Masson 1985:272)*

In a footnote to *The Three Essays on the Theory of Sexuality,* written almost thirty years later, Freud stated:

It has justly been said that the Oedipus complex is the nuclear complex of the neuroses, and constitutes the essential part of their content. It represents the peak of infantile sexuality, which, through its after-effects, exercises a decisive influence on the sexuality of adults. Every new arrival on the planet is faced by the task of mastering the Oedipus complex; anyone who fails to do so falls a victim to neurosis. With the progress of psycho-analytic studies the importance of the Oedipus complex has become more and more clearly evident; its recognition has become the shibboleth that distinguishes the adherents of psycho-analysis from its opponents. *(1905–1915; 1962:130)*

Freud held these views until the end of his life (1940:97). His absolute and unwavering insistence on the universality of the (positive) Oedipus complex had profound consequences for the way in which classical psychoanalysts viewed homosexual development.

Limitations of Freud's Theory of the Oedipus Complex

Psychoanalysis as a system of thought has largely retained the primacy of the Oedipus complex as Freud described it. Thus the vast majority of practitioners today still rely heavily on psychodynamic formulations based on the Oedipus complex construct (Greenberg 1991). Numerous therapists find that their clinical experience is organized and made coherent by such formulations. For the practicing psychoanalyst, oedipal conflict is "experience near."

The "complex" is generally conceptualized in its positive rather than its negative form, and in a relatively unelaborated way. In its basic form, sexual desire for the mother triggers competitive rivalry with the father. Castration anxiety results. Identification with father is associated with repression of the "complex," which, however, can produce unconscious conflict leading to diverse psychological symptoms. The superego results from this identification.

Karen Horney: An Early Dissenter

Even during the early years of psychoanalysis, Freud's theory of the role of the Oedipus complex in psychological functioning had critics among his colleagues.

Arguably the most influential of these was Karen Horney. We devote special attention to Horney not only because of her many contributions to psychoanalysis but also because an overarching theme of this book concerns differences in psychoanalytic ideas about the psychological functioning of lesbians and gay men in particular and women and men in general. It was Horney who exposed Freud's inadequate understanding of girls and women. It is difficult today to imagine the pressure exerted upon the young Karen Horney to accept the views of Freud and of so many in his early circle. What had, in the infant years of psychoanalysis, begun in 1902 as a "Wednesday Evening Discussion Group," meeting at Freud's home (Gay 1988), grew rapidly into a political movement. To say that Freud did not welcome dissent, particularly in areas of which he claimed ownership, would be bland understatement.

Karen Horney was fiery, proud, and independent. She shared with Freud the courage to swim against the tide; however, he was irritated that he happened to be the tide. As early as 1922, in a famous session of the International Congress of Psychoanalysis, Horney openly challenged Karl Abraham, her ex-analyst, and Freud, the presiding chairman, regarding the validity of Freud's view of female development and psychological functioning.

Horney stated that Freud's theory of psychoanalysis was replete with incorrect and biased assumptions about female psychology and suggested the specific ways in which Freud's developmental ideas were incorrect (Horney 1924, 1926). Horney argued that women did not feel inadequate because they lacked a penis. In fact, their biologically determined feminine attributes were virtues, not deficits. If women seemed to envy men, it was because Western European culture was biased against women and women's sense of being unfairly treated relative to men was expressed symbolically in penis envy. Men were also envious of women specifically their reproductive capacity. She suggested that men's anxiety about feminine power caused them to demean women.

Horney also disagreed with Freud's view that the Oedipus complex, even in boys, is the result of biological determinants and is the core dynamic influence in all neuroses. Horney suggested that the intensity of oedipal conflicts is variable and depends on intrafamilial relationships. In insisting on the biological determinants of the Oedipus complex as opposed to sociocultural influences, Freud had made an important error (Horney 1937, 1939; Quinn 1987).

Loewald's Ideas About the Oedipus Complex

The voluminous psychoanalytic literature on the Oedipus complex has been reviewed extensively (Greenberg 1991) and its application to homosexuality discussed in detail as well (Wiedemann 1995; Friedman 1988; Lewes 1988). The articles tend to share common features, however, and we have selected a particularly influential discussion by Loewald for commentary, as an illustration of relatively recent psychoanalytic thought about the topic. Loewald's article, "The Waning of the Oedipus Complex" (1978), was initially delivered as a plenary lecture to the American Psychoanalytic Association. Loewald made an analogy between the developmental stages of the infant and the biblical account of the fall of man suggesting that the early mother-child bond is experienced as "sacred" but doomed to be "violated" by oedipal sexual and aggressive desires (393). Loewald agreed with Freud that during the oedipal phase incestuous and parricidal fantasies are universal. He proposed that the formation of psychological autonomy, central for the synthesis of identity, depends on destruction of parental authority, which is equivalent in the unconscious to murder of the father.

> Assumption of responsibility for one's own life and its conduct is in psychic reality, tantamount to the murder of the parents, to the crime of parricide, and involves dealing with the guilt incurred thereby. Not only is parental authority destroyed by wresting authority from the parents and

taking it over, but the parents, if the process were thoroughly carried out, are being destroyed as libidinal objects as well.   (389)

The organization of the superego, as internalization of narcissistic transformation of oedipal relations, documents parricide and at the same time is its atonement and metamorphosis. . . . The self in its autonomy is an atonement structure.   (393)

Loewald's conclusion that the development of psychic autonomy is based on a parricidal fantasy is expressed as literal fact; there is no suggestion that it is meant to be thought of metaphorically. No empirical support for this conclusion is presented; rather, the reader is asked to suspend critical judgment about it, as one might while reading a paper by Kierkegaard or, perhaps, Loewald's teacher, Martin Heidegger.

Loewald's essay is not only nonempirical, it is anti-empirical. For want of a better term we consider its style to be an example of "romantic authoritarianism." Many psychoanalysts seem to react to it positively, as sympathetic humanists, not skeptical scientists. Its rich evocative qualities strike a responsive chord. A problem with this type of reading of the psychoanalytic literature is that confusion and erroneous reasoning about psychological development and the treatment of patients has resulted from the application of standards that are basically literary and aesthetic to articles about human psychology. It is not likely that many child psychoanalysts today actually believe that the synthesis of the self-concept depends on a parricidal fantasy. The influence of Loewald's paper on modern psychoanalytic thinking is difficult to gauge. Its basic ideas appear to have been neither accepted or rejected but rather absorbed by a culture that appears to tolerate contradictory ideas similarly to the way a clinician would tolerate ambivalence in a patient.

Science, Psychoanalysis, and the Oedipus Complex

Recent observations in the behavioral and neurosciences have raised questions about the ubiquity of the Oedipus complex as well as about its significance for psychological development. These new findings have led us to reexamine Freud's original Oedipus complex construct.

In a review of extrapsychoanalytic research, Mark Erickson recently summarized evidence that secure bonding during infancy is associated with incest avoidance later in life (Erickson 1993). Erickson pointed out that, contrary to a belief widely accepted during Freud's lifetime, nonhuman primates rarely mate incestuously, and incest is rare among other mammals as well. Mounting and sexual exploration of the mother animal may occur but tends to disappear as animals reach sexual maturity. Erickson cited observations by Westermarck that avoidance of sexual intercourse is common among men and women who had lived in prolonged intimacy during childhood. He reviewed studies indicating that sexual avoidance often develops between Israeli men and women who had been raised on kibbutzim together. The same sexual aversion has been observed among Chinese married as children and reared together. Only when early bonding is disrupted is incest likely to occur. Although Erickson did not review studies of fantasy, he pointed out that Freud viewed castration anxiety as the major motivation for incest avoidance. Erickson questioned Freud's emphasis on innately determined incestuous desire and suggested that the motivation to commit incest might not in fact be intense, or even present, among children who have experienced consistently secure early bonding. Incestuous motivations and fantasies might be evidence of disruption of early bonding and the psychopathology that results.

Evolutionary theory supports Erickson's ideas. For example, a sociobiologist recently commented:

> Incest often produces deficient offspring, and it's not in the son's genetic interest to have his mother assume the risks and burdens of pregnancy to create a reproductively worthless sibling. (Hence the dearth of boys who try to seduce their mothers). *(Wright 1994:315–316)*

The same author emphasized that *childhood* scenarios of competition between father and son for mother usually do not have sex as the goal.

> "Why would boys want to have sex with their mothers and kill their fathers? Genes that specifically encourage this aren't exactly destined to spread through a hunter-gatherer population overnight?
>
> When boys reach adolescence, they may, especially in a polygynous society, find themselves competing with their fathers for the same women. But among these women is *not* the boy's mother. *(Wright 1994:315)*

A number of modern psychoanalysts have also criticized Freud's oedipal theory. Chodoff (1966) pointed out that Freud's ideas about childhood sexuality were not based on solid empirical evidence. He doubted the accuracy of Freud's psychosexual developmental theory, and he raised serious questions about whether erotic attraction to parents should be considered a norm for children. Lidz and Lidz (1989) recently discussed cultural influences on the Oedipus complex and questioned its universality.

A particularly detailed critique of oedipal theory was recently published by Albert Schrut, a child psychiatrist and psychoanalyst (Schrut 1993). Schrut observed that many psychoanalysts still believe that all dimensions of Freud's theory remain valid. For example, as recently as 1991, Rangell reaffirmed Freud's conviction that castration anxiety is a universal developmental event, occurring exactly in the way and for the reasons that Freud had originally suggested (Rangell 1991). Schrut's experience, however, suggested otherwise:

> My longitudinal observations and psycho-analytic work with many children over the period of the oedipal years have failed to discover objective evidence that would tend to confirm that castration anxiety is present in most small children. Nor to my knowledge after searching the literature are there any long-term studies involving a sufficient number of children that demonstrate this. *(Schrut 1994:737)*

Another reason for taking a fresh look at the Oedipus complex derives from research on the etiology of psychopathological disorders. Freud (1940) hypothesized that unresolved oedipal conflicts were major if not determining influences in the etiology of neuroses. Among the conditions once considered "neuroses," however, are a variety of anxiety and depressive disorders as well as other psychiatric illnesses. Genetic, constitutional, neurophysiological, and psychosocial influences on the etiology of these diverse disorders have been elucidated recently. The Oedipus complex does not appear to be as central in the etiology of mental disorders as Freud thought.

The same type of criticism applies to the concept of the superego. Freud emphasized the mechanism of identification with the same-gender parent as necessary for oedipal conflict resolution, believing that this identification results in the formation of the superego (Freud 1923, 1933, 1940). Today, the model of superego functioning generally accepted by psychoanalysts has been modified: identifications with both parents as well as other cognitive and psychosocial influences lead a child to develop moral values (Gilligan et al. 1988; Kagan 1984; Kohlberg 1976, 1981; Tyson and Tyson 1990), which contribute crucially to superego development. Revision of Freud's hypothesis concerning superego formation parallels criticism of his model of female development and psychosexual functioning (Schafer 1974).

Freud's psychosexual developmental theory was further weakened by empirical research in the area of gender identity development. Stoller (1968) and Money and Ehrhardt (1972) established that core gender identity—the sense of being male or female—is established before the onset of what was traditionally thought to be the oedipal phase. Gender identity is a psychological construct, yet influenced by constitutional biological factors, cognitive development, and psychosocial learning. The relationship between core gender identity and genital knowledge is complex (Bem 1989). Formation of core gender identity, however, is not dependent upon perception of the genital difference in the way that Freud thought, nor is it primarily motivated by castration anxiety (Fagot 1985; Fagot, Leinbach, and Hagan 1986; Yates 1993). It is likely that establishment of core gender identity precedes and organizes the way in which a child experiences oedipal conflict, not the reverse (Tyson 1982).

Another area of profound change in psychoanalytic theory in recent years has been in the areas of sexual orientation. Modern American psychoanalysts do not view homosexuality as inherently pathological. Nevertheless, despite widespread rejection of the pathological model of homosexuality, most American psychoanalysts continue to believe in the fundamental importance of the Oedipus complex in psychological functioning. The new ideas about homosexuality raise fundamental questions about the role of the Oedipus complex in development. How can "normal" resolution of oedipal conflicts result in homosexuality?

Thus, superego development, gender identity, sexual orientation, personality structure, the etiology of the neuroses (and the psychoses)—all seem to be subject to influences other than oedipal conflict resolution or failure thereof. The questions then are, What specifically is the role of the Oedipus complex in development? Is the Oedipus complex biologically determined, or even strongly biologically influenced, or not?

Although it is not possible to answer these questions completely at this time, we next discuss recent developments in the behavioral sciences that indicate the need for revision of the Oedipus complex as proposed by Freud and his followers.

6

Toward a Revised Formulation of
Male Oedipal Aggression

In the last chapter we discussed evidence indicating that many of Freud's ideas about the role of the Oedipus complex in male development are invalid. Psychotherapy sessions, dreams, and childhood stories and imaginative play are often organized around oedipal themes, however. How can we account for the conundrum?

We conjecture that the aggressive component of oedipal themes is much more prevalent than the erotic component and that the competitive-aggressive motivations of oedipal-aged boys do not occur as a consequence of sexual desires for the mother. Rather they are experienced and expressed as a result of the influence of prenatal androgens on the brain. The fantasies resulting from these prenatal hormonal effects *are* often incorporated into oedipal triangular scenarios, however, and we discuss one way of thinking about this below. We also discuss the significance of this for boys on a gay developmental pathway.

Biology and Psychoanalysis

Even today many psychoanalysts continue to view biological influences on human experience and activity in terms of Freud's instinct theory. Freud characterized instincts as forces representing somatic demands on mental life and creating tensions that are experienced as needs of the id (Freud 1940).

During the latter half of the twentieth century, however, psychoanalytic sophistication about many areas of psychobiology has increased, including the psychobiology of attachment, nonverbal representation, affect regulation, cerebral lateralization, memory, evolutionary psychology and genetics (Kandel 1999). It has become apparent that Freud's instinct theory cannot provide an adequate theoretical framework to integrate psychobiological observations that have occurred since his death.

In chapters 6 and 7 we call attention to an aspect of psychobiology underemphasized by psychoanalytic theory to date—the development and significance of gender-differentiated childhood play. Research findings about this dimension of human development are important for psychoanalytic theory, particularly with regard to oedipal and postoedipal development. Consideration of the significance of childhood play necessitates a more complex model of psychological functioning than that posed by instinct theory and complements that of other areas mentioned above (such as attachment, memory, etc.) and of psychoanalytic developmental theory as traditionally conceptualized to date.

Childhood Play: An Underemphasized Area of Psychoanalytic Theory

To the best of our knowledge, no major psychoanalytic theory, including structural theory (Freud 1923), self psychology (Kohut 1971, 1977), object relations theory (Fairbairn 1952; Jacobson 1964; Kernberg 1976; Greenberg and Mitchell 1983); ego psychology (Hartmann 1964), interpersonal theory (Sullivan 1953), relational theory (Mitchell 1988), or Lacanian theory (Roudinesco 1990) has fully considered the origins or significance of *gender-differentiated* childhood play.

Of the many psychoanalysts who have written about childhood play, one of the most influential has been Winnicott. He considered play between the infant and mother to be fundamentally important in development, particularly for the capacity to be creative. Winnicott discussed the concept of a metaphorical potential space between mother and child that also occurs in the psychoanalytic/therapeutic situation. He likened the therapeutic situation to play in which free association and dyadic communication occurred creatively in such a way as to facilitate health and self-authenticity of the patient. Winnicott thought of play as an activity of the ego and not primarily motivated by sexual or aggressive drives (Winnicott 1967). Winnicott's contributions emphasize the importance of childhood play for the development of fantasy, creativity, mother-infant attachment, and the capacity to respond positively in the psychotherapeutic situation.

Melanie Klein theorized about the unconscious meanings of childhood play (Klein 1937). Klein's contributions and those of other psychoanalysts were discussed in an extensive review of the origins of childhood play and play therapy as a form of treatment by Kanner in 1940. Kanner noted that Groos had speculated, at the turn of the century, that childhood play was instinctually motivated and served the function of rehearsal for adult activities (Groos 1896). He also cited Mitchell and Mason's observation: for children, play is "the serious business of life" (Mitchell and Mason 1935). Anna Freud also discussed play, stressing the distinction between play and work, the former being governed by the pleasure principle, the latter by the reality principle. She discussed the developmental significance of play, from the infant's play with the mother's body to the cooperative play of later childhood (Freud 1965).

Child psychoanalysts routinely use play in their therapeutic work with young children. Yet neither the many psychoanalysts who have discussed play nor the early psychoanalytic pathfinders have conceptualized it as a psychobiologically determined phenomenon, integral not only to the experiential world of children but also in facilitating development of boyhood and girlhood cultures fundamentally different from adults and from each other (Maccoby 1998). In this chapter we consider the relevance of boyhood play for revising oedipal theory. In the following chapter we discuss its significance for late childhood developmental differences between boys and girls.

Psychological Functions of Play

Whereas mammals differ in many aspects of their social, aggressive, and sexual behavior, their young share with the young of birds the capacity to play. The play of young animals, including human beings, is distinctive, exuberant, and seems to be motivated by a primary type of pleasure that children and behavior scientists alike term "fun." Children in all societies play (unless they have been abused or neglected) and have done so throughout recorded history. As human beings grow and develop increasingly sophisticated cognitive capacities and complex social relationships, the capacity to play is expressed in fantasy, art, creativity of all forms, and other diverse ways. Many adults lose their capacities to play for one reason or another, though many do not. Childhood play, however, is distinctive in its intensity, in the frequency with which it is expressed, and in the meaningful space it occupies in a child's inner life. "Do you want to play?" is a universally recognized introduction of one child to another. The process of play itself, particularly play between children, is not taught to them by adults. Nor does it appear to occur as a result of some type of identification with adults.

The term *play*—somewhat difficult to precisely define—connotes certain types of locomotor and/or social behaviors that have multiple functions. Play fosters the development of many types of physical abilities, stimulates exploration of the environment, animate and inanimate, facilitates bonding, structures certain types of social relationships, teaches complex behaviors and skills (which, in other contexts, have survival value), and fosters behavioral flexibility and the capacity to cope with the novel and unexpected (Fagen 1981; Bekoff and Byers 1998). In human beings, play enacted and in fantasy serves as role rehearsal for complex social behaviors required later in the life cycle.

Biologists generally consider the term *play* to connote a few specific types of behavioral patterns. These include mother-newborn play, solitary motoric exercise, as in "kicking up the heels," leaping, somersaulting, and doing backflips, exploratory play with inanimate objects, nonagonistic play fighting and play chasing, and semi-agonistic rough-and-tumble play in which the goal is not to hurt the other participant but during which threatening expressions and overtly aggressive behavior may occur as part of the overall pattern. The type of activity often termed horseplay usually consists of hitting, shoving, pushing, wrestling, kicking, and striking with objects (Fagen 1981). As noted in chapter 4, these behaviors plus competition for territory or for hierarchical rank are commonly termed rough-and-tumble play (RTP).

Rough-and-Tumble Play

In humans, as well as many other mammalian species, sex differences in social play occur. The behaviors that we label RTP constitute one category of childhood play in which sex differences have been reported in most cultures studied and that to a large degree are independent of rearing practices (Maccoby and Jacklin 1974; Pelligrini and Smith 1998; Meaney 1989). With regard to questions about the interaction of nature and nurture and the role of endogenous, biologically influenced motivations in development, considerations of this category of behavior is enlightening.

There is considerable overlap between males and females in most sex role behaviors, including RTP. With the exception of core gender identity and, possibly, neonatal caretaking and interactive activities, most behaviors that occur more frequently in one sex than the other differ in *quantity* of expression but not in quality. Thus males and females both engage in RTP, but males do so more frequently. A particular female may do so with great frequency, however, and a particular male hardly at all. The sex difference in behavior thus refers to group differences but not necessarily to differences between individuals. This illustrates a general principle about the concept connoted by terms such as *endogenous* and *innate*. These terms refer to the likelihood that certain traits will occur in specified environments rather than to the inevitability that they will occur in all individuals. Moreover, it is not necessary for every single individual in a given population to manifest a particular trait in order for it to be considered innate (Wilson 1978).

Hormonal Influence on Sex Differences in RTP

Unlike many other forms of behavior, including sexual activity, RTP behaviors of early life are strikingly *similar* across different species, not only in their expression but also in the neuroendocrine mechanisms that influence their expression and in their psychosocial consequences. Games like "king of the mountain" or wrestling contests are typical ways in which the tendency toward RTP is expressed. It is perhaps sobering to acknowledge that, in addition to human beings, young monkeys, baboons, gorillas, horses, zebras, goats, sheep, deer, pigs, rats, guinea pigs, gerbils, and the young of numerous other species all participate in versions of such activities (Fagen 1981; Meaney 1989).

Sex differences exist in RTP in large measure because of the effect of androgens on brain differentiation during critical periods of embryogenesis (Gorski 1991; McEwen 1983). Prenatal androgens *organize* the differentiation of the brain in such a way as to influence childhood RTP. The "hardwiring" of male and female brains differs as a result of the prenatal effects of androgen, and this difference leads to postnatal behaviors that are expressed at a time when no sex differences in circulating blood androgens exist (Gorski 1991; McEwen 1983; Maccoby and Jacklin 1974; Bekoff and Byers 1998).

In thinking about child development from a psychoanalytic perspective, we find it helpful to keep comparisons of human and nonhuman RTP in mind. The idea that there is an innate tendency for boys to engage in certain types of play *complements* but does not replace the role of identification in development. It does suggest, however, that identification not be viewed in a unitary way. It is but one of many factors that influence behavior. The mental experience of identification itself might sometimes be the product of other influences including those of prenatal androgens on the embryonic brain and genetic influences.

Nature, Nurture, and RTP

In a discussion of sex differences in the social play of mammals, Meaney (1989) states:

> In many social mammalian species, the demands on the animals differ as a function of gender. The sex differences in the social play of the juveniles appear to reflect these differences, such that young males and females engage in behavior from which they are most likely to benefit developmentally. In the case of play-fighting, the early hormonal environment increases the tendency to engage in play-fighting. For the males of several species this is likely to be of considerable adaptive significance. Thus, perinatal androgens appear to influence selectively the type of interactions from which social learning is derived. *(Meaney 1989:259)*

Juvenile play behavior, especially RTP, is a good example of an interaction between biological and social events. As a result of exposure to androgen perinatally, an animal is predisposed to participate in play fighting. This behavior in turn is utilized socially to facilitate the formation of dominance hierarchies. Much social development of young animals occurs within the context of these hierarchies.

This view of developmental biology emphasizes the way in which behavior and biology are integrated to facilitate social adaptation during development. It is quite different from Freud's emphasis on the adversarial relationship between biology and culture (Freud 1930). For example, establishment of mammalian dominance relationships leads to social organization that allows large social units to function effectively. In the natural world, males that compete during their juvenile years are rarely wounded or killed. Even later in life, although mature males of many species may in fact be fatally injured during battles for dominance, death is the exception rather than the rule.

103

Neuroendocrine Influences on Childhood Fantasy

Biological factors that predispose to RTP not only influence activities that may be observed and even quantified, but also influence *fantasy* as well. Fantasies in boys that are based on competition between males, usually involving arduous physical tasks or heroic performances at athletic or dangerous activities, are, in our view, the elaborated experiential manifestations of central neurobiological influences. Obviously, the particular environment that a child is raised in shapes his or her fantasy life to a great degree. Yet the contribution of prenatal hormonal influences is also great. It is safe to conclude that boys are generally innately predisposed to be attracted to the superhero role. Indeed those "superheroes" who do not possess magical attributes, such as the capacity to fly, for example, but who are heroic by virtue of character and athletic endowment (such as Tarzan) may be thought to be the perfect products of the prenatal and pubertal influence of testosterone.

RTP, Competition, and Cooperation

"Purely" altruistic behavior is relatively rare among human beings, unquestionably less prevalent than various forms of aggressive destructiveness (Wilson 1978). In humans, as in social insects and mammals, altruism usually involves close kin or members of one's tribe. Because of the experience of transference, however, we humans may have feelings toward nonrelatives that are similar or identical to those we have toward close kin. Perhaps for that reason, we seem to be capable of more altruism than most mammals.

The play behaviors that we have called RTP do not always lead to acts of competition and aggression. Sometimes they may be precursors to social behaviors based on cooperation and even altruism later in life. For example, hierarchical social organizations that are similar to or elaborated versions of those of juvenile males on athletic teams exist in many areas of adult life. Some social functions seem best carried out by such organizations. Teams of various sorts (not only athletic) are only examples of this. In these social units competition for a particular niche may be viewed as being in the service of "higher" form of cooperation. Destruction of one of the participants in the competition would weaken the social unit. Struggles for dominance in this type of situation may be a way of establishing expertise at roles that are required by the larger society.

It is also important to realize that a strong predilection toward RTP on the part of an individual should not be equated with destructive aggressiveness. For example, several years ago a well-known professional football player, John Offerdahl, carried out a heroic rescue of an aged couple whose car skidded into a lake. He explained that as he was carrying it out he had had the thought "that she's someone's mother, or grandmother, so you picture your mom and your grandmom. It makes you realize how precious life is" (Offerdahl 1993:48). Nonhuman mammals rarely, if ever, put their lives at risk to help nonkin in this fashion. Many other instances of human altruism toward nonkin have been documented (Oliner and Oliner 1988). Offerdahl's remarks implicate transference as a mechanism influencing motivation in that regard. His altruistic acts required athletic abilities, and he was bold enough to carry out such acts because of his long-standing affinity for RTP. The psychosocial effects of rearing would appear to influence the adaptive function to which RTP abilities are put later in life. In nontechnical parlance, children who have been loved are prone to behave lovingly toward others. In fact, childhood RTP may have important functions that are not necessarily related to social dominance at all. Development of psychomotor skills need not be in the service of competitive struggles. Similarly the scene of two children tussling, giggling, and thoroughly enjoying themselves suggests possible bonding functions of RTP.

Clinical Considerations

Without claiming to be comprehensive, we review below some common situations in which the endogenous predisposition to RTP may present as a major component of the total clinical picture. In these situations constitutional predispositions influence the way in which oedipal enactments are expressed in the family. For example, the "setting" that regulates the motivation toward RTP may be extremely different between father and son, and either may be more inclined toward RTP. This type of imbalance *in itself* is not necessarily problematic. Countless fathers and sons negotiate their differences about these and other matters successfully. Some do not, however, and we first consider a father-son pair in which the father has the higher motivation to participate in RTP.

This type of father experiences a consistent feeling of pressure to participate in RTP activities, even during adulthood. A weekend athlete, when friends and family socialize, he spontaneously organizes "touch" football games. This father follows organized sports and may have a season ticket to the games of his favorite team. He identifies with the athletes and relishes the dramatic competitive struggles in which they are engaged.

The son in this family is not particularly motivated to participate in RTP. The father is disappointed that his son does not share his enthusiasm for athletic activities. He spends much time attempting to teach his son how to throw a ball, swing a bat, and be proficient at other athletic tasks. Despite good intentions, the father usually becomes irritable in reaction to his son's awkwardness. His pedagogical style is hypercritical, demanding, and tough-minded. Between ages five and twelve or so, the son tries to better himself at activities that his father enjoys. After that, he gradually loses interest in them. Father and son (both heterosexual) drift apart, and by the boy's teenage years they spend very little time together. The son grows older and increasingly prefers intellectual pursuits. Both father and son feel deprived. The father wishes that he had a "pal" who could be more "normal" like him. The son wishes that he had a father who could understand and accept him.

In this type of situation both father and son are likely to feel alienated and depressed in their family setting. The father devalues his son, for not being athletic, but also secretly devalues himself for not being "intellectual." The son is likely to have internalized his father's standards for masculine behavior. Despite a self-contained facade, he secretly feels inadequate.

During the son's childhood, the father's problem was his rigidity and his narcissism. Seeing his son as an extension of himself, he assumed that the son's RTP profile should be the same as his own. The facts were otherwise, but the father was unable to interpret the son's innately low motivation to participate in RTP as anything but a defect. A father who was better able to tolerate difference would not have made his relationship with his son conditional on RTP performance.

Let us now consider a situation in which a son is at the higher end of the RTP spectrum and his father is at the lower end. Once again we focus only on the parent-child pairs not able to tolerate such disparity.

In this hypothetical case the father is a sedentary professional who devalues RTP, which he considers "barbaric." His wife shares his values. They have scholarly ambitions for their young son and are put off by his competitive, physically adventurous temperament. From earliest years he has been drawn to RTP. Despite all admonitions and criticism, he careens through childhood with abandon. By the time he is ten or twelve years old, he is embattled with his parents. As his autonomy has increased with age, so have their punishments and constraints. A hero to his peers, he is a "problem child" in his family. Because he does poorly in school, despite being intellectually gifted, his parents seek psychiatric consultation. All three members of this family are angry and depressed. As far as the son is concerned, he participates in athletics as a "natural" way of life. "I was born this way," he says, and he is more or less correct. Careful history taking reveals that the entire behavioral repertoire that is unacceptable to his family is confined to RTP. The boy has no symptoms of antisocial behavior, no learning disability, no impulse disorder. He feels guilty that he is unable to be the kind of son his parents desire. His peers relate to him as a dominant male; hence he does not consciously view himself as being unmasculine. In his father's eyes, however, the boy is not en route to becoming a "complete" man. With his father's values internalized (despite himself), the son has low self-esteem and a persistent sense of masculine insecurity.

Gay Youth

With regard to the development of gay youth, their temperamental aversion to RTP is often part of a more general tendency toward cross-gender sex stereotypic interests. Fathers often react to this by withdrawing from them or attempting to change their temperaments, with unfortunate consequences for the father-son relationship. The chasm between the gay teenager, and his well-intentioned, conventional heterosexual father, is often even greater than in the first case discussed above and cannot be bridged by the ordinary methods that such fathers might use to reach heterosexual sons who are more like themselves. The poignancy of the situation is often increased because both father and son may have loving feelings for each other but are unable to create a communication bridge built on shared interests. Particularly with preteen sons, fathers sometimes insist that their sons play catch with them or participate in little league baseball. They feel that persistence and insistence about this are requirements for being an involved, caring parent. The son in these situations is likely to feel tortured, and the father bewildered. Misunderstandings tend to be compounded by the fact that the son may only recently have recognized that he is gay, or may not yet even fully realize it himself. Sometimes these fathers are frankly homophobic, but not always. Many a father believes that the reason his son retreats from team sports is that he lacks skill. The father presents himself as role model and tries to foster skill development, believing that this will increase his son's popularity with peers. The son, on the other hand, realizes that his interests are innately different from those of most other boys. If his father insists that he pursue sex-stereotypical masculine activities, the son is likely to develop secondary symptoms of anxiety and depression. Situations of misunderstanding such as these are discussed more extensively in the clinical section of this volume.

The scenarios outlined above are meant to illustrate only some of the ways in which the constitutional motivation to participate in RTP enters the clinical situation. Understanding the origins and manifestations of these behaviors is necessary in order for a clinician to be optimally helpful to his or her patients. Because of limitations of space, we did not describe the other parent's role in the family system. Obviously, the mother's input can ameliorate or exacerbate difficult situations. Our purpose here, however, is not to discuss family dynamics but simply to make the point that the endogenous motivation to participate in RTP has direct clinical relevance.

RTP Versus Destructive Aggression

In distinguishing RTP from aggression we have essentially taken one subgroup of behaviors that Freud would have considered to be manifestations of "activity, mastery, dominance" out of the aggression category, leaving other subgroups having destructiveness as their goal. Thus, we would go so far as to suggest that it is "instinctive" to be motivated toward RTP and "instinctive" therefore to be motivated toward physical competition with another male. Unlike Freud, who assumed that oedipal father-son competition was associated with unconscious *homicidal* fantasies, we raise the possibility that oedipal-age competitive feelings sometimes stem from an impulse to *play* and to compete. We speculate that parricidal fantasies become more common during late childhood and adolescence and, even then, are not universally experienced.

The term *aggression* generally connotes *destructiveness*. Moyer (1976) has suggested that the term *aggression* be applied to behavior leading to damage or destruction of some target. He has proposed a classificatory system based on characteristics of the stimulus that evokes aggressive responses. The categories (which are not mutually exclusive) are predatory, inter-male, fear-induced, irritable, territorial, defensive, maternal, instrumental, and sexual. We agree with the usefulness of defining aggression in terms of *motivated destructiveness*. In human psychological functioning the concept of destructiveness must, however, include both actual and *fantasized* damage to an object.

There is no question that homo sapiens is an innately aggressive species, and therefore many find it intuitively appealing, as Freud did, to conceptualize an aggressive instinct. There has never been a time in all recorded history without war and violent crime. Our species appears to have an omnivorous appetite for destruction. We are the "natural enemies" of each other, of most other mammalian species, including those who have no other natural enemies, and even of other diverse life forms that constitute the planetary ecosystem.

E. O. Wilson (1978) has written:

> Human aggression cannot be explained as either a dark angelic flaw or a bestial instinct. Nor is it the pathological symptom of upbringing in a cruel environment. Human beings are strongly predisposed to respond with unreasoning hatred to external threats and to escalate their hostility sufficiently to overwhelm the source of the threat by a respectably wide margin of safety. Our brains do appear to be programmed to the following extent: we are inclined to partition other people into friends and aliens. In the same sense that birds are inclined to learn territorial songs, and to navigate by the polar constellations, we tend to fear deeply the actions of strangers and to solve conflict by aggression. These learning rules are most likely to have evolved during the past hundreds of thousands of years of human evolution and thus to have conferred a biological advantage on those who have conformed to them with the greatest fidelity.

Boyhood and Adult Aggression

There is substantial evidence that the same prenatal organizing hormonal influences that predispose *most* boys toward RTP also predispose *many* to be truly aggressive.

Psychological investigators have studied aggression in diverse ways using structured paper and pencil tests, semistructured interviews, projective tests, observed, naturalistically occurring social interaction, social psychological experiments, epidemiological studies of specifically defined acts of aggression, studies of environments in which aggressivity is common, tape recordings of psychotherapeutic sessions, psychiatric examinations of violent criminals, neuropsychiatric studies of violent patients and brain-damaged patients, postmortem studies of the brains of violent people, and effects of drugs that amplify or inhibit aggressive behavior (Glick and Roose 1993; Goodman et al. 1993; Lewis 1989 [1967]; Maccoby and Jacklin 1974; Moyer 1974; Prentky and Quinsey 1988; Valzelli 1981). Across all measures in all studies, and in all cultures studied and throughout recorded history, males have been found to be more aggressive than females (Moyer 1974, 1976). Of course, just as females engage in RTP, so they also may be violently destructive. Most violence, however, is enacted by postpubertal males. This is true despite the fact that substantial childhood violence goes unreported since its victims are other children. Sex differences in prepubertal aggressivity, however, also occur in the expected direction (Gilligan 1982; Maccoby and Jacklin 1974)—that is, males are more likely than females to engage in it.

Despite these observations, the relationship between aggression and male sex steroids is not simple. At postpubertal physiological levels testosterone does not "cause" aggressive activity. Children as young as age four who have the disorder known as precocious puberty experience the biological effects of adult levels of testosterone. They are not innately hyperaggressive, however, just as the majority of physiologically normal men are not (Money and Ehrhardt 1972). Many interactions involving testosterone exceed the scope of this article (Rose 1985). In adults true aggression appears to be expressed as a result of intricate interactions between absence of constraints, stimulating social circumstances, and constitutional predispositions of various types. In children true aggression appears to be expressed as a result of similarly complex interactions. Thus many children undoubtedly have the capacity to be truly aggressive and therefore to harbor destructive and even homicidal fantasies.

Parricidal Fantasies in Boys

Given the great prevalence of true aggressiveness, even in childhood, there is no great difficulty in finding parricidal fantasies among oedipal-aged boys. Whether such fantasies are truly normative or merely constitute the expression of a specific subgroup of an even larger group predisposed to competition but not necessarily to *mortal competitiveness in fantasy* seems uncertain. What is more important, in our view, is that the fantasies of aggression and dominance in the relationship between son and father do not necessarily derive from the erotic desire for the mother (or in the case of those so programmed, erotic desire for the father) but are a manifestation of an independent psychodevelopmental line. Even when parricidal fantasies and wishes are expressed by oedipal-aged boys, they should not necessarily be understood as a wish for the actual death of the father.

The child psychoanalyst Albert Schrut has pointed out that fantasies of sex and death by three-to-six-year-old children are quite different from those of adolescents and adults. Here it is important to keep in mind the idea of a spectrum of psychopathology from normal to severely disordered. The more a child has experienced sexual and/or physical abuse and/or neglect, the more likely his fantasies take on an adultlike quality with homicidal and erotic fantasies toward others, including those in his family. On the healthier end of the spectrum, however, this is much less likely. For example, Schrut observed:

> For young children death often means a brief disappearance. Death fantasies and other hostile fantasies are often voiced towards fathers, mothers, and especially toward siblings during periods of rivalry. These may be accompanied in some children by varying degrees of "anxiety" or "guilt" but generally, such reactions are apparently transient and minor except in children where pathology already exists. *(Schrut 1994:736)*

In chapter 5 we summarized evidence that erotic desire for the mother should not be taken as a universal developmental norm. We now further explore relationships between sexual and aggressive experience and fantasy during development. We begin with developmental differences in the hormonal regulation of sexual and aggressive realms of experience.

Neuroendocrine Determinants of Sexuality Versus RTP and Aggressiveness

We have a number of reasons for believing sexuality and RTP fall along different developmental lines. From a neurobiological perspective, the RTP testosterone-dependent system is influenced by biological mechanisms that are fundamentally different from those that determine and control erotic activity. Space permits only a brief summary of the relevant differences here. Those who wish a more inclusive discussion are referred to recent reviews (Byne and Parsons 1993; Friedman and Downey 1993a, b; Gorski 1991; LeVay 1993; Meyer-Bahlberg 1993; Collaer and Hines 1995; Paredes and Baum 1997; Herbert 1996; Breedlove 1994).

In brief, there are two major biochemical pathways by which androgens organize the structure of the central nervous system. In one major pathway, androgens are converted to estrogens intraneuronally, and the biochemical response of the cell is actually to the estrogens. In the other major pathway, the cell responds directly to androgens, and these are *not* metabolized to estrogen in order to exert their effect. Sex-stereotypical mating behavior, which in rats includes mounting, intromission, and ejaculation in males and lordosis in females, and other forms of sexual activity in primates, appears to be influenced by both pathways. In contrast, RTP is influenced only by androgen that is *not* metabolized to estrogen. Moreover, the anatomic sites that regulate mating behavior are distinct from the anatomic sites that influence RTP (Meaney, Dodge, and Beatty 1981; Meaney and McEwen 1986; Oomura, Yoshimatsu, and Aou 1983; Perachio, Marr, and Alexander 1979; Valzelli 1981).

Childhood Sexual Development

Let us return here to the topic of the psychology of the Oedipus complex itself. Even if children do not normally experience sexual desire for their parents, might not the complex be based on their erotic desires for other objects? Consideration of this possibility necessitates a closer look at childhood sexuality.

As we mentioned earlier, sexual behavior occurs in immature animals but not in its full form. For example, in nonhuman primates immature animals typically carry out some but not all of the sequences necessary for adult-type copulation (Harlow 1986). The nonhuman animal data has some interesting parallels in the sexual activity of children. Thus a recent investigation of the frequency of various sexual behaviors in normal four to six year olds revealed that touching genitalia or displaying sex parts of each other occurred reasonably often. Behaviors characteristic of adult sexuality were rare, however, and when present generally signified sexual abuse (Yates 1993).

The important psychoanalytically informed research of Galenson and colleagues demonstrated that children frequently engage in intentional genital self-stimulation *prior* to the "oedipal phase" of development (Galenson 1993; Galenson and Roiphe 1971, 1976, 1980; Roiphe and Galenson 1972, 1973, 1981). Galenson's research also suggested that at least some of these children probably experience early forms of erotic fantasy. Although the importance of this research cannot be overemphasized, it should not be taken to mean that erotic fantasy and activity during childhood—whether oedipal or preoedipal—is *normative*. Orgasm may occur during very early childhood. How frequently it actually does, during naturalistic circumstances, is another question, however. Even Galenson's careful observational research has not established that orgasm *usually* occurs during most early childhood sexual activity.

Freud extended the meaning of what is usually considered to be erotic to include many related but not specifically sexual dimensions of behavior and experience including gender identity role, attachment behaviors, and feelings of sensual pleasure. If we adopt a more circumscribed use of the term *erotic*, limiting it only to those experiences that are associated with feelings of sexual desire and arousal (i.e., erotic affect as opposed to diffusely pleasureful feelings), there is good reason to believe that only some children—by no means all—and boys far more frequently than girls experience meaningful erotic arousal during or prior to the oedipal phase of development. We hypothesize that even when such arousal is experienced, sexual desire for a *parent* (as a primary stimulus) is highly variable and in fact rare in families that are not dysfunctional. What little evidence exists seems to us to suggest great diversity in the emergence of childhood sexuality. The age at which the various components of erotic motivations become more salient probably varies substantially between children, and important differences between boys and girls are present.

In any case, in boys *and* girls as well, we hypothesize that the erotic component of the Oedipus complex is not a normatively occurring, innately determined event during the oedipal phase of childhood as Freud had proposed.

Castration Anxiety

The years during which oedipal-like conflicts are experienced are crucial for integration and representation of the body image. Consistent with our belief that incestuous wishes are *not* universal and biologically determined, we do not accept the theory that the symbolic representation of bodily damage, even including genital damage, is necessarily and inevitably triggered by such wishes. We hypothesize that many types of fears are symbolically represented somatically by young children and that diverse wishes are experienced as unacceptable and therefore likely to provoke severe punishment. In taking this position, we explicitly disagree with Freud's theory and that of classical psychoanalysts such as Rangell (1991) that castration anxiety is universally experienced as a concrete reality during the oedipal phase of development.

Adult Sexual Fantasy

During adulthood erotic activity and imagined or fantasized erotic activity seem to function as a series of acts, depicted, as it were, on a canvas. As is true with other areas of motivated patterned activity, however, sexual activity that appears to be a single, unitary behavior actually consists of components of smaller behavioral units that under usual, natural circumstances connect seamlessly with each other. To put this somewhat differently, the story line, whether sexual or otherwise, consists of connected frames, each of which, in turn, is made up of subframes, smaller mental units. One can liken this to chemical compounds composed of molecules that are themselves composed of elements.

In adults erotic stimuli are processed according to personal narratives (called "sex scripts" by Stoller) composed of "impulses, desires, defenses, falsifications, truths avoided and memories of past events, erotic and nonerotic-going back to infancy" (1979:viii). People tend to return over and over again to the content of a quite specific erotic narrative theme that includes the fundamental features of sexual object and situation. In our culture the concepts of the triangular and of the forbidden are both important influences on the structure of sexual narratives. In adult sexuality the past is always conflated with the present. The condensation of past objects and situations, and imagined (forbidden) objects, situations, and part objects, with present actors in erotic narratives provide dramatic and endlessly fascinating dimensions to personal scenarios of lust, passion, and desire. It is probably never possible for someone to recall his or her childhood sexual life without its being colored by the condensation, or fusion, between childhood and adult affects, images, and self and object representations (Stoller 1975, 1979, 1985; Kernberg 1995; Person 1995).

The Development of Erotic Fantasies

Since investigation of childhood sexuality is so frequently discouraged for political and cultural reasons, knowledge of the mechanisms by which sexual fantasies are fashioned during development is limited. Child psychoanalysts have much to offer in clarifying open questions, but a major limitation of their contribution is that their patients understandably tend to come from pathological groups. With these qualifications in mind, we speculate that, as children grow, those that experience erotic arousal/desire (most boys and some girls by late childhood) construct ever more elaborate sexual fantasies. These fantasies depend, to some degree, on cognitive growth, social development, and knowledge acquisition. For example, an oedipal-age child might experience erotic arousal in response to a heterosexual or homosexual stimulus consisting of a nude body. Cognitive processes that adults take for granted, but which are actually rather complex, are required for people to integrate coitus, mutual masturbation, fellatio, and anal intercourse into their sexual repertoires. How these processes are experienced and expressed during development is presently not clear. The creation of dramatic scripts that organize fantasy and integrate erotic desire, competitive hostility, and terror also depends on complex cognitive processes. We conjecture that substantial variation exists between children with regard to the age when these "oedipal-like" scripts are constructed.

The Oedipus Complex and Gay Development

Of all aspects of oedipal psychology the role and manifestations of the Oedipus complex in gay development must be considered the most speculative and least empirically supported. The reason for this is that there is no data base on the Oedipus complex of children who grow into gay adults—other than in deviant samples, such as children with gender identity disorder (American Psychiatric Association 1994).

With that qualification in mind, let us turn our attention to the "complex" as a whole. Just as has been reported in the psychoanalyses of heterosexual men, memories of having been sexually attracted to a parent—in this case, the father—have been reported in the psychoanalyses of gay men (Isay 1989). Although this sometimes occurs, there is no evidence that it is normative. We suggest that most boys whose sexual object is male are not primarily sexually attracted to their fathers but to peers, siblings, fantasized figures, imaginary playmates, movie stars, and others. Thus, just as with boys on a heterosexual developmental track, the childhood erotic fantasies of boys on a homosexual path consist of components that await integration and elaboration later in development. During the oedipal age range, we speculate that these fantasies are present in only rudimentary form.

What about fears of retaliation—e.g., castration anxiety? We propose that all boys—regardless of their sexual orientation—are likely to be frightened of adult males. Thus it is common for gay men to be anxious about retaliation for erotic impulses, which they unconsciously view as unacceptable, from adult male authority figures, symbolically representing their fathers. They also depict jealousy of mother for father's attention in oedipal-like terms, as might be expected, and in this situation the retaliatory figure in mental scenarios is the mother (e.g., internal maternal representation). We view the need for paternal attention as a yearning for paternal love and attachment that is usually not primarily sexually motivated. Although this point may seem obvious from the perspective of a modern clinician, it is important to emphasize because it is fundamentally different from Freud's model of castration anxiety. Children on a homosexual development track are likely to fear bodily damage, represented, sometimes but not always, in their minds as genital damage, in the same way that children on a heterosexual developmental track are, but not as a specific way of depicting retaliation for erotic wishes.

The impetus for chapters 5, 6, and 7 comes from our study of the psychoanalytic theories of homosexuality. Many psychoanalysts had believed (and some continue to believe) that erotic desire for the mother is biologically programmed to be intensely experienced in mid childhood. Homosexual orientation therefore must inevitably represent developmental derailment. In recent years most American psychoanalysts have revised their ideas about homosexuality and now see gay people as developing along different lines than the heterosexual majority. The significance of this for Freud's theory of the Oedipus complex, however, tends not to be addressed as we have done here. Having been drawn to a consideration of oedipal developmental theory by our work on the psychoanalytic theory of homosexuality, it soon became apparent that a more sweeping and inclusive revision of the theory was needed.

We find it helpful to keep in mind that the theory of the Oedipus complex was formulated by an adult, who looked back at his development during his self-analysis. The Sophoclean plays about Oedipus Rex are also about the reconstruction of the past by an adult. Although the fantasies of children are replete with oedipal-like themes, they are qualitatively different from those of adults. The fairy tales of the brothers Grimm, for example, or the early films of Walt Disney evoke terror, fear of bodily damage, punishment and retaliation by vengeful adults, loss, and grief. They are not, however, based on the kind of erotic sexuality that Freud suggested all children experience. Parents, therapists, and teachers have ample experience with oedipal-aged children who have expressed wishes that their parents would die. These same children still want their parents to put them to bed, however, as Albert Schrut observed (Schrut 1994).

The more pathological the family environment, the greater the likelihood that sexual and aggressive abuse and neglect have occurred, the more probable it is that the fantasies of children take on the insistent urgent qualities of adult fantasies. Thus we suggest that children who express oedipal wishes in the specific concrete form proposed by Freud are likely to have been abused and/or neglected. Perhaps our more important criticism of classical psychoanalytic theory is that the Oedipus complex (composed of erotic desire for the mother, parricidal wish, and resulting castration fear) should not be considered an integrated, irreducible psychological unit that appears as a unified mental structure during mid childhood. We have discussed evidence supporting the view that childhood competitive-dominance and sexuality develop along different pathways and suggested sexual and aggressive themes that are integrated into oedipal-like narratives during the latter half of childhood in ways that differ from child to child.

7

Late Childhood: The Significance of Postoedipal Development

In this chapter we discuss postoedipal development in boys and girls. The fact that their developmental pathways are asymmetrical has been underemphasized in psychoanalytic theory and is important for understanding the origins of adult sexuality. In boys intolerance of cross-gender behavior in peers, homophobia, and homosexual orientation have their origins in late childhood. In girls late childhood is a time during which themes emphasizing emotional closeness, particularly in familial settings, become elaborated in fantasy. This provides the context for romantic and sexual development throughout life. Girls, anchoring their self-esteem in intimate relationships to a much greater degree than boys, are also much more tolerant of gender-atypical behavior and less liable to be homophobic or become so later in life.

The Juvenile Male Peer Group: Origins of Homophobia and Homosexuality

Childhood play marks the beginning of developmental lines that differ between the sexes. The two pathways are dramatically evident during late childhood during which peer relationships are organized so differently that developmental psychologists have suggested that boys construct a culture organizing male behavior, and girls a culture organizing female behavior (Maccoby 1998).

Juvenile Peer Relationships and Social Play

In early childhood social play is primarily intrafamilial; children play with their parents and siblings. Some peer play occurs during toddlerhood and more by mid childhood. During mid and late childhood social play becomes predominantly a form of peer interaction. Meaney, Stewart, and Beatty have observed that this is true of humans and other mammals as well:

> In most (mammalian) species the most predominant form of peer-peer interaction is that of social play. In many species, peer-peer interactions may almost be equated with social play. Considered another way, it is the tendency of young animals to engage in social play that leads to peer-peer contact.   *(Meaney, Stewart, and Beatty 1985)*

Children's Play Is Sex Segregated

A striking fact about human development, empirically established and unanticipated by psychoanalytic developmental theory, is that during mid and late childhood boys tend to play with boys and not girls, girls with girls and not boys (Maccoby 1998). Although some cross-gender play occurs, it is far less common than same-gender play. A developmental psychologist summarized this phenomenon as follows: "Gender segregation is an almost universal phenomenon, found in all cultural settings in which children are in cultural groups that permit choice" (Fabes 1994).

It is notable that, as a general rule, *gender-segregated play* occurs regardless of the attitudes and values of parents toward it and presumably among children who differ with respect to the degree of resolution of their oedipal conflicts. There is a good deal of evidence indicating that it is initiated and perpetuated by children themselves (Fagot 1994) and does not occur as a result of identifying with adults or complying with their directives for appropriate behavior.

The Peer Groups of Boys and Girls

Boys' peer groups tend to be cohesive, bounded both from girls and from adults, and organized hierarchically. Dominance rank governs much group behavior. In free play juvenile boys tend to be territorial, competitive, unaccepting of participation by girls, and devaluing of behavior that is deemed feminine or girl-like. Their verbalizations tend to be confrontational and replete with challenges, mockery, and bravado. In interactions within the group, and outside the group as well, boys tend to resist the influence of girls and women. Unlike girls, who tend to solve problems by stressing reason and emphasizing the importance of polite behavior, boys tend to solve problems through giving orders, attempting to gain dominance and physically intimidate others. They are difficult to influence with polite suggestions (Gilligan, Lyons, and Hamner 1989). Interestingly, boys' groups tend to be larger than girls.' Whereas girls gravitate to dyadic interactions and those between dyads and relatively small groups of peers, boys are drawn to groups of five to eight individuals or even more. Throughout childhood girls seem to be more drawn to the company of single other females—peers and adults, including their mothers—than boys to the company of single males. When with others, girls tend to be more verbal, sharing of experience and feelings, confessional, expressive, and empathic. Girls' interactions stress mutuality and something we term relationality (Gilligan, Lyons, and Hamner 1989; Gilligan 1982; Maccoby 1990). As many journalists and behavioral scientists have observed, boys tend to be more instrumental and, when in groups, to be drawn to coordinated group athletic activities.

Girls are less aggressive, more affiliative in fantasy and in observable behavior than boys, and their groups tend to be less bounded. Girls alone, in dyads or in groups, are more responsive to suggestions by adults of both sexes. They are also much more tolerant of gender-role behavior that is atypical. Thus, juvenile girls are less likely to exclude boys from joining their play than boys are to exclude girls. Girls playing with boys or pursuing activities that are generally considered "masculine" are less likely to be condemned by other girls than are boys who become involved in stereotypically feminine activities. Both juvenile-aged boys and men have a pronounced tendency to negatively categorize boys who become engaged in female-like behaviors.

Gender-Coded Object Hunger in Boys

We speculate that both juvenile-aged boys and girls experience phase-specific motivation to participate in same-aged peer behavior. In the case of girls, however, this need is less likely to be rigidly gender-coded, and probably less likely to be rigidly age-coded as well. That is, if same-aged girls are not available, juvenile-aged girls are more able than boys are to substitute activities with boys, or with older women, without paying a psychological penalty. We believe that boys experience a more intense, persistent, insistent need for same-sexed peer relationships. When not available, boys are more likely to experience something that we have termed gender-coded object hunger—they yearn for same-sexed playmates and fantasize about them. Although boys in this situation will participate in social activities with girls, if available, they are more likely to pay a penalty. This comes in the form of condemnation from other boys and males, if such behavior becomes public knowledge, and from their own fantasy constructions, if it remains private.

The Functional Significance of Boys and Girls' Interests and Cultures

Eleanor Maccoby raised a question about the adaptive significance of juvenile male play.

> Why should a young male who will later seek to father many children avoid girls and engage in male-male rough play during his childhood years? To ask this question makes us aware how little we know about the adaptive functions of play in childhood for later childhood functioning.
>
> *(1998:93)*

We suggest that a possible answer to this might come from evolutionary theory. Certain types of group activities enhance the likelihood of survival of individuals and require highly coordinated activities. We are impressed by the similarity between juvenile male group behavior, as it occurs naturalistically in many societies, and the attitudes and conduct of men in the military. Let us explain by first discussing research on boyhood behavior carried out by an anthropologist who sat in on the activities of little league baseball teams and studied their verbal and nonverbal behavior (Fine 1987). Little league baseball involves more than five hundred thousand children nationally and internationally and its participants are usually intensely involved not only in a sports activity but in a world with moral and dramatic components different from that experienced or taught in their families. Little league baseball players, mostly boys, enter a domain whose rules are taught by adult coaches (almost always male) and by other boys and whose motto is "Character, Courage, Loyalty." This motto captures something of the difference between boys and girls' cultures. Girls would not be likely to relate to such a slogan. In fact, it is similar to the motto of men in military organizations, in which the central principles involve being loyal to comrades in arms, having courage to adapt to adversity, and having moral integrity. This type of morality places the fate of the team, or the group, above that of particular individuals. In contrast to the mother-infant and peer-peer dyadic relational model prototypical for girls, this model is hierarchical and oriented toward conformity to the norms of the group.

The Culture of Soldiers

The military historian John Keegan has observed that, despite substantial differences in nation of origin and historical epoch, soldiers often share a behavioral code (Keegan 1994). Although different in certain respects from that of boys, we are nonetheless impressed by its similarity in others. Of course, the universe of adult warriors is darker, and, unlike boyhood athletes, soldiers face immediate danger to life and limb. Nevertheless, like juvenile boys, soldiers are hierarchically organized and live within a bounded male society. Loyalty, honor, stoicism, courage, and obedience to leaders are highly valued. The fate of the group is placed above that of the individual. This creates a cohesive social organization composed of comrades in arms, each of whom adheres to a code of conduct and trusts the others to do so. In the world of soldiers:

> Admiration derived from something other than his badges of superior rank. It came from the reputation he held as a man among other men. . . . An officer might be clever, competent and hard working. If his fellow soldiers reserved doubt about him none of these qualities countervailed. He was not one of the tribe. *(Keegan 1994:xv)*

Keegan discusses what he calls "warrior values" in English, French, Arab, German, American, and many other soldiers throughout history: "exponents of a code of courage and duty that belongs to the origins of their republic" (1994:xvi).

In speculating along these lines we are not advocating that males should so develop. Our perspective is descriptive, anthropological and mindful of evolutionary theory as well. We have noted that play fighting is not actual fighting—its intent is to have fun and it seems to foster bonding. However, as children grow, their behavior becomes incrementally more complex. Play fighting and associated activities grow to be associated with the formation of social dominance structures. *These are organized in specific ways and carried as cognitive maps in the minds of the individuals who are part of the group.* The similarity in social organization and moral belief systems between many hierarchical juvenile male groups and adult military organizations invites the speculation that the two are functionally related in some fashion.

An Anthropological View of Masculinity

In discussing masculine psychology from an anthropological perspective, David Gilmore observed that androgynous cultures do in fact exist but are rare (1990). An overview of all societies suggests that so-called manly codes occur along a spectrum, from those that might be called extremely macho, to those that are much less so, to the relatively few that are not organized around masculine roles but nevertheless sanction physical protection of the social unit as a male responsibility. "In most societies, however, three moral injunctions exist for men: to impregnate women, to protect dependents from danger, to provide resources for kin" (Gilmore 1990:223). The concept of manhood is a cultural construction, one that is adopted by individuals who grow and develop in a particular cultural context.

Interestingly, Gilmore notes that in societies with strongly defined traditional norms for masculine behavior altruistic behavior toward the welfare of the group as a whole, including women and children, is often positively sanctioned:

> One of my findings here is that manhood ideologies always include a criterion of selfless generosity, even to the point of sacrifice. Again and again we find that "real men" are those who give more than they take, they serve others. Real men are generous even to a fault. . . . Non-men are often stigmatized as stingy and unproductive. Manhood therefore is also a nurturing concept. . . . It is true that this male giving is different from and less demonstrative and more obscure than the female. It is less direct, less immediate, more involved with externals; the "other" involved may be society in general rather than specific persons. *(229)*

In any case, the notion of altruism toward the society as a whole, among those who are capable of defending it from predators, is also compatible with the perspectives of evolutionary psychology.

Gilmore considers modern American society to fall in the mid-range on a hypothetical "macho-gender neutral" spectrum. However, developmental psychologists observe that juvenile-aged children are probably the most sexist of all social groups (Maccoby 1998; Thorne 1993). Their sexist values are maintained even when their parents and teachers sanction cross-gender role behavior—and boys are far more sexist than girls. As we explain below, the developmental problems for gay and prehomosexual boys are different from those of lesbians and prehomosexual girls: a consequence of the naturalistically occurring distinct childhood cultures of boys and girls.

The Aversion to Sex Atypical Behavior by Juvenile Boys

The study of little league baseball players referred to earlier revealed how negatively boys value what might be construed as feminine behavior in their peers.

The boys were discouraged from expressing feelings of vulnerability and, in fact, from discussing feelings generally. Empathic and confessional discussions were frowned upon. To be considered feminine or girl-like was a grave insult to be responded to with contempt. Gary Fine, the researcher who studied the behavior of these juvenile boys, observed that antihomosexual remarks were freely expressed: "The world view of these boys stressed male domination, female submission and the importance of presenting an adequate image to male peers. "Being like a girl" was scorned—and in that context, being homosexual was a grave insult" (Fine 1987:115).

The boys used terms such as *homosexual, queer, gay, faggot* to connote behavior they considered feminine-submissive, not sexual orientation. In fact, most seemed not to know what homosexuality actually was or what gay people were really like. This research was carried out in the 1980s, before positive images of gay people began appearing in the media. We doubt that these images, which have had a positive effect on the culture at large, have permeated the culture of juvenile-aged males, even now.

Homophobia

The negative sanction toward activity that is labeled homosexual is strong during the juvenile phase of development and seems part of the moral values of many male peer groups. This moral framework is asymmetrical for boys and girls. This has consequences for the development of boys and girls who are on a homosexual developmental track. Boys are likely to exclude and/or abuse other boys perceived to be homosexual. Gender-nonconforming boys, however, are likely to be acceptable to girls, who are much less governed by sex-role stereotyped moral values. The topic of juvenile-aged girls accepting or excluding other girls perceived to be homosexual has received only scant attention. It seems that girls appear much less likely to label other girls homosexual and to negatively value them because of this. We do not suggest that all juvenile male groups are homophobic, rigid, hierarchical, and xenophobic. Many are, however, and this has significance for developmental and clinical psychology, both in theory and practice.

We hypothesize that homophobia begins among boys during the juvenile phase and that later forms of even more malevolent antigay attitudes arise from this phase of life. Since its origins appear to be associated with the conduct of juveniles in naturalistically occurring peer groups, whose attributes include being bounded from and resistant to the influence of adults, those who seek to ameliorate homophobia in the general population are faced with a difficult task. The little league study suggests that antifeminine attitudes among male juveniles are probably common.

These attitudes exist among boys across the entire spectrum of normalcy and psychopathology. They occur in those whose families are organized traditionally and are not deviant as well as in those whose families are pathologically disorganized. Child abuse, neglect, and diverse other stressors are regrettably common, however, as are diverse traumata that occur early in life. We conjecture that these have an amplifying effect on normally occurring juvenile male gender-role insecurity and that this leads to extreme and malevolent manifestations of homophobia.

Male Homosexual Development

Both homosexuality and homophobia are rooted in male juvenile development. Neither can be understood without understanding the other. The underlying psychological factors that influence the way in which the two forms of behavior unfold involve the attitudes that boys have about gender role behavior.

As the developmental psychologist Eleanor Maccoby observed, boys and girls form different peer cultures during mid and late childhood (Maccoby 1998). In boys the sexual fantasies that determine orientation as homosexual-bisexual or heterosexual tend to be in place by late childhood (Herdt and McClintock 2000). An important covariant of those on a homosexual track concerns their gender role behavior and pattern of peer relationships. Children on a homosexual developmental pathway are drawn toward gender nonconformity. Many are ostracized by other boys or find interacting with them so aversive

that their only same-aged friends are female (Saghir and Robins 1973). The research of developmental psychologists discussed earlier in this book indicates
that boys joining female peer groups, or who even have dyadic relationships exclusively with girls, are quite age-atypical. We believe that this contributes to the
self-labeling of being different experienced by such children. They experience
themselves as different not only from the heterosexual majority because of their
sexual fantasies but also from their male peers because of their gender role behavior. Bem posed a causal connection between the onset of homosexual desire
and the sense of being different from other boys (Bem 2000). Here we emphasize other consequences of the sense of being different from peers.

Difference, Shame, and the Juvenile Peer Group

Same-sexed peer groups construct norms for behavior that are different from
each other. These norms then become *internalized and part of the code of ideal
behavior against which actual behavior is measured by children.* This process of
internalization of peer values and attitudes is part of childhood moral development. Boys who become part of female groups are likely to be labeled
"sissies" by other boys, and the literature on male homosexuality reveals that
this has indeed frequently occurred during the childhood of countless gay men
(Saghir and Robins 1973; Friedman 1988; Zucker and Bradley 1995; Hanson
and Hartmann 1996). Failure to live up to internalized gender-coded male
peer group standards is likely to be responded to with shame (Morrison 1989;
Lewis 1992; Pollack 1998). This painful feeling is not unique to those on a gay
developmental track but is unfortunately experienced quite commonly.

For many boys anxiety about becoming sexually aroused in the company
of other boys may exacerbate the sense of being different. Such anxiety may
influence them to avoid male peer activities that involve showering or changing clothes in a locker room, for example. The two domains, gender-role nonconformity and homoerotic fantasy, thus overlap in development but are not
congruent. Each may contribute to a boy's sense of difference from peers, but
the influence of each varies from child to child.

Girlhood and the Psychobiology of Maternalism

In comparison to boys, girls are more nurturant, relational, and accepting
of others, particularly of those who are gender-nonconforming. We suggest

that they are predisposed to be this way from birth. We begin our discussion of girls with discussion of the psychobiological influences leading them to be on a different developmental pathway than boys. We then discuss how different their late childhood peer groups are from those of boys, and comment on the significance of these differences for psychoanalytically oriented clinicians.

Maternal Doll Play—Maternal Interest

Although the evidence for biological influence on maternal interest in humans is less substantial than on RTP, it seems to us to be compelling, nevertheless. Girls throughout the world are more interested in infants and in playing with dolls representing infants than boys are. This interest occurs by mid childhood and probably is attributable to hormonal influences that are prenatal, since there are no differences in sex hormone levels between boys and girls at that time. They parallel the interest shown by juvenile nonhuman female primates in interacting with infants of their various species (Meaney, Stewart, and Beatty 1985).

Also supporting the prenatal hormonal hypothesis is that girls who are exposed to androgenizing hormones prenatally evince much less interest in doll play and express less maternal interest in fantasy, even if they later become wives and mothers (Money and Ehrhardt 1972). This effect occurs whether the excessive prenatal androgens are endogenous and due to the disorder congenital adrenal hyperplasia (CAH), or exogenous and administered to mothers during pregnancy and transmitted across the placenta to the fetus (Ehrhardt and Baker 1974; Hines 1998; Berenbaum and Snyder 1995; Berenbaum 1990). Although these girls have different play preferences than controls, their *gender identity* is normally female. They know that they are girls and experience themselves as feminine without desire to change sex (Zucker 1999).

In chapter 4 we discussed the syndrome of complete androgen insensitivity (AIS): genetic males whose cells are completely impervious to the effects of androgen because of a genetically determined disorder. These individuals have female-appearing external genitalia and are raised as girls. They have more interest in doll play and infant care when they are children than boys do, comparable to or even greater than normal girls (Money and Ehrhardt 1972). This line of research is also compatible with investigation of lower mammals indicating that males castrated at birth and therefore deprived of androgen become more responsive than normal to their young whereas females given androgen become less responsive (Stern 1989).

An hypothesis integrating the above research is that prenatal androgen influences the embryonic brain in some manner yet to be determined so that maternal interest is suppressed or extinguished. Without such influence, and with appropriate psychological input, maternal interest and play is experienced and expressed directly and in fantasy. A qualification is necessary at this point, lest it seem that all that is necessary for women to be adequate mothers is that they not be prenatally androgenized. In discussing the developmental behavioral capacities of girls and women, we refer to fantasy construction, preference for certain activities, and predilection toward particular interpersonal styles. We do not refer to maternal competency—a complex area of its own—here.

The Line of Development of Girls

From an evolutionary perspective it makes sense that females have an innate tendency to care for their offspring (Fisher 1999). By mid and late childhood, themes of childcare, expressed in the play and fantasy of girls, are usually embedded in narratives involving familial relationships and tasks carried out in family groupings, such as food preparation, for example. These themes may be found in fantasies expressed in stories and art from children all over the world, and are quite different than those of boys. Girls' narratives tend to involve intrafamilial relationships, and drama is provided by threatened or actual loss of relationships. Boys' narratives, on the other hand, usually involve heroic combat with powerful adversaries. Whereas the themes expressed by girls frequently involve parenting and home-care activities, those of boys rarely do but rather are centered on events that occur outside of the home (Nicolopoulou 1997; Nicolopoulou, Scales, and Weintraub 1994; Sheldon and Rohleder 1995). It would appear that innate tendencies are reinforced by social experiences in such a way that mutually reinforcing behavioral sequences and cascades become part of the repertoire of boys and girls from early childhood. Girls are naturally drawn toward interaction with infants and infant surrogates. The more experience they have, the better they get at the actual care of children. Young boys, less drawn to infants, remain less interested in home-care activities throughout later childhood as well. Whereas girls are socialized to be parents, a role that stimulates their imaginations as well, boys are much less so.

Girls and Sports

In our era girls commonly engage in athletic team sports such as soccer, softball, and basketball. We have failed, however, to find documentation that teams of girls exhibit the same type of rigidly hierarchical groups that boys do in which negative traits are *gender-coded*. Girls do not spontaneously tend to rebuke others for being "queer" or "dykey." Of course, one reason for this might be that male activities tend to be more highly valued than female activities in the general culture. For girls, participation in boy-like activities may involve status gain, and for boys, participation in girl-like activities may involve status loss (Maccoby 1998). We do not think this entirely explains the lack of symmetry in the gender-coded condemnation of out-group behavior that we describe. We believe that the contrast is attributable to intrinsic differences between the cultures of the two sexes. Females throughout the life cycle are more likely to respond to atypical gender-role behavior in an accepting and nonthreatened way than are males. Femalelike behavior in boys triggers the emotions of anxiety and anger in other males. Whereas malelike behavior might do this in women, it has to be far more extreme.

The Female Peer Group

Girls do not seem to form the rigidly bounded, hierarchically structured type of late childhood peer groups as frequently as boys do. Although, as toddlers, girls initiate gender-segregated play, their approach to gender segregation appears to be more flexible than boys as development proceeds. They seem less threatened by gender-role nonconformity, and their groups are not as walled off from the world of adults as those of boys are. They gravitate toward each others' company in smaller groups than boys do, and their behavior is much more organized around empathic emotional communication in durable relationships. To be sure, girls are not immune from status ambitions. Alliances are made, cliques are formed, and politics is practiced in girls' groups. The influences that shape these interpersonal transactions, however, are quite different from those we have described among boys.

Although girls develop romantic interests in parallel with boys, these are much less likely to be focused on erotic sexuality. Rather, they emphasize intimacy and commitment (Gilligan 1982). We earlier suggested that the moral development of boys includes the internalization of the attitudes and values of all-male peer groups. We conjecture that the moral development of girls is quite different. It continues along lines of development present earlier and emphasizes nurturance, caring, and protofamilial relationships (Gilligan, Lyons, and Hamner 1989). Thus the moral development of boys and girls is asymmetric, in keeping with their asymmetric peer development.

Boys and the All-Male Group: Clinical Implications for Therapeutic Work with Heterosexual Men

The juvenile male peer group is a powerful organizer of the representational world of boys. It becomes the basis for elaborated fantasy later in life and, for many men, is the primary referent that regulates feelings of honor, respect, pride, and shame. Men frequently see themselves as actors in an all-male world—a fact appreciated by the writers of much great fiction such as *Moby Dick*. The conflict between the yearning for honor, among men, and for acceptance by women and families is the substance of myth.

It is not uncommon for the preoccupation of men with their place in the world of men to be a reason for difficulties in the functioning of heterosexual couples. In this situation the woman feels that her partner, although he may be decent and sexually adequate, is often not "emotionally present." Rather, he is invested in sports and perhaps competitive business activities and other pursuits that involve him with other men—in actuality or in fantasy. He is perfectly happy to have his partner passively share such events with him from time to time. However, he resists participation in truly mutual activities. His female partner *feels* excluded because she *actually is excluded* not only from his social life but from an important domain of his inner life. Thus the myth that has organized his development from late childhood, and still does, conflicts with the myth of romance, sharing, and intrafamilial intimacy that has organized hers. In our experience, men with this profile are often raised in families lacking warm, affiliative relationships with girls. They may not have sisters, for example, or their mothers may be unavailable or frankly neglectful and uninterested in their late childhood development. Space does not allow us to discuss clinical techniques for influencing this type of problem therapeutically here—except to emphasize that when it is present it is important that it be recognized.

Male Abuse of Females

Pathological elaborations of their gender-specific interpersonal style may lead men to abuse women in various ways.

Whereas women tend to stress reasonable cooperation in resolving disputes, men tend to be confrontational and to respond to frustration with threats. Valuing a hierarchical model of interpersonal functioning, the possibility of being subservient to a woman tends to trigger anxiety and anger in many men.

A common pathological pattern occurring in heterosexual relationships is one in which the woman struggles to find common ground. The man sees her efforts to construct partnership as a threat to his dominant (e.g., alpha) status. He responds with threats, menacing behavior, and, in more extreme situations, physical abuse.

Space does not allow us to discuss patterns of dysfunctional relationships here. We have found it helpful in couple therapy, however, to intervene swiftly when a man attempts to structure communication of the couple, and in the therapeutic situation, along stereotypically masculine lines. Therapeutic interventions generally include psychoeducation about behavioral gender differences and, when necessary, overt protection of the woman from gender-role abuse.

Gender-Role Abuse of Boys by Women

Women, too, may carry out gender-role abuse. One way in which such abuse is expressed is via the mislabeling of RTP in boys as a form of male aggression. There are no studies documenting the frequency with which this occurs, but our clinical experience suggests that it is reasonably common. We have pointed out elsewhere that the tendency to RTP varies within genders and the interaction or "fit" between child and family members often shapes familial interactions (Friedman and Downey 1995).

Aggressive activity has destructive intent and is motivated by hostility. In contrast, RTP is a form of play that has many adaptive functions including the facilitation of peer bonding. Parents may mislabel RTP as a form of male violence, however. In these situations the parent, often the mother, projects hostility onto a son who is then devalued because of a strong temperamental predisposition toward RTP. There are many reasons for this type of mislabeling and scapegoating. Some women who do this are borderline and experience RTP as threats to already fragile self-boundaries. Others have been traumatized by men and see the exuberant child as a potential future sexual offender or wife abuser. Sometimes such mothers are radical feminists who believe that the behavior of offspring should be influenced to be as gender-neutral as possible. Some women displace their hostility from abusive mates to their sons. Often multiple factors interact to lead to the final form of the behavior. We consider such activity on the part of mothers as much an example of gender-role abuse as overt homophobic activity on the part of males who devalue other males labeled as being feminine or unmasculine.

Childhood is bounded by two gender-specific types of relationships. Virtually all infants are cared for by women—their mothers and female caretakers. As many psychoanalysts have pointed out, this creates different adaptive tasks for boys and girls during toddlerhood. Whereas girls identify with this mothers (in the process of forming an adequate psychological skeleton), boys must disidentify (Greenson 1968). Chodorow (1989, 1994) and Gilligan (1982) have suggested that this is a reason that women feel strengthened by emotional intimacy, and men weakened and threatened.

The asymmetry in gender-self security mechanisms that boys and girls experience and express becomes pronounced as childhood progresses. Let us now turn our attention to the different pathways in the relational patterns of children during late childhood. Girls tend to continue the types of relationships they have had earlier, except that they preferentially relate to other girls much more than boys. Their relationships are affiliative, emotionally expressive, nonaggressive, and organized in the same way that their earlier relationships were. For girls the dyadic relationship with the mother serves as the prototype for future relationships, including those with peers during late childhood.

For boys the developmental pathway is quite different. Boys must adapt to greater discontinuity than girls. Interpersonal relationships with male peers are not organized in the way they were in their families. Mothers, and often sisters, continue to influence familial communication patterns. Girls, women, and even adult males are excluded from juvenile male peer culture, however. Juvenile males tend to form all-male peer groups whose rules of operation seem to be set by themselves. From a developmental perspective, boys are likely to be faced with the requirement of gaining entry to such groups at a time when their gender-self security systems may be fragile. Retreat from this requirement back to the security of their familial relationships may come with a price—a sense of shame. Boys who are accepted by their peers experience increased gender-self security. Those who are rejected, or assigned an extremely low status in the group, experience a sense of shameful masculine inadequacy. In this chapter we noted that, in our culture, the gender insecurity experienced by juvenile males motivates them to be homophobic. The roots of adult male homophobia are to be found in the juvenile male peer group.

Some qualification is necessary here. Some girls' cliques operate similarly to boys' groups, and some girls therefore experience similar developmental pathways to those of boys. Boys do so more commonly, however. The phenomenon of the juvenile male peer group occurs with substantial variability. We do not suggest that this is a uniform experience that *all* boys must cope with; rather, it is a common experience affecting many—probably most—children.

Implications for Psychoanalytic Psychology

Psychoanalysis is a depth psychology concerned with the way in which meanings and messages are represented in the mind, and not just with observable phenomena. We now comment on the significance of late childhood gender asymmetry for psychoanalytic psychology.

Psychoanalysis presently suggests that during the first half of childhood self-representation is synthesized, self-cohesion established, and the structure of the mental apparatus created (Engel 1962; Moore and Fine 1995). According to most psychoanalytic schools of thought, it is during the preoedipal and oedipal phases, from infancy to age six or so, that the unconscious and conscious templates are created that permanently structure interpersonal relationships. Afterward, their contour is largely determined by unconscious symbolic representations and narratives depicting the person's relationships, primarily with mother and father but sometimes with key significant others as well. These early relationships determine the form and content of transference as it is expressed in the psychoanalytic relationship. Even if the Oedipus complex is taken metaphorically and not literally, its format of symbolically representing *intrafamilial* relationships and conflicts is seen by most psychoanalysts today as valid. Subsequent interpersonal relationships are viewed as repeating these conflicts—in elaborated and/or disguised ways, perhaps, but repeating nonetheless. Later phases of life, such as adolescence, for example, are seen as occasions where the underlying Oedipus complex is reexperienced, reworked, and coped with anew (Blos 1967, 1968).

The developmental perspective that we put forth here is somewhat different than that of traditional psychoanalytic developmental theory. We suggest that intrafamilial (e.g., caretaker) representations are in fact mentally encoded consciously and unconsciously prior to the age of six or so. Following that, however, development diverges dramatically for the two sexes. By late childhood the inner representational worlds of boys and girls are fundamentally different. The difference in their conscious and unconscious psychological functioning becomes more pronounced with subsequent development.

Unconscious Representation in Boys and Girls

In boys the juvenile per group influences their moral development and the way in which they mentally process the feeling of shame. Perhaps even more important, we suggest that the juvenile male group occurs for psychobiological reasons and is similar in its functioning to the similar groups of nonhuman primates (Friedman and Downey 1993). Let us return to the topic of representation here. One way of thinking about the development of representationality in boys is to make an analogy with biology. In this analogy boys develop male peer group "representational receptors," in similar fashion to cells developing hormone receptors. This analogy is a way of expressing the fact that the individual child has a psychological need for a gender-specific type of peer relationship and a mental way of representing that need. In girls, in contrast (staying with the same analogy), so-called representational receptors are the same as they have always been. The representational receptors of boys—and not of girls—are an additional new component, added to their mode of representationality used in the past.

Let us now consider the mental mechanism of *condensation* originally described by Freud in his discussion of the primary process (Freud 1900). We conjecture that the way in which the juvenile peer group is mentally represented tends to be condensed with earlier developmental phases. Thus the mental representations of the father figure may be condensed with those of male peer figures in dream scenarios. We find it helpful from a therapeutic perspective to dissect these two developmental phases—early and late childhood—during psychoanalysis. Because psychoanalysis is a *dyadic process*, the expression of conflicts pertaining to a *group* may be particularly camaflouged in the transference.

In this chapter we have particularly emphasized that the origins of certain psychological difficulties—gender insecurity and homophobia—appear to be located in late childhood of boys much more frequently than girls. Psychotherapists work with individuals, however, and we are mindful that many children develop along lines different from the mainstream. Our clinical experience indicates that late childhood is a crucial phase for the development of gender-valued self-regard in both sexes and that working through conflicts specific to this developmental phase is usually necessary for an optimal therapeutic result.

8

Female Homosexuality:
Classical Psychoanalytic Theory Reconsidered

In this chapter we discuss the status of "classical" psychoanalytic thought about female sexual orientation. Taking a historical perspective, we reassess key areas in light of advances in a number of extrapsychoanalytic disciplines. We use the words *traditional* or *classical* to refer to a body of psychoanalytic work published in such journals as the *International Journal of Psychoanalysis,* the *Journal of the American Psychoanalytic Association,* and in scholarly monographs and books. We distinguish between contributions from "psychoanalysis proper" and from psychoanalytically informed psychology, which tends to be discussed in different scholarly publications.

The psychoanalytic theory of female homosexuality occupies an unusual position in modern psychoanalytic thought because it continues to be influenced by models of the mind that have largely been discarded in other areas of psychoanalytic psychology—even those pertaining to male homosexuality.

Freud's Masculine Bias Revisited

Although much has been written about the limitations of Freud's phallocentric perspective (Bardwick 1971; Fisher 1973; Walsh 1987), curiously little attention has been devoted to its continuing influence on the psychoanalytic theory of female sexual orientation. Freud paid far greater attention to male than female homosexuality. In contrast to extensive discussions of homosexuality in men, he devoted only one paper explicitly to the topic in women (Freud 1920). An early letter of Freud to Fleiss is instructive with regard to his gender bias:

Oct. 17, 1889
Bergasse 19
Dear Wilhelm
What would you say if masturbation were to reduce itself to homosexuality, and the latter, that is, male homosexuality (in both sexes) were the primitive form of sexual longing? (The first sexual aim, analogous to the infantile one—a wish that does not extend beyond the inner world.) If moreover, libido and anxiety both were male?
Cordially,
Your
Sigm (Masson 1985:380)

Freud's greater interest in male than female homosexuality was expressed in other ways as well. In the *Three Essays on the Theory of Sexuality,* for example, arguing that "inversion" is not a form of degeneracy, he commented: "It must be allowed that the spokesmen of 'Uranism' are justified in asserting that some of the prominent men in all recorded history were inverts and perhaps absolute inverts" (Freud 1905).

The paradigm of the negative Oedipus complex and the relationship between paranoia and unconscious homosexual conflicts were both illustrated by psychobiographies of men: the Wolf Man (Freud 1918) and the Schreber case (Freud 1911), respectively.

Throughout the history of psychoanalysis substantially greater attention has been devoted to male than female homosexuality, a trend that has continued up to the present (Panel 1983; Friedman 1988; Lewes 1988; Isay 1989). In contrast to the psychoanalytic literature on male homosexuality, the literature on female homosexuality is extremely sparse. The major psychoanalytic contributions on the topic are listed in table 8.1.

The handful of patients described in the traditional psychoanalytic literature to date can hardly depict the different psychological profiles of homosexual and bisexual women in the general population. As we discuss more extensively below, the diversity of developmental pathways leading to homosexuality in women may be even greater than that in men. Many psychodynamic configurations associated with female homosexuality have yet to be described in the psychoanalytic literature.

Table 8.1 Analytic Literature on Female Homosexuality

Reference	Number of Cases
Freud 1920	1
Flügel 1925	1
Ferenczi 1926	1
Jones 1927	5
Fenichel 1929	1
Saussure 1929	1
Deutsch 1932	11
Brody 1943	1
Thompson 1947	1
Bonaparte 1953	0
Bacon 1956	0
Bergler 1958	1
Lichtenstein 1961	4
Khan 1962	1
Socarides 1978	3
DeFries 1979	16
McDougall 1980	4
Stoller 1985	1
Siegel 1988	12
McDougall 1989	1
Quinodez 1989	2
Total Cases	68

The Traditional Psychoanalytic Literature Portrays
Female Homosexuality As Inherently Pathological

Most psychoanalytic articles, until quite recently, have presented female homosexuality as resulting from developmental derailment, which leads to global character pathology. Thus Bacon described homosexuality as a "perversion" resulting when a "normal instinct for heterosexual learning or sexual dependence" is turned from its true path." She suggested that a common homosexual dynamic was for the little girl to turn from her father to sexual attraction to females. This served as a defense against the oedipal wish. Bacon portrayed homosexual relationships as unsatisfying, since they developed as a result of fearful avoidance of heterosexuality (Bacon 1956).

Socarides (1978) characterized female homosexuality as the mirror image of male homosexuality—a perversion due in most cases to preoedipal developmental failures with inability to resolve separation-individuation phase conflicts. Socarides's female homosexual patients are in flight from men because childhood fears of being poisoned and devoured by mother made them unable to cope with real or imagined oedipal disappointments from father. Fears of merger with the homosexual partner and murderous aggressive and masochistic fantasies of injury from sexual intercourse plague these women. Socarides proposed that the treatment goal of any lesbian patient must be the change of sexual object from same to opposite sex (Socarides 1963).

In an unusually influential discussion of a single case, Kahn conceptualized a homosexual relationship in a young woman as an attempt to repeat and elaborate conflicts from an archaic relationship with a depressed, hypochondriacal mother. Castration anxiety, penis awe, body-ego distortions, and unresolved oedipal conflicts contributed to the dynamics of the case (Kahn 1962).

Joyce McDougall elaborated the same etiological mechanism for the genesis of homosexuality in women as Socarides had suggested (McDougall 1980). According to this theory, women are homosexual because of severe preoedipal psychopathology, specifically, difficulties in the separation-individuation phase. The woman hypothetically copes with penis envy by internalizing parts of the father and transforming herself into the phallus. She then finds a female partner with whom she acts out her rage and desire for love from the inaccessible, narcissistically isolated and controlling mother. This solution is seen as a perverse "third structure," neither psychotic nor neurotic but clearly character disordered. The four case histories McDougall described all depict women with severe character pathology including poor object constancy, intense depression and anxiety with projected paranoid rage, fantasies of murder and being murdered, impaired identity development, and episodes of depersonalization.

More recent authors have echoed the major themes outlined by Bacon, Socarides, Kahn, and MacDougal, albeit with some variations. Thus Quinodez (1989) proposed that, rather than identification with the father's penis, the primary characteristic of lesbianism is identification with the baby. Quinodez speculated that homosexuality blocks regression toward psychosis and simultaneously blocks progression toward the oedipal situation, a more advanced developmental level (Quinodez 1989).

Elaine Siegel presented an additional twelve cases of homosexual women who received analytically oriented psychotherapy for diverse symptoms including incomplete body image, lack of stable object relations, poorly developed gender identity, suicide attempts, sadomasochistic interpersonal interactions, and micropsychotetic episodes. Siegel speculated that the homosexual orientation of these patients was a consequence of their severe psychopathology (Siegel 1988).

The assumption that homosexuality is associated with global character pathology had dominated the older psychoanalytic literature about men as well, but was revised (Panel 1983; Friedman 1988; Isay 1989; Lewes 1988). A perspective about the sexual orientation of women similar to the modern psychoanalytic perspective about men has been expressed by psychodynamically oriented psychotherapists (Boston Lesbian Collective 1987; O'Connor and Ryan 1993; Stein and Cohen 1986), but from within the psychoanalytic "establishment" this has been done in only a limited way. Thus, the glossary of *Psychoanalytic Terms and Concepts* of the American Psychoanalytic Association (Moore and Fine 1990) introduces the entry on homosexuality with a discussion that disavows the older pathological model.

> Hence, while psychoanalytic observations that consider childhood sexuality conflict, defense, and compromise formation have furnished basic data on psychosexuality, the determinants of homosexual object choice are not yet clearly delineated. Unconscious biases for homosexual and heterosexual object choice differ. They are not necessarily correlated with a particular clinical picture but are recognizable only through psychoanalytic investigation.
>
> Many homosexual individuals appear capable of living well-adjusted lives and show no evidence of significant psychopathology. Homosexual men and women, like heterosexual, are capable of mature, lasting attachments, although individuals of both sexual orientations may be masochistic, narcissistic, depressed, borderline, or psychotic.
>
> *(Moore and Fine 1990:86–87)*

While the material quoted above is not biased toward a pathological model, a subsection of the article headed "Female Homosexuality (Lesbianism)" emphasizes that homosexuality in women results from profound psychological defects and developmental derailments. The entry begins by noting that "female homosexuality (lesbianism) has been much less explored and reported by analysts than male homosexuality, and the formulations regarding it are more questionable" (Moore and Fine 1990).

Following this qualification, the defect theory of homosexual orientation in women is presented historically. In the older psychoanalytic literature conflicts of the phallic-oedipal phase are stressed. Psychodynamic configurations discussed include defensive regression to the preoedipal mother-daughter relationship, incestuous strivings, fear of retaliation from imagos of mother and sisters, castration anxiety, penis envy, and masculine identifications. The more recent literature, while continuing to emphasize unresolved oedipal conflicts, stresses developmental disturbances in the child-mother relationship during the preoedipal separation-individuation pha se as being significant influences on the genesis of same-sex erotic object. Both maternal and paternal neglect and abuse are cited as reasons for the developmental derailment of the prototypical girl who ultimately becomes a lesbian.

> Congenital defects, repeated medical procedures, and the mother's physical or emotional absence may contribute to such disturbances and may distort sexual identity. . . . Significant contributions to a homosexual orientation may be found in a father who shows contempt and criticism toward men who take an interest in his daughter, frightening or painful heterosexual encounters, disappointments in heterosexual love experiences or marriage, or the unavailability of heterosexual objects.
>
> *(Moore and Fine 1990:87)*

Although the glossary asserts that complex biopsychosocial interactions lead to homosexual orientation in women, in fact only traumatic psychosocial causes are discussed. Regarding the possible role of biological influences, the glossary states:

> Attempts to establish somatic (chromosomal and hormonal) factors in sexual orientation have not been convincing. While somatic factors determine the anatomical sex, especially prenatally, object choice appears to be environmentally determined. Psychoanalysts have postulated that conflict either during the separation-individuation stage or during the oedipal stage may lead to identification with the parent of the opposite sex and homosexual object choice.   *(Moore and Fine 1990:86)*

We conclude that the so-called classical or traditional psychoanalytic literature on homosexuality in women continues to emphasize a psychopathological perspective. This is true to a much greater extent than in the comparable psychoanalytic literature on homosexuality in men.

Martha Kirkpatrick: A Dissenting Psychoanalytic Voice

In 1984 the American Psychoanalytic Association sponsored a panel entitled "Toward the Further Understanding of Homosexual Women." It followed upon a similar session devoted to homosexual men that was presented the year before. Taking exception to traditional or classical psychoanalytic views, Martha Kirkpatrick, a panelist, expressed alternative ideas about homosexuality in women based on psychoanalytically informed research on lesbian mothers. She observed that "many assertions about homosexuals—hatred of the opposite sex, regression from oedipal disappointments, inability to tolerate the discovery of sexual differences—can be applied equally to many heterosexuals" (Wolfson 1984).

Kirkpatrick suggested that the male model, which has led psychoanalysts to identify genital release as the major organizing and motivating factor in psychological development, may be inadequate for female development. Intimacy, and the quest for intimacy, play a greater part; the fantasy life of girls is less organ-directed and more interpersonal and varied than that of boys and men. Kirkpatrick later observed that feminine identity and self-esteem, maternal interest and capacity, and sexual orientation appeared to be dimensions of behavior that vary independently. Elaborating on her ideas about the role of intimacy in female psychosexual functioning, she speculated that in some women homosexuality might result as a variation of a need for intimacy rather than of erotic sexuality. She suggested that a woman might prefer another woman as a sexual partner because of feelings of profound intimacy, although she might have more intense orgasms with a man (Kirkpatrick 1989).

Kirkpatrick's emphasis on separate developmental lines for male and female self development and actualization is in keeping with recent psychoanalytic (Tyson 1982) and extrapsychoanalytic contributions to the psychology of women.

Psychoanalysis, Psychopathology, and the *DSM*

The traditional psychoanalytic literature on female homosexuality was written, for the most part, prior to publication of the third edition of the *Diag-*

nostic and Statistical Manual (*DSM*) of the American Psychiatric Association (American Psychiatric Association 1980). The previous edition of the manual (American Psychiatric Association 1968) had been based on psychoanalytic perspectives about psychopathology, but *DSM-III* was not. Originally many psychoanalysts objected to the diagnostic format posed in the *DSM-III* because it was exclusively based on manifest experience and observable behavior. Influenced to a far greater degree by the descriptive psychiatrist Kraepelin than Freud, the *DSM* in its present form (American Psychiatric Association 1994) was generated in order to increase reliability of diagnosing mental disorders, and accomplished that goal. Psychoanalytic and psychoanalytically oriented clinicians have found it not only helpful but necessary to utilize a psychodynamic and a descriptive frame of reference simultaneously. The utility of multiple models of psychological functioning was made evident by recognition that advances in psychopharmacology were often helpful to psychoanalytic treatment and posed no threat to psychoanalytic psychology. For instance, modern psychoanalytic clinicians routinely use lithium carbonate in addition to psychoanalytically oriented psychotherapy or psychoanalysis in the treatment of bipolar patients.

It is striking that not a single article in the classical psychoanalytic literature on female homosexuality has utilized the diagnostic schema of the *DSM* in addition to traditional psychoanalytic models of psychopathology. This is important since many discuss patients who have symptoms of major mental illnesses. Rather than conceptualize psychopathology as part of Axis I and Axis II psychiatric disorders, the authors attribute it to the patient's homosexual orientation, or they attribute both the sexual orientation and the mental disorders to common etiological factors. Of course, most of these articles were written prior to the publication of *DSM-III*. Although there appeared to be solid clinical rationale for their perspective at the time they were written, the approach they take toward psychopathlogy has been invalidated by advances in descriptive psychiatry. We note, moreover, that many homosexual and bisexual women function at a well-integrated psychological level and never seek assistance from mental health professionals. They should not be included in etiological formulations about disturbed patients as they have in the traditional psychoanalytic articles on female homosexuality. As a general rule, modern gay and lesbian patients seek psychological treatment because of Axis I and Axis II mental disorders and/or personal and relational difficulties, often stemming from the effects of homophobia in its various guises. We further discuss psychopathology in lesbians in part 2 of this volume. The topic of homophobia is crucial to understanding psychopathology in all nonheterosexual people. We discuss this in part 2 as well.

Diversity of Developmental Histories of Homosexual and Bisexual Women

The life history narratives of lesbian and bisexual women are certainly as diverse as those of gay and bisexual men, and probably even more so. A trend across classical psychoanalytic papers has been to ignore crucial developmental differences and assume that the homosexual and/or bisexual orientation of all women resulted from a common set of psychodynamic influences. From a descriptive perspective, however, a variety of groups of homosexual women have been discussed, some of which have no parallel among men. This is hardly surprising since the recently emergent field of sex differences in behavior has identified many areas of psychological development and functioning that are more commonly experienced by one sex. Some experiences of each sex have no mirror image in the life cycle of the other.

Although development pathways are often different between the sexes, they sometimes do resemble each other. Thus Ponse (1978) and Golden (1987) described women who have "always felt different" and who appear to have been on a basically homosexual developmental track from early childhood. This type of developmental pathway is similar to that experienced by many gay men.

A different group of women find their way to homosexual orientation despite feeling themselves to be heterosexual throughout their early years, sometimes until mid adulthood. These women have usually had sexual experiences with men, have been married, and are often mothers. During adulthood, however, they realize that despite sexually satisfying experiences with men their needs for emotional intimacy and empathic communication remain unfulfilled. Often to their surprise, they find that sexual feelings emerge when these needs are met by another woman. Frequently these women are not consciously aware that they have ever before experienced homosexual desire (Kirkpatrick 1984). We have described homosexual feelings in such women as having been "kindled" in a setting of emotional trust and closeness. Sometimes these women evolve a lesbian identity and social role. Others may become involved in a homosexual relationship without experiencing the need to define their identity as "heterosexual," "lesbian," or "bisexual." Although more research is needed to place our ideas about this on a solid empirical foundation, we believe that these types of developmental sequences occur much more commonly in women than in men.

Yet another group of homosexual women are so-called political lesbians. These women are a subgroup of feminists who believe that discriminatory treatment of women is fostered by patriarchal social organizations and that heterosexuality and heterosexual coitus symbolically express domination and subjugation of women by men. In the context of this belief system, homosexual feelings may be experienced and expressed in relationships (DeFries 1979). Although these three groups have received some scholarly attention, far greater diversity exists among women of homosexual orientation than is represented by these groups alone.

Diversity of this scope suggests multiple etiological mechanisms and psychodynamic motivational pathways. In fact, no single theory of the origins of the sexual object can be valid for all women or men, whether homosexual, heterosexual, or bisexual. Apparently there are many different sequences of biopsychosocial interactions, occurring during different life cycle phases, whose final common pathway is the manifest experience of homosexual desire and activity.

Female Gender Identity Development

The concept of primary femininity is now generally accepted among psychoanalysts, partially as a result of the influence of the new knowledge about embryogenesis of sex differences in anatomy, physiology, and behavior mentioned above. Stoller coined the term *core gender identity* to signify the enduring awareness that one is either male or female. Stoller distinguished core gender identity from feelings about how "masculine" or "feminine" a person feels. He pointed out that once core gender identity was established, it functioned as a stable personality trait, in contrast to feelings about masculinity and femininity, which fluctuate with self-esteem and with intense mood states (Stoller 1968). Independently, Money speculated that gender identity, the awareness of being either male or female, was a psychological "differentiation" that occurred prior to what psychoanalysts term the oedipal phase of development. He suggested that gender identity was part of an orderly linear sequence of distinctions—beginning with prenatal differentiations of the tissues of the genital tract and central nervous system. He defined gender identity as the private awareness that one is male or female, and gender role as the expression to others of gender identity (Money and Ehrhardt 1972).

At present it appears that differentiation of gender identity occurs as the result of biological, psychological, and social influences. Space does not allow for extensive discussion of the interactions that lead to the differentiation of gender identity, and the reader who wishes more information is referred to Zucker and Bradley (1995). It is clear, however, that differentiation of gender identity does not depend on recognition and response to genital differences between males and females as Freud had suggested. Moreover, gender identity is established prior to the occurrence of the oedipal phase of development.

We return at this point to the topic of female homosexuality proper. The classical papers on the subject are based on drive-conflict theory and generally accept Freud's views that "penis envy" and "castration anxiety" are part of the biological "bedrock" that underlies psychological organization. Those classical articles that were written after Margaret Mahler's contributions tend to supplement the Freudian paradigm with a Mahlerian one that stresses failure of separation-individuation from the mother (Socarides 1978). None of this literature utilizes a developmental paradigm that includes the modern concept of primary femininity. The omission is crucial, particularly in light of Kirkpatrick's theories about intimacy and female homosexuality.

For example, Gilligan (1982) and Chodorow (1989, 1994) have discussed differences in the relationship between the meaning of gender identity and interpersonal intimacy in the development of boys and girls. As a developmental life task, both sexes must develop a sense of self and, associated with this, separate and individuate from the mother. Only boys, however, must *disidentify* with their mothers, a developmental task necessary to achieve a firm sense of male gender identity (Greenson 1968). Because of the differential consequences of disidentification from the mother, boys are prone to respond to interpersonal intimacy with insecurity stemming from a sense of threatened gender identity. Girls, by contrast, are prone to respond to interpersonal intimacy with security stemming from a sense of strengthened gender identity (Gilligan 1982).

The association of intimate connection with another person to enhanced gender identity in women and threatened gender identity in men suggests differences in the way the two sexes experience the emotion of love. Thus women are more likely to experience feelings of love, attachment, and connection even as young girls, with the linking of full sexuality to romantic love taking a longer time to develop over adulthood. Contrastingly, males start out with strong sexual feelings in adolescence and over the course of adult development (if it occurs normally) become progressively able to experience attachment and love with the same partner with whom they feel sexual excitement, passion, and release. (These observations apply to the groups as a whole; exceptions to the pattern will always be found.) The significance of this sex difference in rates of development of the different capacities for love and sexuality in women and men has yet to be fully appreciated by psychoanalytic theory. It has surely been inadequately elucidated in the special case of lesbians and gay men. The difference would help explain, for example, why the intense need for intimacy experienced by many women is not met by male sexual partners. It also suggests, as Kirkpatrick implied, that in some women positive cycles become established between strengthened feelings of womanliness and sexual intimacy with other women.

The importance of sex differences in the relationship between intimacy and sexual orientation is perhaps best illustrated by a clinical vignette.

Clinical Vignette

Consider the psychology of each partner in a marriage in which each experiences a loss of passionate vitality. The fifty-year-old wife is struggling to cope with feelings of "emptiness" that have become insistent and persistent in recent years. At work she experiences loss of ambition and energy, a tendency to withdraw from social interactions, and irritability. Although her appearance has not outwardly changed, she feels unattractive. Her efforts to obtain solace and support from her mate are frustrated by his attitude toward her. She experiences him as emotionally "unavailable" and feels lonely in his presence. She complains that his idea of "being together" is to participate in activities at the same time, such as watching television or socializing with friends. He offers her little sense of emotional connection or empathic understanding.

The husband experiences his wife as increasingly clinging, dependent, and self-preoccupied. He feels bewildered by her criticism that he is emotionally "not present" when he is physically in her company. His attempts to hug and hold her are angrily rebuffed when he becomes sexually aroused. She interprets his initiating physical intimacy as manipulative. "All you want is sex," she tells him. She begins to find intercourse invasive and intrinsically devaluing. He interprets her sexual withdrawal as "infantile" and frustrating. He complains that she wants him to relate to her as if she were a child.

The husband spends more and more time at work, where he is perceived as being energetic and effective. It seems to his wife that the more she complains about her loneliness, the more he withdraws. Soon he begins a sexual affair with one of his women colleagues. At this point, his wife begins to have lengthy conversations with a widow who lives nearby. The women meet each other frequently and commiserate about sex differences in behavior. Each feels that the other is warm, supportive, understanding, empathic, expressive, and caring. The friendship deepens and the women discover sexual feelings for each other. Their emergence is a surprise to both. Each is heterosexist in attitude, has never experienced homosexual desire before, and never engaged in homosexual activity. After a period of shock, turmoil, and mutual revelation, they realize that they have fallen in love and allow themselves to express their feelings sexually. Although their love relationship becomes fully sexual, and deeply satisfying to each, neither considers herself a lesbian. In fact, neither feels it necessary to label their same-sex passionate relationship in terms of a particular "sexual orientation" social role.

In this example, intense intimacy in the setting of emotional isolation from husbands kindled sexual desire in two women. Once this occurred, each felt attractive and desirable. The depression experienced by the first remitted. This type of kindling rarely occurs in men except in special situations. A lifelong heterosexual man may develop intensely close friendships during middle or later life, but these are not likely to alter the sex of the object of his erotic fantasies.

Love, Sex, and Psychological Development: The Importance of Sex Differences in Sexual Orientation for a Psychoanalytic Developmental Model

The extremely diverse types of women who experience homosexual desire and become involved in homosexual activity is striking. Included among them are women whose psychological functioning appears to have no parallel with that of men.

Thus, as a general rule, sexual fantasy in males emerges as a conscious experience prior to puberty and acts as a limit throughout the remainder of the life cycle. The people that a man forms sexual partnerships with years after the onset of his sexual fantasy life tend to be restricted to those that fall within the boundaries prescribed by his sexual fantasies. Childhood experiences and events therefore seem to be unusually important—even determinative—for male sexual orientation development. The sexual orientation of most men is, as it were, in place many years before their most important experiences with sexual intimacy and sexual love. It does not appear likely or even possible that the *capacity* for a man to be erotically stimulated by men exclusively, women exclusively, or both, would itself be a direct immediate function of love and intimacy occurring during adulthood.

Among men who have experienced erotic responsivity toward males and females, either the homo- or heterosexual component may be augmented by loving feelings. Men who are exclusively homosexual in fantasy, however, rarely (if ever) become exclusively or predominantly heterosexual in fantasy as a result of loving feelings for a woman. Men who are exclusively heterosexual in fantasy rarely (if ever) become exclusively or predominantly homosexual in fantasy as a result of loving feelings for a man.

Temporal relationships between the emergence of childhood sexual fantasy and the experience of childhood psychosocial trauma (when such exists) are linked much more tightly in the life cycle of most homosexual men than most homosexual women. In traditional Freudian terms preoedipal and oedipal traumata theoretically derail normal heterosexual development and lead to homosexual orientation. Psychoanalysts have no difficulty finding countless patients in whom such traumata occurred coincident with or immediately prior to the emergence of homosexual fantasies. The theory that homosexual fantasies were a direct response to the traumata achieved credibility in psychoanalytic clinical theory partially because of temporal contiguity. For example, consider a homosexual man who has always felt "different" from peers. As a child, he was drawn to aesthetic rather than rough-and-tumble pursuits and preferred to play stereotypically girls' games such as "house" and "jacks" with girl playmates rather than boys' games with male peers. His father was harshly critical, even abusive, his mother overly protective. He experienced homosexual desire from about ages four to five when he developed a "crush" on a male movie star. Shortly thereafter he noticed that he thought about boys in his class when he developed erections and sexual feelings.

A classically Freudian psychodynamic formulation would propose that this man's homosexual fantasies were a symptomatic response to oedipal fears. If the patient had additional "borderline" symptoms, the formulation would stress preoedipal merger fantasies with an overprotective mother. In any case, the hypothesis would be that he identified with his mother, relinquishing her as a sexual object because of fear of his father.

In this hypothetical case the boy's fear of his father (presumably associated with intense castration anxiety), closeness with his mother, feminized gender-role behavior, and homoerotic fantasies all seemed to occur at about the same time. We are not suggesting that this necessarily illuminates questions about etiology. In fact, we have criticized this model in detail elsewhere (Friedman 1988; Friedman and Downey 1993, 1994). Nonetheless, the life history of the patient is such that speculation about maternal identification and castration anxiety, while not necessarily valid, is not inherently unreasonable.

In women, however, the temporal sequences involving homosexual fantasies are much more diverse. Certainly, some women probably experience the same type of temporal sequences between erotic object, psychosocial trauma, and gender role behavior as has been reported for so many male patients. However, many women do not. It is much less plausible for women than for men to invoke a model of early childhood trauma leading to an apparently new psychosexual experience—homosexual fantasies—during middle or even late adulthood. This does not mean that theories linking early childhood fears and fantasies to experiences of mid and/or late adulthood are incorrect, only that they do not appear, at least to us, to be intuitively obvious. Many intervening events and experiences would have to be elucidated for such theories to be compelling. A radically different way of interpreting historical data is that the experience of newfound homosexual orientation during later adulthood is a result of psychological growth, at least in many women. If this is so, it seems to suggest that women have more plasticity with regard to the sexual object than men.

This in turn raises the possibility that the psychoanalytic theory that the first half of childhood provides the basic building blocks and model relationships for all later psychological development may be more true for males than females. To be sure, the theory has been somewhat weakened for men as well, in light of the recently discovered plasticity of the central nervous system in response to psychosocial experience throughout the life cycle (Elbert et al. 1995). Psychoanalysts have tended to adhere to the theory that mental structures, and particularly those that provide meaning to object relations and self-representations, are in place prior to age six or so. We conjecture that the natural history of sexual orientation in women at least raises the possibility that, contrary to the traditional paradigm, many women are capable of mental growth in ways not predicted or expected by traditional psychoanalytic theory.

Pathological Sexualization

Experienced clinicians agree that there are subgroups of patients in whom sexual orientation is itself the result of pathological psychodynamic interactions. By pathological psychodynamic interactions we mean products of unconscious conflict that are inherently maladaptive. Our emphasis in this chapter has thus far been on pathways toward homosexuality that may be termed "positive" in the sense that they are theoretically in the service of love and growth. There are obviously other types of pathways, however, including pathological ones. How are these patients best conceptualized?

We would like to make a comment about sociopolitical influences on clinical psychoanalysis before going further. In the present sociopolitical climate the suggestion that sexual orientation itself might in fact be an end point of pathological psychological interactions smacks of being politically incorrect. In the service of simplicity, and with the hope of diminishing prejudice, some theoreticians have argued that sexual orientation is innocuous and never symptomatic. This perspective seems to us to perform a disservice to many patients, and to be out of keeping with clinical realities. Keeping in mind that sexual orientation, however defined, is not a unitary entity, we note that simply because the group defined as lesbian or gay is not inherently pathological does not mean that homosexual fantasies and/or activities are never symptomatic. They obviously can be and, in some patients, frequently are.

The same observation is applicable to heterosexual fantasies and acts in other patients. The pervasive heterosexist bias of our culture sometimes makes it difficult for clinicians to detect that culturally approved behaviors such as the wish to marry, become pregnant, raise children in the context of conventional family structures, become a homemaker, experience orgasms resulting from vaginal coitus may all be manifestations of psychopathology. These wishes may be maladaptive end products of unconscious irrational conflicts and may produce distress and disability. The great diversity of consciously experienced motives that may be pathological but are not necessarily so dramatically illustrates that psychoanalytically oriented clinicians carry out their therapeutic work with patients rather than "symptoms." Motives are embedded in the context of personal life narratives and, with the exception of the grossest examples of wishes whose enactment would endanger life and limb, cannot be understood out of context.

We do believe it is helpful to conceptualize homosexual and/or bisexual orientation in some women resulting from the very type of unresolved preoedipal, separation-individuation, and oedipal conflicts described by the psychoanalysts whose work is listed in table 8.1. The fact that traditional psychoanalytic constructs appear useful in a particular population of patients does not lead us to infer that such constructs are applicable to all women or even all female patients.

In contrast to these patients are women who are irrationally committed to heterosexist ideals for pathological reasons. To the best of our knowledge this population of patients has not previously been discussed by psychoanalysts. The rubric under which many layers of unconscious conflicts are condensed in these patients is best described as *homophobic-heterosexist*. The usual final common psychodynamic mechanism for this is identification with the aggressor. The life histories of these patients reveal layers and layers of identifications and partial identifications with authority figures who were heterosexist in their values and behavior.

If one takes an overview of all women who experience this type of psychodynamic-psychopathological interaction, many do not experience homosexual desire or become involved in homosexual activity. From a descriptive perspective, however, it is possible to select a subgroup of patients who repress and suppress homosexual fantasy because of such dynamic-pathological interactions. To their detriment, women in this subgroup attempt "through willpower," as it were, to be heterosexual or asexual in order to maintain such self-esteem as they can from adherence to and compliance with ideals that for them are maladaptive. Such women may be involved, for example, in repetitive relationships with men that are characterized by exploitation, abuse, and/or neglect. Among them are some who pathologically sexualize fantasies of submitting to powerful and dominating male authorities. These women experience sexual arousal with men for reasons that are primarily masochistic, in keeping with lifelong self-destructive patterns of sexual and social relationships with men. The treatment of these patients, whose self-destructive fantasies are enacted in abusive and exploitative heterosexual relationships, is every bit as difficult as the psychoanalytic treatment of tenaciously self-destructive patients in general.

Masculine Identification and Penis Envy

Of psychodynamic mechanisms frequently referred to in the traditional psychoanalytic literature as influencing homosexual motivation in women, masculine identification and penis envy have received particular attention.

Beginning with Freud (1920), traditional psychoanalytic theorists have emphasized that homosexual fantasy in women is generated by a heavily masculinized self-representation. To express this in simplified formulaic terms, the patient unconsciously thinks, "I am much more like a man than a woman. It is therefore appropriate for me to experience sexuality like a man, and to act like a man as much as possible in sexual encounters." The unconscious belief of being "male-like, or masculine" stems from irrational conflicts about being a woman. The conflicts, in turn, derive from traumatic and painful interactions with both parents during childhood. These ultimately lead to identification with the parent of the opposite sex rather than of the same sex. In addition to idealizing a masculine sexual role, the patient devalues her own representation as a woman. She believes that to be penetrated by a man during the act of sexual intercourse is to be violated, debased, humiliated, and injured.

The equation of homosexual orientation with cross-gender identifications, whether in women or men, has been criticized by many. For example, Domenici and Lesser recently observed:

> Anti-homosexual theory building went in another direction as well when it followed Freud's lead in "Psychogenesis of a Case of Female Homosexuality" (1920). Here Freud posited that his lesbian patient had to turn into a man to love another woman. Following this model, analysts theorized a gendered split between identification and desire (O'Connor and Ryan 1993). Identification and desire came to be viewed as opposed: one cannot have and be the same sex at the same time. By positing identification and desire as binary opposites, the normative structure of heterosexuality was buttressed and essentialized.   *(Domenici and Lesser 1995:3)*

That there is an association between cross-gendered identifications and homosexuality, critics have suggested, is a manifestation of prejudice and bias resulting from psychoanalytic phallocentricism, bourgeois conventionality, and inadequate cultural and historical relativism (Domenici and Lesser 1995; Drescher 1998). As tempting as it might be to adopt this stance, we cannot, since the situation is more complex than would be the case if these criticisms were entirely valid.

On the one hand, it is true that there is no demonstrable association between homosexuality and cross-gendered behavior among adults who are reasonably psychologically well adjusted and who do not meet *DSM-IV* criteria for psychiatric disorders. We interpret this to mean that there is no inherent, necessary psychological association between homosexuality (no matter how defined) and cross-gendered behavior and, presumably, cross-gendered identifications.

In both men and women, however, *childhood* cross-gender preferences and activities are powerful behavioral predictors of adult homosexual orientation. This conclusion is based on numerous retrospective studies of patients and nonpatients and prospective studies of children with gender identity disorders (Green 1987; Whitam and Mathy 1991; Whitam and Zent 1984; Bailey and Zucker 1995).

Thus the idea of some type of association between sexual orientation and gender stereotypic childhood behavior is not simply the product of bias but also derives from extensive empirical research.

Of course, association does not indicate causality. Discussing gay men, for example, Richard Isay has suggested that their childhood cross-gender behaviors result from and are reactive to primary homosexual orientation rather than the reverse (Isay 1989). The same could be true of many homosexual women.

The developmental associations between cross-gender behavior and adult homosexual orientation should not be taken to mean that in every instance such an association exists. The concept of association is a statistical one and refers to the probability of occurrence of a specified behavior in comparison with a defined comparison group—in this instance, people whose sexual orientation is heterosexual. Psychodynamic and statistical frames of reference are quite different. Even though statistical associations indicate behavioral effects in groups of individuals, they rarely suggest effects that involve all individuals. Thus it is entirely in keeping with the known empirically established "facts" that a particular woman who is totally homosexual in fantasy and activity, and has always been so, has never experienced meaningful cross-gender interests. It is possible to be faithful to the empirically established data on the development of people who become homosexual in orientation and not suggest a "gendered split between identification and desire" (O'Connor and Ryan 1993).

We turn our attention now to penis envy, a concept that overlaps with masculine identification. As Ernest Jones put it in 1927: "I cannot possibly desire a man's penis for my gratification since I already possess one of my own, at all events I want nothing else than one of my own" (Jones 1927).

Socarides summarized the contributions of Raymond de Saussure in this regard, as follows:

At the root of homosexual fixations there is always a warped bisexuality arising from the fact that the woman has not been able to accept her femininity. The refusal derives from castration fear and consequent penis envy. In some of his patients an identification with the mother becomes impossible and the girl identifies herself with her father in order to give a child to the mother.

He noted that homosexual fixations correspond to the patient's projections.

Frequently the patient may project her femininity onto the mother and then onto other women who continue to represent the mother. Almost as often, the patient thwarted at not being able to satisfy her own masculine tendencies exaggerates her feminine qualities, becomes excessively narcissistic, and sees herself mirrored in some way in other women who have a high degree of feminine narcissism.   *(Socarides 1978:122)*

Elsewhere, Socarides writes, "In homosexual women there are intense desires for revenge and uncontrollable aggressive feelings. . . . Strong penis envy components are mixed with intense oral wishes." (1978:135)

This brings us to the broad theoretical question Is there in fact an association between penis envy and female homosexuality? And, if so, is there a causal connection, as some psychoanalysts have suggested? We first consider the concept of penis envy in relation to the psychosexual development of women. Continuing a discussion we began in chapter 1, most modern psychoanalysts agree that intense and persistent penis envy is a pathological phenomenon (Moore and Fine 1990). In contrast to Freud, modern psychoanalytic theories do not assume that girls normally view themselves as castrated boys or that the onset of the sense of femininity in girls is associated with a sense of self-defect. Persistent penis envy is associated with intense and chronic feelings of anger, depression, and anxiety. The girl wishes to obtain a penis by castrating a male, thereby depriving him of an instrument of power and repairing her sense of inadequacy. Accumulated clinical experience suggests that penis envy appears to be a meaningful psychodynamic constellation in certain types of patients. There is no valid evidence, however, that this psychodynamic configuration is associated with any type of sexual orientation.

We now turn our attention to mental disorders that some theorists have suggested are associated with homosexuality and, in women, with pathological penis envy.

In the history of psychoanalytic ideas, particular attention has been given to possible association between unconscious homosexual wishes and paranoid delusions. The connection was originally suggested by Freud in his discussion of the Schreber case (Freud 1911). Although Freud's original case was that of a man, his point that paranoid delusions might be a defense against unconscious homosexual wishes was subsequently extended by other psychoanalysts to women (Socarides 1978). Inspection of data from clinical research, however, reveals an interesting sex difference in the delusional and hallucinatory constructs of paranoid psychotic patients. Clinical observation indicates that the delusions and hallucinations of paranoid psychotic men more often have homosexual content than do those of nonparanoid psychotic men (Socarides 1978). This is not true of paranoid psychotic women, however, who are apt to experience themselves in terms of negatively valued heterosexual, not homosexual, imagery. Thus a paranoid psychotic man might hear voices calling him "queer" or "cocksucker" whereas a woman would be similarly likely to hear voices calling her "slut" or "whore."

Research comparing homosexual and heterosexual women has not established that any type of paranoia is more common among either group than the other (Saghir and Robins 1973). In addition, manifest homosexuality, no matter how defined, has not been demonstrated to occur more frequently among paranoid than nonparanoid patients.

Before we leave the area of paranoid psychotic symptoms in relation to unconscious homosexual motivations, we note that, even with regard to men, Freud's original speculations have not been validated (Friedman 1988).

Other psychotic patients provide an additional window on psychodynamic-psychopathological interactions. Women with psychotic depressions sometimes have delusions involving their reproductive organs. Interestingly, these somatic delusions are generally of degeneration and decay—as, for example, that the uterus is being devoured by rats. Delusions that seem to involve the mechanism of penis envy rarely occur.

These data are important because they indicate that when women experience their genitalia as defective, it is not usually in comparison to the genitalia of men but rather to the functional genitalia of women. Furthermore, when the genitalia are embedded in a symbolic way in a fantasized narrative, the story line does not involve revenge, retaliation, and extraction of a penis from men but rather the wish-belief that the patients are using their genitalia to attract men sexually. Because of this they experience guilt of psychotic intensity.

Before leaving the topic of descriptive psychoanalytically informed research that might shed light on the penis envy hypothesis about female homosexuality, we note that there are no published studies indicating that girls with intense and persistent penis envy later become homosexual women. There are also no empirical data that even support the hypothesis that most girls with childhood gender identity disorder actually experience intense penis envy. (One way of gathering data about this would be from projective psychological tests, another from psychoanalytically informed interviews, yet another way from the psychoanalytic situation itself.) Not only have there been no research studies of these issues but there has not even been a substantial body of published case reports supporting the association.

Because of space limitations we are unable to adequately consider the interesting question of whether mild and transient penis envy should be considered a normative phase in the development of girls, as some psychoanalysts suggest (Moore and Fine 1990). Our own opinion about this is negative. We believe that the issue of envy should be distinguished from that of cross-gendered identifications. An essential component of the paradigm of penis envy is the idea of genital defect associated with self-insecurity, fragile self-esteem, and anger. In our view so-called mild and transient penis envy seems nothing more than one way in which the trial partial identification with the other sex is experienced. Such processes of internalization occur in both sexes and are not confined to early childhood but continue throughout the entire life cycle. For reasons that are outside the scope of this paper, males are more likely to identify with other aspects of the female than her genital organs. In any case, we do not believe that the concept of even mild and transient penis envy as a psychological norm is valid.

During Freud's lengthy career his attitude toward putting aside old formulations as he moved to new paradigms was less than enthusiastic (Gay 1988). He frequently added theory to theory, like an architect who changes styles as he builds new rooms on previously existing structures without altering them. The end result might be dazzlingly brilliant but not necessarily coherent or valid. While of great interest to psychohistorians, Freud's reluctance to discard old ideas has provided substantial difficulties for clinicians.

Perhaps because of Freud's unique role as the creator of psychoanalysis, the field as a whole still retains some of his idiosyncrasies. It seems very difficult for psychoanalytic theoreticians to completely and utterly abandon outmoded ideas. This is unfortunate, since a number of psychoanalytic ideas about female homosexuality need to be discarded. One of these, as we have pointed out, is that female homosexuality is a response to pathologically intense unconscious penis envy.

Two additional types of developmental derailment cited by traditional psychoanalytic theorists as contributing to homosexual motivations are pathologically intense fantasies of fusion with an ambivalently perceived maternal imago and unresolved oedipal conflicts leading to identification with the parent of the opposite sex. Concerning the first, we note that feminist critics of traditional psychoanalytic theory have commented that Freud's heterosexist bias led him to overvalue competitive striving and autonomy as signifiers of psychological health. They have observed that terms such as *fusion* have sometimes been used to describe lesbian relationships in a disparaging way and have stressed the significance for healthy psychological development of intimate connection, mutual engagement, mutual empowerment, empathy, and relational authenticity. For example, of traditional psychoanalytic thought Jessica Benjamin observed that "it treats experiences of union, merger, and self-other harmony as regressive opposites to differentiation and self-other distinction" (Benjamin 1988). In addition to this type of criticism by feminists, we would add that intense fantasies of merger with the maternal imago have been invoked as important in the genesis of borderline syndromes overall (Stone 1986). We find no theoretical or empirical rationale for believing that this dynamic is specific even to those forms of homosexuality that are generally considered to be pathological.

With regard to oedipal issues, heterosexual, homosexual, and bisexual women provide abundant evidence of unresolved oedipal conflicts during uncovering psychoanalytically informed treatments.

In thinking about the role of unresolved oedipal conflicts in the origins of a particular sexual orientation, it is important to keep the distinction between etiology and psychodynamics in mind. Thus two patients might be similar with regard to unresolved oedipal conflicts. In one instance, however, these may be the result of primary genetic and/or psychoneuroendocrine influences, in the other, primary interpersonal traumata whose consequences have been internalized. Furthermore, as is generally true of psychodynamic theories of behavioral influence, unresolved oedipal conflicts are not specific. Theoretically, one female patient might identify with an obese father and become homosexual but not obese. Another, with similar psychodynamics, might become an obese heterosexual woman.

Faced with competing paradigms, and many gray zones of psychodynamic interactions on the border between adaptation and maladaptation, clinicians must live with substantial anxiety-provoking ambiguity. We believe that meticulous session-by-session psychodynamic formulation allows for data-based speculations about repressed, warded off, and conflictual material. Often the interpretive work must follow a here-and-now path in light of a road to early development that is not clearly delineated. In fact, we suggest that in order for clinicians to adopt a suitably professional and helpful clinical stance, they must often be able to tolerate ambiguity without resorting to a premature need for closure about sexual orientation in numerous specific situations. This is not to suggest that such closure is never indicated but simply that exploration and the type of empathic, painstaking dissection of motivations that psychoanalysts are skilled at often reveals defenses that allow patients to discover relationships between values and impulses that are most accurate and valid for them. In that sense the psychoanalytic theory of female sexual orientation is likely to be informed by the treatment and investigation of every patient, as it was at the very inception of psychoanalysis.

Afterword to Part 1

At the time this book was being written, psychoanalysis had radically revised its models of gender identity development and of the psychological development and functioning of women. These modifications in psychoanalytic theory occurred primarily because of extra-analytic research carried out by Masters and Johnson (1966) and the work of gender identity researchers and clinicians (Money and Ehrhardt 1972; Stoller 1968). The dramatic changes in theory were followed by vast changes in psychotherapeutic practice. Countless psychoanalytically oriented clinicians responded to new knowledge about psychosexual development and functioning by revising their approach to the treatment of women and of patients with diverse sexual disorders and other types of difficulties as well. The experience of psychoanalysis with homosexuality was somewhat different. As we discuss in the final chapter of this volume, following the lead of American psychiatry, psychoanalysis altered its ideas about homosexuality for many different reasons. A major emphasis of the American Psychoanalytic Association, and of organized psychoanalysis in the United States since then, has been to ameliorate antihomosexual bias in psychotherapeutic practice and psychoanalytic education. We consider clinical issues pertaining to prejudice and discrimination against gay/lesbian people in the second part of this book. Other modifications in the way that psychoanalytic psychotherapists think about sexual orientation seem necessary in addition to those involving prejudice, however. Perhaps the most far-reaching implication of extrapsychoanalytic and psychoanalytic experience with gay/lesbian individuals involves sex differences in behavior. Males and females, alike in some ways, are quite different in others. The differences involve all aspects of their psychosexual functioning. Although there has been scant psychoanalytic literature suggesting that these differences might involve unconscious mental functioning, we conjecture that sex differences exist in this area as well. The precise psychological processes involved in such differences remain to be clarified in the future.

We focused on mid and late childhood development in the preceding chapters because our primary goal was to critically assess the significance of the Oedipus complex in psychological development. We omitted the vast literature on attachment, the mother-infant relationship, the acquisition and differentiation of gender identity. These topics all require detailed review of psychological functioning during the first three years of life. To adequately carry out such a task would require an additional book. Although we discussed sexuality, we barely touched on the topic of love. We felt that there was no way of accomplishing this without considering so many additional topics that publication of this volume would have been greatly delayed.

In the introduction to part 1 we emphasized the need for all behavioral scientists and clinicians, including psychotherapists, to utilize a systems approach to conceptualizing human behavior. This requires active interdisciplinary communication, today honored more in spirit than in practice.

To better understand sexual orientation the need for bridge building and integration across diverse disciplines is substantial. Psychoanalytically oriented therapists have much to learn from other disciplines but much to contribute as well. Therapists work with patients and clients who experience disability and distress to a greater degree than that found in the general population. Nonclinicians often note that patient populations are biased and the usefulness of information obtained from patients is therefore limited. Although this drawback must be acknowledged, psychotherapeutic work leads to knowledge of patients in great depth—greater depth, in fact, than is obtainable by any other means. Psychotherapists are not only privy to the private thoughts and wishes, feelings, and fears of people, their clinical work is based on close observation. They routinely observe the ways in which the inner experience of people changes over time. Collaborations between psychotherapists, social scientists, and bench researchers seems necessary to acquire models that are complex enough to describe human experience and activity. It is in the service of such collaboration that part 1 of this volume was written.

Part Two

Clinical

Introduction to Part 2

The clinical half of this volume focuses on homophobia and internalized homophobia. We discuss women and men across a wide range of ages and adaptive capacities and different psychotherapeutic approaches including psychoanalysis and exploratory and supportive psychotherapy. The area of sexual orientation is broad, and we hope to consider many topics in the future—other than homophobia and internalized homophobia—that we could not here.

Throughout most of the twentieth century heterosexual orientation was conceptualized as the norm and nonheterosexual orientation as deviant, even pathological. Psychoanalysis, if not totally responsible for this view, certainly contributed to it heavily. American psychoanalysis has abandoned this idea, however, and a number of recent meetings of the American Psychoanalytic Association have focused on the deleterious effects of heterosexism and homophobia (Panel 1998).

In the first part of this volume we discussed evidence suggesting that the determinants and meanings of sexual orientation are quite complex. Men and women experience sexuality (including sexual orientation) differently. There are important behaviors and experiences that the genders share, however, including—in the case of nonheterosexual patients—painful interactions that result from antihomosexual prejudice. These can produce immediate distress and disability, but their traumatic effects can be internalized and experienced chronically thereafter, unless treated with psychotherapy. The discussions of the psychological processes and manifestations of internalization that contributed so richly to psychoanalytic psychology were, for the most part, written prior to the 1970s (Schafer 1968; Meissner 1981). Many of these insights are relevant to understanding and treating homophobia, as we illustrate in these chapters.

Our final chapter critically considers the history of organized psychoanalysis and sexual orientation. What has the field, as a whole, learned from the profound changes in understanding human sexuality that have only recently occurred? Hopefully, this chapter will stimulate debate and discussion about the organization of psychoanalysis and facilitate bridge building between psychoanalysis and the many extrapsychoanalytic disciplines with which it shares common borders.

9

Homophobia, Internalized Homophobia, and the Negative Therapeutic Reaction

The many new developments in psychoanalytic ideas about homosexuality have led to a need for revised psychodynamic formulations about the causes and treatment of psychopathology, particularly in gay/lesbian people. The most important influence on symptoms that cause distress and disability in gay/lesbian people recognized only recently is homophobia. In fact, it is not possible to understand clinical problems involving sexual orientation without understanding homophobia. Whereas specific aspects of homophobia vary to some degree across ethnic, religious, socioeconomic, and geographical groups (e.g., countries of origin or areas of origin within countries), common themes occur that are rooted in history. The clinical issues we discuss later in this chapter and the scientific concepts reviewed earlier are best understood within the context of an intellectual tradition shaped by the civilizations of ancient Greece and Rome and by the ideas of the Bible, elaborated and expressed in religion, art, philosophy, political science, and legal policy.

We first consider Greece and Rome. In Greece there was a marked contrast between pre-Platonic ideas about homosexuality and those adopted, late in his life, by Plato and by Aristotle.

In ancient Greece homosexual activity was common, and generally accepted (Dover 1989). Avoidance and negative responses toward people who participated in such activity were not the norm and, apparently, not as common as has been recently the case in many modern countries. However, the concept of "sex-typical behavior" seems to have been endorsed throughout the Greek city-states. Males were supposed to behave in certain ways, and females in other specific ways. As has been true in many societies throughout history, males that behaved like females were disparaged. Simply participating in homosexual activity, however, was not generally taken as evidence of such cross-gender behavior.

Erastes-Eromenos

There is no question that overt homosexual activity was widespread in Greece by the early part of the sixth century B.C. By way of historical landmarks: homosexual activity is extensively depicted in vase paintings, most of which were made between 570 and 470 B.C. (Dover 1989). A specific type of homosexual relationship was idealized in Archaic (before 480 B.C.) and Classical Greece—that between the eromenos, a mid or late adolescent, and an erastes, an older male lover. An eromenos may have been involved with one or more erastes and also with women.

The characteristic configuration of homosexual courtship in vase painting is one in which one of the erastes' hands touches the eromenos's face—the other reaches toward or touches the genitals. The eromenos passively participates in the sexual act but himself is not sexually motivated or sexually aroused. The type of intercourse was intracrural—the erect penis of the erastes thrusting between the thighs of the eromenos—both standing and facing each other. The eromenos does not have bodily orifices penetrated by the erastes. Homosexual fellation is usually not depicted in vase paintings, for example, in contrast to scenes of heterosexual fellation (often enforced).

The erastes was mentor, tutor, and suitor of the eromenos. It seems to have been this idealized relationship that was analogous to our concept of romantic "love." (It was of course different in important ways as well, since our own attitudes were influenced by the medieval notion of heterosexual courtly love.) The ancient Greeks "fell in love" with some frequency, however, and when they did the object often appeared to be a youthful person of the same sex.

The erastes-eromenos relationship was entirely voluntary, and the courtship by the erastes could be rejected by the eromenos without social penalty. The relationship was also temporary. It was discontinued when the eromenos grew into late adolescence or early adulthood. He graduated from pupil to friend and the continuance of an erotic relationship was socially disapproved of and usually ended.

Although most vase paintings depict male homoerotic activity, some depict sexual acts between women. Indeed, one of the earliest lesbian poets, Sappho, wrote homosexual poetry during the Archaic period. Sappho seems to have been a teacher more or less in the erastes/eromenos tradition. Her voice is unusually important in a tradition that so heavily emphasizes men. She was a poet much admired in the ancient world and is a presence and inspiration for poets today.

Although the erastes-eromenos relationship was idealized, other forms of homosexual activity also occurred and appear to have been accepted (Dover 1989).

Plato and Aristotle

In his famous letter to a mother of a homosexual, Freud, attempting to diminish the mother's antihomosexual prejudice, mentioned Plato as one of history's illustrious homosexuals. (The letter is reproduced in chapter 16.)

Plato's ideas about sexuality seem to have changed during the course of his life, however. In the *Symposium*, his famous discourse on love, homosexuality was idealized:

> Those that enjoy lying with men and embracing them . . . are the best of boys and lads because they are naturally bravest. . . . When they grow up such as these alone are men in public affairs. And when they become men, they fancy boys and naturally do not trouble about marriage and getting a family but that law and custom compels them; they find it enough to live unmarried together. . . . When one of these meets his own proper half whether boy-lover or anyone else, then they are wonderfully overwhelmed by affection and intimacy and love.
>
> *(Warmington and Rouse 1984)*

Plato's prohomosexual attitude had changed by the time he wrote the *Laws* at the end of his life. Here he expressed the view that it was desirable for citizens to reduce to a bare minimum all activity of which the end is physical enjoyment in order that the irrational and appetitive element of the soul may not be encouraged and strengthened by indulgence. An argument was made that homosexual pleasure was unnatural and homosexual activity, a crime caused by failure to control the desire for pleasure. This latter position anticipated views of homosexuality that recurred during the late Middle Ages and subsequently (Dover 1989; Boswell 1980).

Aristotle, too, endorsed matrimony, condemned homosexuality, and considered it a manifestation of a morbid disposition. Given Aristotle's enormous influence, it is important to emphasize how little he knew about the biological facts of human sexuality, however. For example, the basic facts of reproductive physiology taken for granted today—by virtually everyone, regardless of educational level—were unknown during Aristotle's time. Aristotle was unaware of the way in which conception occurred. He theorized that the role of the sperm was active and that it, somehow interacting with the menstrual blood, which functioned as a passive receptacle, created an embryo. Similarly, in propagating the species the role of the mother was entirely passive; she was a receptacle for the active material, donated by the father, that led ultimately to a child (Canteralla 1992).

Homosexuality and Homophobia in Rome

In discussing Roman sexuality, Boswell cited Edward Gibbon who observed that "of the first fifteen emperors, Claudius was the only one whose taste in love was entirely correct—meaning heterosexual. If Gibbon was right, the Roman Empire was ruled for about 200 consecutive years by men with considerable homosexual interests" (Boswell 1980:61).

Prior to the third century A.D. homosexuality and homosexual relationships were seen by Romans as part of the diversity of human behavior. There was one important exception, however—participation by adult male citizens in passive sexual behavior, in today's jargon, being a "bottom." This was looked upon with scorn and was equated with behaving like a woman, boy, or slave, all people excluded from the political power structure.

The Greeks had not believed that a single God revealed to mankind a code of conduct that included regulation of sexual behavior. The emergence of Judeo-Christian monotheism has influenced attitudes and laws about homosexuality from the Roman Empire to our own times.

In the third century A.D. antihomosexual attitudes and laws emerged. Society became less urbanized and more rural. There was pressure throughout for sexual asceticism as a reaction against what was perceived to be moral decadence, and there was increased governmental regulation of personal morality.

Christianity became the official religion of the Roman Empire during the fourth century A.D.. In A.D. 342 gay marriages were outlawed. By A.D. 533 the emperor Justinian decreed that those found guilty of homosexual relations were to be castrated and executed. After Rome was sacked twice in the sixth century, Christianity became the only organized force to survive the disintegration of Roman institutions. It soon became the focus of organized morality throughout Europe (Boswell 1980; Greenberg 1988).

Homosexuality in Medieval Europe

The antihomosexual attitudes of the latter Roman Empire abated during the early Middle Ages. Progressive urbanization occurred and, by the tenth, eleventh, and first half of the twelfth century, learning surged. During this time interval there seemed to be a revival of positive attitudes toward the homosexuality of the early Roman Empire and the pre-Classical Greeks. Knowledge of the ancient world was valued, and sexuality between same-sexed partners was not only tolerated but sometimes celebrated. This soon changed.

The historian John Boswell has written:

> During the 200 years from 1150 to 1350 homosexual behavior appears to have changed in the eyes of the public, from the personal preference of a prosperous minority, satirized and celebrated in popular verse, to a dangerous, antisocial and severely sinful aberration. Around 1100 the efforts of prominent churchmen . . . could not prevent the election and consecration as bishop of a person well known to be leading an actively gay life-style, and much of the popular literature of the day—often written by bishops and priests—dealt with gay love, gay life-styles, and a distinct gay subculture. By 1300 not only had overtly gay literature all but vanished from the face of Europe, but a single homosexual act was enough to prevent absolutely ordination to any clerical rank, to render one liable to prosecution by ecclesiastical courts or—in many places—to merit the death penalty.
>
> *(Boswell 1980:295).*

By the mid thirteenth century European countries decreed harsh penalties for homosexual activity. For example, a thirteenth-century Spanish royal edict stated:

> Terrible sins are sometimes committed and it happens that one man desires to sin against nature with another. We therefore command that if any commit this sin, once it is proven, both be castrated before the whole

populace and on the third day after, be hung by the legs until dead and their bodies never be taken down.   *(Boswell 1980:288).*

In France a code was issued specifying castration for a first offense, dismemberment for a second, and, in the unlikely event of survival, burning for a third offense. Female homosexual activity was forbidden as well, and the punishments were dismemberment for the first two offenses and burning for the third.

What accounts for the radical change in attitude? There are many theories about this but no definitive answer. A trend toward centralized authority and ecclesiastical power developed throughout Europe. The Inquisition violently retaliated against dissidents and deviants from established mores, many of whom were not homosexual, of course. Centralized control of sexual behavior was viewed as appropriate and in keeping with centralized control of moral behavior. Theological and legal frames of reference were fused, and resultant antihomosexual attitudes became influential, remaining so in many areas of the world to this day.

The *Summa Theologica* of St. Thomas Aquinas became the standard of Roman Catholic dogma. Homosexuality was viewed there as an unnatural sin, along with masturbation, nonprocreative heterosexual coitus, and intercourse with animals.

Later European and American attitudes toward homosexuality remained strongly influenced by its status during the late Middle Ages. In England "buggery," defined as "carnal knowledge by mankind with mankind or with brute beast or by womankind with brute beast," was deemed a capital crime. From the fifteenth through the nineteenth century execution for homosexual activity was practiced throughout Europe.

In the American Colonies homosexuality was generally treated as a capital offense as well. Many states, after independence, adopted sodomy laws; many still carry these on "the books" (Posner 1992).

Condemnation of Nonprecreational Sex

In the late Middle Ages sexual lust that went beyond what was then interpreted as "natural" was condemned as moral vice. This tendency continued throughout the nineteenth century in Western European countries and the United States. In the eighteenth and nineteenth centuries physicians joined those whose voices were raised against unrestrained sexual lust. By and large, this was thought to be a problem of males, in whom both sodomy and masturbation were condemned. A particularly influential antimasturbation tract was written by Lord William Acton. According to him, the boy who masturbates becomes debilitated:

> The frame is stunted and weak, the muscles undeveloped, the eye is sunken and heavy, the complexion is sallow, pasty or covered with spots of acne, the hands are damp and cold, and the skin moist. . . . If his habits are persisted in, he may end in becoming a driveling idiot or a peevish valetudinarian. Such boys are to be seen in all stages of degeneration but what we have described is but the result toward which they all are tending.
>
> *(Acton 1995 [1875]:273)*

Homosexuality and Medicine

Two mutually incompatible ideas about homosexuality became popular in the nineteenth and early twentieth centuries, both based on the idea that homosexuality is somehow biologically caused and innate. Some physicians and writers such as Ulrichs (Kennedy 1980–1981), Hirschfeld (1914), Ellis (1897), and others (Bullough 1976) argued for a medical view of an innate homosexuality that some even saw as a third sex. In their opinion homosexual people really practiced a different kind of sexuality than the heterosexual mainstream but were, in their personalities and general attributes of functioning, just like everyone else. They were opposed to the criminalization of homosexuality and did not see homosexual behavior as pathological or evidence of moral weakness. Opposed to this, however, was the popular idea that homosexuality was a manifestation of hereditary degeneracy.

Degeneracy

In American and European society the nineteenth century witnessed the progressive growth of the status and influence of physicians. Physicians in charge of mental asylums sometimes used their newfound influence to lecture the public on mental illness. There was a tendency to emphasize reciprocal effects of psychological disease, vice, and the decline of civilization.

A French asylum director, Morel, outlined a theory relating vice to mental illness that was highly influential in Europe and America. Like Lamarck, Morel

173

believed that acquired characteristics could be inherited. According to Morel's paradigm, a noxious environment leads to vice and psychological deterioration that can be transmitted genetically. Afflicted offspring are predisposed to unhealthy lifestyles characterized by alcoholism, malnutrition, and poverty. This further influences the genetic endowment. Thus, progressive degeneration of people in a particular social class could occur from one generation to the next. Many social theorists in the nineteenth century considered homosexual activity, along with alcoholism and violent criminality, to be a form of hereditary degeneracy (Morel 1857, 1860; Greenberg 1988).

A particularly influential publication in this area was Krafft-Ebing's *Psychopathia Sexualis*, which included homosexuality with sexual deviations. Although Krafft-Ebing did not argue that homosexual people should be treated as criminals, or that they were morally inferior, he was, nonetheless, one of a number of physicians who suggested that homosexual acts were symptomatic of an illness of some type (Krafft-Ebing 1965 [1886]).

Greenberg has pointed out that the term *homosexual,* coined in the later nineteenth century, marked an important point of departure in modern thought about homosexuality since it involved classification of people rather than conduct. This term emerged from publications that were sympathetic to homosexual people. Moreover, the word *homosexual* began to be employed in a new way, as a noun. There were negative consequences to this (Greenberg 1988), since it became possible to discuss "the homosexual" in medical terms, facilitating stigmatization and discrimination (Bullough 1976; Goffman 1963).

The medicalization of homosexuality was later to have grave consequences. In the twentieth century, for example, in the United States, until the 1970s it was believed that homosexual people suffered from sociopathic personality disorder or were sexual deviants, similar to pedophiles and exhibitionists. As a result of these ideas people who today would be called lesbian or gay were not allowed to emigrate to the United States, or adopt children, or work in governmental positions and were subject to other forms of discrimination. The interested reader is referred to Gonsiorek and Weinrich (1991), Bayer (1981), and the Group for the Advancement of Psychiatry monograph (2000).

Heterosexism

Heterosexism refers to the assumption that sexual life should be organized around traditional heterosexual monogamous relationships whose primary goal is procreation and child rearing (Herek 1996). Such familial organization is believed to deserve special cultural/legal privilege and status as opposed to all other forms of sociosexual organization. The tendency for heterosexism to become extreme, used in the service of antihomosexual bias, has been present since the late Middle Ages, although a more liberal perspective is currently emerging.

Homophobia

It is apparent even from this brief overview that antihomosexual attitudes, however irrational, are deeply rooted in ideas that have been influential for many hundreds of years. Nevertheless, they were not given the name *homophobia* until the late 1960s. A psychologist-educator coined the term to signify an irrational aversion to homosexuality and to homosexual people.

Dr. George Weinberg was shocked by the intensity of negative reactions he encountered when he attempted to lecture to audiences about the unfairness of the (then) prevalent attitudes toward homosexuality.

> In Chicago I needed an escort to get from a radio station to my hotel. Later, in Baltimore, a caller to a radio program threatened my life and was encouraged by the interviewer. In New Jersey, a bomb threat emptied out the church in which Merle Miller and I were scheduled to speak. A reaction this explosive needed to be understood, so I gave myself the assignment of studying it. . . . Out of my study came the recognition that I was up against a phobia—an irrational revulsion so widespread that it had gone unrecognized by most people. . . . In 1967 I invented the term "homophobia" to describe this irrational reaction. *(Weinberg 1972:introduction)*

The word *homophobia* has come to be accepted in the mental health literature, and we continue to use it in this book. From a psychoanalytic perspective, however, the term has limitations. Phobic people tend to be anxious, dependent, and retreat from feared situations to the comfort of supportive human relationships. Thus a phobic patient tends to be able to tolerate a dreaded situation when in the presence of a trusted, idealized partner. Phobic people do not devalue or ragefully attack phobic objects. They do not inspire fear in others.

The projection of rage and malevolent intent is a characteristic of paranoid psychological functioning. The person experiences others as harmful, motivat-

ed by malevolent intent, and is full of hostility toward them. Such paranoid individuals feel entitled to their hostility: "You deserve to be hurt because you
wish to hurt me." Paranoid people engage in endless combat and retreat from
other people (Cameron 1959). They often have histories of abuse and neglect
and may also have family histories of paranoia in some form. In his famous discussion of Dr. Schreber, Freud suggested that paranoid delusions were a defense
against unconscious homosexual wishes (Freud 1911). This can occur in individual cases, but extensive scholarship and clinical research indicates that this
hypothesis of the etiology of paranoia in general is incorrect (Shapiro 1981;
Friedman 1988; Lothane 1992). Paranoid people do tend to have feelings of insecurity about their gender identity/role, however. The combination of rage,
gender role insecurity, and projection can lead paranoid males to the belief
"He wants to screw me, therefore, I have to hurt him." If one takes an overview
of people who experience intense antihomosexual prejudice, we suspect that
they manifest paranoid tendencies much more frequently than phobic tendencies. From a descriptive perspective, people with antihomosexual attitudes
tend to be authoritarian, conservative, come from religious backgrounds in
which homosexuality is viewed negatively, and tend to have little or no contact with homosexual people (Herek 1985).

Both men and women may be homophobic. In men developmental influences include early childhood gender/role insecurities stemming from a
need imposed by adaptation for boys to disidentify with certain aspects of
their female caretakers (Greenson 1968; Gilligan 1982; Chodorow, 1989,
1994). Conflicts about gender role and gender self-esteem may be amplified
later by oedipal conflicts in mid and late childhood and by conflicts resulting
from abuse by male peers during later childhood. We discuss these mechanisms in other chapters. Yet another possible influence was elucidated in a recent study. Heterosexual men were divided into two groups, homophobic
and nonhomophobic, on the basis of self-report. They then were exposed to
sexually explicit videotapes while penile circumference was monitored. The
nonhomophobic men did not manifest erection in response to tapes of male
homosexual activity. The homophobic men did—to some degree—and also
tended to deny subjective feelings of arousal, even though laboratory measures indicated such (Adams, Wright, and Lohr 1996). Although there is no
reason to believe that this mechanism is the rule in homophobia, it obviously sometimes occurs and is important for clinicians to consider.

In women mechanisms leading to homophobia are more diverse. They
include factors that cause people to condemn homosexual activity generally

(e.g., religious fundamentalism, stereotypic false beliefs about the personalities of homosexual people, etc.) as well as particular idiosyncratic development influences experienced by individual women. For example, in either sex homophobia might stem from identification with a homophobic parent.

Internalized Homophobia

In the early 1970s generally accepted clinical ideas about homosexuality changed radically. The most important reflection of such change was deletion of the category Homosexuality from the *Diagnostic and Statistical Manual* (*DSM-III*) of the American Psychiatric Association (1980). The profound consequences of this decision have been discussed in many forums (Bayer 1981). At about the same time a set of observations and inferences about the origins and treatment of psychopathology in gay patients began to emerge, which came to be labeled gay affirmative ideas about psychotherapy. In a carefully reasoned and highly influential article that focused on "internalized homophobia" in gay men, Malyon (1982) noted that socialization involves internalization of values, attitudes, and beliefs. Because children who ultimately become homosexual adults are raised in heterosexist and homophobic settings, their socialization leads to internalization of negative attitudes and beliefs about homosexuality. Malyon pointed out that negative internalizations influence "identity formation, self-esteem, the elaboration of defenses, patterns of cognition, psychological integrity and object relations. Homophobic incorporations also embellish superego functioning and in this way, contribute to a propensity for guilt and intropunitiveness among homosexual males." Negative attitudes and beliefs about homosexuality become part of the self and negative attitudes and beliefs about the self come to be signaled by homosexual desires.

Importance of Late Childhood in the Development of Internalized Homophobia

The concept of internalized homophobia is applicable to psychosexual development as well as current mental functioning. For example, Malyon has emphasized the consequences of internalized homophobia for identity formation during adolescence. Since Erik Erikson's contribution in the late

1950s, adolescence has been recognized as being a phase of critical importance for identity development. Erikson noted that identity formation involved mental processes that organize the representational world and preserve a sense of self-cohesion and continuity over time. Another aspect of identity concerns the integration of the young person into specific social groups. Family, ethnicity, race, religion, gender, and sexual orientation all provide opportunities to "identify" with group attitudes and values. When group attitudes, values, and other attributes are internalized, they contribute to the sense of identity (Erikson 1959).

We pointed out previously that traditional psychoanalytic theorists who have considered internalization have focused on early childhood as a critical period during which processes of incorporation, introjection, and identification influence personality development (Meissner 1981; Schafer 1968). Relatively sparse attention has thus far been devoted to late childhood as a time of particular importance with regard to the genesis of internalizations, such as the negative ones that influence internalized homophobia.

Internalized homophobia may develop during late childhood as well. An important psychological process that leads to internalized homophobia during late childhood is identification with the aggressor, a mental mechanism common in victims of abuse. The boy adopts the same view of himself that is communicated by aggressive peers who have tormented him. The tendency to form cliques and to exclude or scapegoat others who are "different" may be manifested by girls as well. The feeling of having been "different" and alienated from peers during middle and later childhood is also reported by lesbians. In girls, however, the experience often appears to be less toxic than for boys, as the public humiliation is less aggressive.

The Self and Its Objects: Attribution of Self-Hatred to the Homoerotic Fantasy

In discussing self-hatred, Freud (1917) emphasized the importance of introjection of an ambivalently perceived object. He suggested that loss of such an object triggered the mental mechanisms that lead to the taking of that object into the representation of the self. Because the hostility felt toward the object has been repressed, the patient is not aware that the lost relationship was suffused with hostility as well as love. The hatred of the "other" now directed toward the self leads to decreased self-esteem and melancholia. Although Freud initially focused on loss resulting from death, many other types of losses may trigger this psychodynamic process as well (Bowlby 1980).

Other psychological processes in addition to introjection of the ambivalently held object may lead to negative self-valuation. Whatever its intermediate mechanisms are, however, negative self-valuation *may come to be attributed to homosexual desires or to temperamental characteristics associated with such desires.* Thus, although its origins may be rooted in phenomena that are quite different, the patient may consciously believe that he hates himself because he is homosexual.

The attribution of negative self-valuation to homosexuality is often the result of a condensation of different symbolic narrative representations in a person's mind. Each component of this condensation may be composed of elements that are internalized representations of different ambivalently experienced formative relationships that have occurred during early childhood with parental figures. These early occurring psychodynamic constellations may be condensed into later occurring frankly homophobic personal narrative segments. They may be "packaged," as it were, in the conscious mind under the rubric that therapists term internalized homophobia.

Internalized Homophobia Resulting from Unresolved Childhood Traumatic Stress Reaction

Case Example 1

A gay man of thirty-four years had feelings of inferiority in dealing with older men in the workplace who were authority figures and whom he presumed to be heterosexual. When he felt that these men were evaluating his performance unfavorably, he experienced nausea and chest pain as well as disabling anxiety symptoms. Medical workup for the physical symptoms had been negative. Because the patient did not appear to have severe psychopathology, the therapist used a supportive approach. He emphasized that the patient's professional performance was superior and that the patient irrationally minimized this because he was gay. The therapist stressed that there was no need to think less of oneself for being gay and that there was actually no evidence that the men to whom the patient responded were in fact homophobic. The patient's response to this strategy was to become paralyzed by anxiety, and consultation was requested.

Review of the patient's history revealed that his father, who had been perfectionistic and hard-driving, had had a myocardial infarction when the patient was eight years old. The father's career was cut short by his sudden illness, and, although he survived, he became bitter that his ambitions had not been fulfilled. The patient was present during his father's heart attack and had vivid memories of his father complaining of crushing chest pain and becoming diaphoretic and nauseated. Hovering for many hours at his father's bedside during the convalescence, he had experienced an intense sense of his father's loss of power and status as a result of the illness.

Later this patient's father remained hypercritical toward him—involved but unaffectionate—and the patient had conflicting feelings of anger at his father's controlling behavior and guilt to be angry with a man so debilitated. He also thought that his father might be more satisfied with him if he were more "macho"—better at sports and other interests such as military history enjoyed by the father. Years later, he decided that his father had really not loved him because he was homosexual.

Actually many of the patient's symptoms, including hypochondriacal worries about his heart and guilty ruminations that he did not deserve praise for performance successes, were not a result of internalized homophobia at all but were rather due to a reaction to a traumatic event and its prolonged aftermath. The patient attributed the origins of his guilty conscience to being homosexual. The primary basis for his childhood guilt, however, was not the presence of early homosexual desire but angry feelings toward his father and the magical believe that he had caused his father's cardiac illness. These feelings and beliefs were disguised and condensed in the conscious perception of conflicted feelings about being gay.

Distinction Between Internalized Homophobia and Early Occurring Masochistic Psychodynamics

Internalized homophobia is so commonly experienced by gay and lesbian psychotherapy patients that many clinicians believe it to be universal in our culture. Guilt and shame at being gay leads to self-hatred and to self-destructive behavior. During early childhood years the families and support systems of many patients who later develop internalized homophobia are nurturant, however, and endow the patient with a sense of positive self-regard. When self-hatred emerges later, it is a consequence of defensive partial identification with aggressors, "layered over" earlier occurring self-acceptance.

The group of patients who come to therapy (and adult life) with this advantage is very large and probably constitutes a majority of those who ultimately are successfully treated with gay-affirmative therapeutic strategies. Such individual enter the therapeutic situation with the basic capacity to love and work preserved, although this may be temporarily hidden by the psychological symptoms associated with profound conflicts about lesbian or gay. The restoration of self-esteem as a result of gay-affirmative therapy, combined with the sense of social integration associated with becoming part of the gay/lesbian subculture generally leads to a favorable therapeutic result.

An Intermediate Group: The Internalized Homophobia Fault Line

In an intermediate group with regard to psychopathology-internalized homophobia are patients who develop along more or less normal (neurotic) lines but in whom intense manifestations of internalized homophobia are triggered by a life stressor of some type. Associated with generalized symptomatic regression are a nucleus of symptoms resulting in and from internalized homophobia.

The following vignette illustrates such a situation in a young woman who was a lesbian.

Case Example 2

T, a thirty-one-year-old teacher living in a five-year relationship with her woman partner N, age forty-two, presented for treatment because of depression and total avoidance of sexual activity with N during the preceding six months. An emotionally traumatic incident had occurred at work involving T when one of her pupils had been abused by a parent and T had failed to recognize it. The case was ultimately detected by a medical team after the child was hospitalized for a head injury. T's superior, her principal, rebuked her for having been negligent. T was assailed with guilt—at first concerning her fantasized neglect of her student, then also for her sexual impulses toward women. Once thoughts about punishment for homosexual behavior were linked with conscious guilty feelings, T was unable to engage in any sexual activity with her partner N. N had made attempts to engage T in sexual intimacies, but when all her overtures were rebuffed she had withdrawn. One to two months after, T developed feelings of diminished self-esteem, ugliness, guilt, and shame.

Exploration in psychotherapy revealed that T was preoccupied with thoughts of God's punishing her by sending her to hell for her homosexual behavior, although she had no conscious belief in God at the time. Actually, T had experienced thoughts of being punished by being sent to hell for her homosexual impulses for many years. These had been transient, and experienced without any accompanying affects, and therefore possible to disavow until the traumatic incident occurred. Despite a significant amount of internalized homophobia, T had nonetheless managed to enjoy a satisfying emotional and sexual life as a lesbian until the reprimand by her principal.

When she experienced the trauma of her student's injury and the resulting criticism by herself and others of her failure to protect the child, the previously isolated internalized homophobia became associated in her mind with conscious feelings of guilt. T then became sexually avoidant of her partner and, as a secondary phenomenon, her partner withdrew sexually from her.

The internalized homophobia had become more burdensome when the patient interpreted the principal's rebuke symbolically. She had placed the rebuke in a narrative context in which she felt guilty about being homosexual and fearful that she would damage others in some way. The injury of her student and her principal's criticism, therefore, seemed to her to be an enactment of dreaded fantasies come true. This occurred even though the reprimand had nothing to do with T's being a lesbian, a fact of which her principal was unaware.

Once insight about these matters became available to the therapist and the patient, it became possible to trace the internalized homophobia back to the patient's father's angry attacks on closeness between T's mother and herself as a child. Her father was recalled as an abusive womanizer, her mother as a depressed, submissive, but loving woman whose favorite child was T. T's experience of internalized homophobia appeared symbolically to represent a partial regressive identification with her father in symptomatic response to a traumatic life stressor. In treatment T acknowledged that her father was an irrational, overcritical man whose values she no longer wanted nor had to live by. Ashamed of her "silliness" to have been so affected by his views, she reached out to her partner N and slowly reestablished a sexual relationship with her. T also found herself "coming out" to a number of family members and friends to whom she had always presented herself as heterosexual and realized in retrospect that her unfounded fear of their condemnation had prevented her from being more honest with them earlier. T's depressive symptoms resolved and did not recur.

In this case T's character organization was essentially neurotic and not borderline (Kernberg 1975). In the descriptive terminology of the fourth edition of the *Diagnostic and Statistical Manual* (American Psychiatric Association 1994) her diagnoses were Axis I-Dysthymia and Sexual Aversion Disorder. Axis II: None. During the course of T's development, internalized homophobia had not been superimposed on earlier severe character pathology. For this reason a relatively brief period of therapy proved helpful.

It is notable that for many years T seemed not to be hampered in her psychological adaptation by hatred of her lesbian self. A psychological vulnerability or "fault line" in the structure of her personality existed, however. When a traumatic life event occurred, latent feelings of guilt and shame that were associated in T's mind with being homosexual surfaced and required intervention. T's loss of sexual desire and associated sexual avoidance are relatively common symptoms experienced by women, whether lesbian or heterosexual, when psychological and relationship difficulties are severe.

LifeLong Self-Hatred

In contrast are patients who experience *lifelong* self-hatred because they have been abused and/or neglected in early childhood. Whatever the reasons for this self-hatred, if these children are on a developmental track to becoming gay or lesbian they may ultimately attribute *all* self-hate to being gay or lesbian. They become unable to condemn themselves for being gay or lesbian without triggering the emergence of self-hate that was not necessarily developmentally associated with homophobic motives in the first place.

The early childhood years of these latter patients were tormented. Later exposure to homophobic social communications result in negative internalizations that follow earlier occurring negative internalizations. Freud pointed out that patients such as these behave as if their self-representations are under constant attack by a sadistic internal agency that debases the self and makes it suffer. He called this a harsh superego and hypothesized that it results from unresolved oedipal guilt (Freud 1924). Subsequent psychoanalytic clinicians have emphasized that earlier occurring traumata also influence this type of dynamic (Asch 1988). A person whose early bonding experiences were abusive or neglectful is frequently drawn to sadistic and abusive relationships later in life. During childhood the tendency to *provoke abuse* from others offers a measure of mastery and control over anxiety-provoking events that may be even more traumatic when they occur spontaneously. This type of person constructs a narrative as he or she develops in which the pattern of provoking abuse from others is repeated in all intimate relationships and often recurs during psychotherapy.

Patients with global and tenacious self-hatred tend to become involved with others with whom they repeat a scenario in which they experience chronic feelings of hostile depression, helplessness, and fantasies of suffering as an "innocent victim." These fantasies have multiple functions including the preservation of a fantasized tie with an ambivalently perceived preoedipal maternal representation and the warding off of attack by a fantasized oedipal father representation. These patients often suffer from the effects of punitive unconscious objects incorporated during childhood. They have an intense and persistent need to atone, and their interpersonal relationships are organized to meet this need (Glick and Meyers 1988). Because their manifest presentation may emphasize homophobic symptoms, their underlying character pathology may *not* be immediately evident.

Gay-Affirmative Therapy

The basic premise of a gay-affirmative perspective is that the deleterious effects of biased socialization may be lessened and even largely eliminated with corrective therapeutic experiences that facilitate and support self-actualization and a sense of pride in being gay. The basic therapeutic models that Malyon applied to his work with gay patients were the notion of "corrective emotional experience" as discussed by Alexander and French (1946) and the stages of interactional psychotherapy as described by Wolmann (1975). Malyon and subsequent therapists have stressed that gay-affirmative ideas do not in themselves constitute a specific system of psychotherapy but rather are meant to provide a framework that informs psychotherapeutic work with gay patients. Moreover, the concept of other pathogenic influences on major psychopathological disorders, such as schizophrenia and manic-depressive disorder, is not discarded by therapists who adopt a gay-affirmative point of view.

As is true of all types and strategies of therapy, some patients appear unresponsive to gay-affirmative interventions. The most important clinical subgroup and the one that we wish to discuss here are those that manifest variants of what Freud (1923) termed the negative therapeutic reaction. This may be associated with symptoms of internalized homophobia at the manifest level.

The Negative Therapeutic Reaction

In 1923 Freud first described the negative therapeutic reaction in patients treated with psychoanalysis as follows:

> There are certain people who behave in a quite peculiar fashion during the work of analysis. When one speaks hopefully to them or expresses satisfaction with the progress of the treatment, they show signs of discontent and their condition invariably becomes worse. One begins by regarding this as defiance and as an attempt to prove their superiority to the physician, but later one comes to take a deeper and juster view. One becomes convinced, not only that such people cannot endure any praise or appreciation but that they react inversely to the progress of the treatment. Every partial solution that ought to result, and in other people does result, in an improvement or a temporary suspension of symptoms produces in them for the time being an exacerbation of their illness; they get worse during the treatment instead of getting better. They exhibit what is known as a "negative therapeutic reaction." (Freud 1923).

Freud went on to explain that these patients appear to "need" their illnesses and to view recovery as a danger. He observed that they seem to have profound unconscious feelings of guilt:

> As far as the patient is concerned this sense of guilt is dumb; it does not tell him he is guilty; he does not feel guilty; he feels ill. This sense of guilt expresses itself only as a resistance to recovery which is extremely difficult to overcome. It is also particularly difficult to convince the patient that this motive lies behind his continuing to be ill. (Freud 1923)

Subsequent psychoanalytic clinicians have elaborated on Freud's clinical findings. In discussing the negative therapeutic reaction, Kernberg (1988) emphasized worsening of the patient's condition at precisely those times he or she perceived the therapist to be a good object. Like Freud, Kernberg observed that the negative therapeutic reaction is frequently a manifestation of unconscious guilt. Kernberg also noted that it may be expressed by patients with narcissistic and sadomasochistic personality disorders, however. In these patients, guilt is reinforced by unconscious envy. They envy the analyst for being free of the tormenting conflicts from which they suffer. Kernberg also noted that certain patients are disturbed to such a degree that they experience any primary love object as destructive. In these patients love can be experienced only as destruction.

Traits Associated with the Negative Therapeutic Reaction

Many other psychoanalysts have discussed the negative therapeutic reaction in their patients and have described traits likely to be associated with it. These patients have histories of either having been success-avoidant or of experiencing successful accomplishment as a trigger for depression. As Freud (1916) wrote years before he reported on the negative therapeutic reaction, the patients seem "wrecked by success." They tend to have difficulty allowing others to be helpful to them. As a result, their histories are replete with instances in which they avoid making relationships with such people or undermine such relationships if they threaten to become established. Although the traits may not qualify for diagnosis as a specific personality disorder (for instance, the *DSM-IV* [American Psychiatric Association 1994] does not include a category for Self-Defeating Personality), they reflect psychodynamic and psychopathological configurations that therapists regularly encounter.

Negative Therapeutic Reaction and Gay-Affirmative Psychotherapy: Further Considerations

Because the negative therapeutic reaction was originally described by Freud, and elaborated on subsequently by other psychoanalysts, certain of its features are stressed more than others. For example, clinicians have emphasized that manifestations of the negative therapeutic reaction occur within the transference in the psychoanalytic situation. Although this is true, the negative therapeutic reaction occurs among patients treated with diverse other therapies. Transferential reactions of varying intensity are, in fact, part of the psychology of everyday life. Psychoanalysis and psychodynamically oriented psychotherapy are the only forms of psychological treatment that attempt to make use of such reactions for therapeutic purposes, however.

Certain types of transference reactions render some patients unable to accept supportive gay-affirmative interventions. Frequently, neither the patient nor the therapist recognizes the occurrence of a specific relational pattern. For instance, the patient diligently applies himself or herself to the therapeutic work. He or she idealizes the therapist and seems to feel involved in the psychotherapeutic process. Symptomatic improvement occurs, and patient and therapist attribute this to the patient's increased self-esteem and sense of integration. Shortly thereafter the patient's clinical condition deteriorates markedly. Even as she or he becomes severely symptomatic, the patient reassures the therapist, "This is not your fault. In fact, you are the best possible therapist for me. The problem is entirely mine!"

Often the therapist finds the patient likable, even admirable, at the beginning of the relationship. The patient's apparent modesty (which hides an underlying tendency toward self-debasement) may be initially confused with true humility. As the repetitive pattern of psychopathology unfolds, however, the therapist is likely to feel progressively more angry toward the patient. These hostile feelings trigger guilt. Particularly anxiety-provoking for many therapists are sadistic fantasies about the patient, which the therapist does not fully recognize are elicited and provoked as a consequence of the patient's psychopathology. Usually, in this type of situation, detailed assessment reveals that the patient's developmental course was one in which early childhood was filled with self-hate, which was condensed into internalized homophobic narratives constructed during later childhood. In situations such as these the treatment strategy generally needs to be changed from supportive psychotherapy to a more exploratory or uncovering approach.

Support Versus Insight

Although both supportive and exploratory psychotherapy may be practiced by therapists who have a gay-affirmative stance, the techniques used to treat patients with similar symptoms differ. For example, a patient who expresses self-hatred because he is gay might be immediately and vigorously challenged by a supportive gay-affirmative therapist. The therapist might observe that there is no logical reason to disapprove of one's homosexuality. He or she might counter incorrect ideas about homosexuality espoused by the patient with psychoeducation and encourage the patient to become involved in homosexual relationships rather than attempt to suppress the need for companionship and sexual expression. In contrast, a therapist using uncovering techniques would seek to explore with the patient the meaning of his or her negative feelings about the representation of him or herself as homosexual. Only following detailed consideration of unconscious motivation would the patient's irrational belief systems about being homosexual be interpreted.

A supportive therapist therefore would use the techniques of confrontation, clarification, and psychoeducation almost immediately. Many patients respond positively to this approach in weeks to months. In contrast, the therapist using an exploratory approach would be more likely to present a relatively unstructured (although empathic and accepting) therapeutic persona. This would facilitate regression and transference distortion. Simultaneously, the therapist would seek to communicate his wish to truly understand the patient, and a therapeutic working alliance would emerge. Within the context of profound trust that usually takes many months to develop, the therapist through interpretation and other techniques would attempt to alter the balance between the patient's unconscious wishes and fears.

Patients with Negative Therapeutic Reactions: Assessment

The presence of a negative therapeutic reaction becomes apparent when deterioration in the clinical condition of the patient immediately follows optimistic expressions by the therapist about the patient's progress or apparent solutions to life's difficulties that emerge in the treatment situation. The pattern is repetitive. The worsening of the patient may be primarily expressed in the relationship with the therapist, in life outside the therapeutic relationship, or in both.

Importance of the Patient's Psychiatric Diagnosis in Assessing Symptom Exacerbation

The specific symptoms that may worsen in the patient are diverse and depend to a large degree on psychiatric diagnoses. Someone with diagnoses of dysthymia, substance abuse, and borderline personality disorder is likely to manifest one type of symptomatic profile, whereas a different patient with, for example, anxiety and avoidant personality disorder would manifest quite different symptoms when his or her course worsened. We have found it helpful in assessing the total adaptive and maladaptive behavior of the patient to describe not only Axis I and Axis II disorders according to the *DSM* but his or her character type as well. By this we mean the traits of specific character types as traditionally conceptualized in psychoanalytic clinical theory—obsessive, hysterical, phobic, paranoid, schizoid, explosive, passive-aggressive, and so on (Stone 1980).

There may be times during the waxing and waning of the patient's clinical condition when his or her character type influences the way in which symptoms are expressed even when no personality disorder is present. For example, a thirty-year-old man responded to openly expressed approval about being gay from members of his psychotherapy group and his psychologist with depression and increased obsessional behavior. The latter did not meet criteria for obsessive-compulsive personality disorder but was confined to increased rigidity, emotional coldness, and hypercritical, oppositional, negativistic behavior. The patient's depression was partially masked by the more dramatic traits of his obsessional character, evidenced by power struggles with his lover and with his therapist. The pattern of his waxing and waning personality symptoms not only impeded progress during treatment but threatened the stability of work and love adjustment. This pattern, not superficially evident, emerged only after meticulous historical assessment.

Level of Personality Structural Integration: An Additionally Important Diagnostic Concept

In addition to consideration of the *type* of character defenses, we have found Kernberg's (1975) concept of *level* of personality structural integration to be helpful in diagnostic assessment. Kernberg pointed out that certain patients, albeit neurotic, have intact representational worlds and retain the capacity for delay of gratification, impulse regulation, and appropriate social behavior. In contrast, others have fragmented representational worlds and lack the capacity to regulate their impulses. Their interpersonal relationships are often episodically explosive. Unlike patients in the first group, the latter patients lack object constancy and experience identity diffusion. Whereas patients in the first group characteristically use defenses such as repression, isolation, and reaction formation, those in the second group are more likely to use projection, denial, projective identification, and splitting. Regardless of the type of character defenses used by patients in the latter or "borderline" group, their basic symptoms are due to fragmented self and object representations and a loss of cohesion in the sense of self. Thus two patients may appear to have identical character defenses, but if they were from groups whose level of personality structural integration differed, their basic problems would be experienced and expressed variably.

We stress these diagnostic concepts because manifestations of the negative therapeutic reaction may appear disguised or masked by dramatic symptoms whose relationship to the stressors that we have described above might not be immediately evident. For example, among patients involved in partnerships the manifestations of the negative therapeutic reaction might be signaled by relationship dysfunction. Both partners may attribute their difficulties to excessive demands made by the other. Actually, the difficulties may be a function of the worsening of borderline symptoms in one partner, which occurs as a consequence of the negative therapeutic reaction. Because of the use of denial and projection by borderline patients, many therapists might not immediately realize that the patient's worsening in the context of the therapeutic relationship itself may not be for reasons other than those perceived by the patient.

Gender Differences in the Manifestations of the Negative Therapeutic Reaction

Because of gender differences based in biology as well as in rearing and in social circumstances, men and women with comparable levels of personality organization, and even similar psychiatric diagnoses and degrees of internalized homophobia, may present clinically in quite different ways. The most dramatic difference the authors have seen is the tendency of the female patient to respond to conflict and anxiety by seeking to fuse with the object, whereas the male patient is more likely to seek distance. The following cases illustrate this difference:

Case Example 3

An emotionally needy woman with a borderline character organization and frequent bouts of depression had been talking with her female therapist about her yearning to find a partner with whom to share her life. Past relationships had ended with furious outbursts on the patient's part after provocations by her. The therapist privately noted that the patient had cut her hair in a comparable style to hers, had bought a similar necklace, and had taken to wearing similar clothing. At this point the patient met a woman at a social event, had sex with her the same night, and arrived at her session three days later announcing that the two were in love and had decided to move to a distant city together. Careful history taking revealed that the patient actually knew very little about her new partner. Among the sparse information available, however, were the facts that the partner had difficulty holding a job, few vocational skills, a history of substance abuse and brief episodes of prostitution, and that she had moved frequently, never living in one place for more than a year. She presented herself to the patient as someone who had endured "hard times" and had put these behind her, but she gave no actual evidence that she had done so. The patient had already given her small sums of money and had tentatively agreed to provide more substantial financial support in the future. The patient herself, however, had limited economic means.

In this case the patient who yearned for closeness with her female therapist, and was secretly angry and disappointed not to enjoy more intimacy with her, first created a physical resemblance, then sought out a surrogate female partner whose appropriateness as a match for her was questionable at best. This relationship was immediately formalized by the decision to share a residence and to sever connections with all persons currently in the patient's life, including the therapist. The therapist saw that the patient had enacted her self-destructive scenario (a replaying of early childhood events in which her mother rejected her for her more physically attractive sister) both in her outside life and in the transference, because her action was a parody of the search for intimacy she had been discussing with her therapist. The therapeutic relationship proved strong enough that the patient was able to remain in treatment and eventually to find a more appropriate life partner.

Case Example 4

A thirty-five-year-old man with similar psychodynamics came for treatment of depression after his partner of five years died of a lingering illness. After he had established a relationship with his older male therapist, he began to have periods of severe anxiety during scheduled separations from him. He dealt with these episodes by cruising and engaging in sexual activity with partners he did not know and whom he never saw again. This was not a pattern of behavior he had ever engaged in before.

The therapist was impressed with the self-destructive quality of this behavior, which developed in the context of a deepening tie between patient and therapist.

Whereas the female patient displaced a wish for intimacy with the therapist and translated it into action with an inappropriate partner, the man defended against such a wish by participating in repetitive, distant interactions with a variety of partners. These gender differences are quite typical.

Men and women are equally likely to engage in a variety of other defensive behaviors, however, while evincing a negative therapeutic reaction. Thus patients of both genders may devalue the object (either in the transference or outside the therapy), demonstrate explosive hostility, provoke the therapist's concern by making puzzling errors of judgment, forget appointments or even the past therapeutic work, and so forth.

Treatment

Once the negative therapeutic reaction has been diagnosed, the therapist must then make a decision-tree concerning treatment. If the negative therapeutic reaction is associated with undiagnosed Axis I or Axis II psychopathology, this should be appropriately diagnosed and treated. The most common example of this is one of the mood disorders.

As a general rule, the therapeutic environment should be altered. Because direct expressions of approval trigger the negative therapeutic reaction, more emphasis should be placed on exploration of meaning and less on direct messages of support and approval.

Many therapists become anxious when the patient seems to experience self-abasement in the treatment situation, and they may label this "internalized homophobia." Although such needs should not be endlessly indulged, a certain amount of expression of symptomatology is often necessary before confrontation and interpretation can have therapeutic impact. The therapist must be able to tolerate the patient's need to express feelings of self-denigration that the patient believes are "caused" by being homosexual. Early in the treatment a simple comment, "You seem to be pretty hard on yourself," is often the extent to which interventions might be made. Only later, when the patient is able to listen to more complete discussion, should the therapist engage in it.

Younger gay therapists who have only recently worked through their own conflicts about being gay are particularly at risk of falling prey to the patient's unconscious need to suffer. Excessively defensive behavior by the therapist in response may take the form of premature expression of support—with such comments as "It's OK to be gay—after all, I'm gay myself." This type of interaction often triggers a cycle of symptomatic worsening in the patient.

Patients who experience the negative therapeutic reaction are among the most difficult to treat with psychotherapy. If the negative therapeutic reaction is embedded in global and lifelong self-destructive character pathology, the course is likely to be lengthy and arduous and the treatment outcome uncertain. Individual cases may always be exceptions, however. It is often not possible to predict the patient's capacity to respond to therapy prior to undertaking this time-consuming and difficult therapeutic work.

10

Internalized Homophobia, Pathological Grief, and High Risk Sexual Behavior in a Gay Man with Multiple Psychiatric Disorders

Male sexual fantasy motivates sexual activity, yet its determinants have not yet been completely described. In this chapter a patient is discussed who experienced the onset of a new erotic fantasy during middle age. This motivated risky sexual behavior during a seven-month period. Although the patient's self-destructive sexual activity ceased as a result of supportive psychotherapy and pharmacological treatment of his psychiatric disorders, his sexual fantasy persists. In order to understand X's history and course it is necessary to have a psychodynamic perspective. The reasons that his treatment included both psychopharmacology and psychotherapy are discussed.

Among gay men a behavioral risk factor for contracting HIV is unprotected receptive anal intercourse with unknown and/or multiple sexual partners. Such unsafe behavior occurs more frequently among individuals who have poor impulse control, particularly if sexual activity occurs while under the influence of alcohol or other substances of abuse (Mann and Tarantola 1996; Royce et al. 1997). Although descriptive and epidemiological studies have been helpful in establishing this, the specificity of the influences leading to high-risk sexual behavior remains to be established. Clarification of the motivation of particular individuals to participate in such activity at a particular time requires a frame of reference based on individual psychology.

An especially salient issue with respect to sexual behavior concerns the influence of unconscious conflicts on consciously experienced erotic fantasy. Fantasies are imaginary stories that endow our inner worlds with meaning and serve many purposes. Some are role rehearsals for the future, some help preserve self-esteem and a sense of security (Person 1995). Erotic fantasies are uniquely suffused with sexual feelings (e.g., "lust") that become more and more intense as the somatic changes of sexual arousal/excitement progress. Sexual activity and fantasy may be endowed with many meanings involving power and aggression, dependency, love and intimacy, self-rebuke, self-punitiveness, and other meanings as well (Ovesey 1969; Kernberg 1995; Person 1995).

Regardless of sexual orientation, some patients experience shame, guilt, and negative self-valuation in response to erotic fantasy and/or activity. This may take a unique form in gay patients, however, when self-condemnation is a reaction to homosexual orientation. The conscious and unconscious conflicts associated with such negative judgments about the self have come to be termed internalized homophobia (Malyon 1982).

Internalized Homophobia

The negative valuing of the self because of homosexual desires/experiences occurs in patients across all diagnostic categories and in nonpatients as well. Even among people with little or no antecedent psychopathology, the effects of internalized homophobia can be dramatic and severe (Friedman and Downey 1995; Downey and Friedman 1996). In many suffering diminishes as a result of the psychological growth associated with the complex processes termed "coming out" in the lay and professional literature. The person labels her or himself lesbian/gay, adopts a lesbian/gay social role, and finds a niche in the lesbian/gay subculture.

In contrast with such individuals are those with primary psychiatric disorders who in addition experience the deleterious effects of internalized homophobia. In order to effectively treat these patients, it is necessary to understand the relationship between internalized homophobia and their diverse psychiatric symptoms. It is also necessary to conceptualize the etiology of component conflicts whose final common pathway is negative labeling of the self because of homosexual orientation. Both groups of patients, those with primary homophobia and those with primary psychiatric disorders and secondary homophobia, may attribute the exclusive cause of their psychic suffering to internalized antihomosexual attitudes. Clinically significant aspects of this attribution may be out of conscious awareness yet have a profound behavioral effect nonetheless.

A developmental psychodynamic perspective is particularly helpful to understand and treat patients with major psychiatric disorders who, moreover, experience the deleterious effects of internalized homophobia. These effects may be expressed in broad areas of psychological functioning leading to impaired interpersonal relationships and vocational performance.

In the man discussed below a new erotic fantasy resulting from unconscious conflicts associated with internalized homophobia and unresolved grief motivated unsafe sexual activity. The vignette illustrates the usefulness of a developmental psychodynamic perspective in addition to a descriptive psychiatric one for establishment of a sound treatment plan.

Vignette

A forty-year-old single businessman who lives alone sought consultation because of depression and a pattern of sexual behavior that he labeled "self-destructive." Openly gay for more than twenty years, X was exclusively homosexual in orientation.

Until the onset of the problems requiring consultation and treatment, he had practiced "safe" sex. By this he meant that he abstained from receptive anal intercourse with all but one partner whom he knew intimately and who was HIV-, insisted that all sexual partners wear condoms no matter what sexual activity was engaged in, and abstained from sexual activity while under the influence of drugs and alcohol.

For reasons unknown to him, approximately seven months prior to the consultation, his pattern of sexual experience and activity radically changed. On weekends, between Friday and Sunday evenings, he would arrange to have sex with men he met at bars and via telephone advertisements. Often snorting cocaine, he had unprotected anal intercourse many times during the weekend with many different partners. A close friend, understandably worried about the patient's safety, finally prevailed upon him to seek professional assistance.

The patient's erotic fantasy life had changed immediately preceding his altered sexual activity pattern. For many years he had enjoyed activities and fantasies of mutual fellatio, masturbation, and intercourse in which he was the penetrator, "the top." The change in sexual fantasy consisted of replacement of his previous sexual fantasies with an insistent, persistent sexually arousing fantasy of having a man ejaculate into his rectum. This fantasy associated with masturbation became a rehearsal for sexual activity. When his partner ejaculated into his rectum, the patient experienced intense orgasm.

X had been tested for HIV five times during the past five years and had learned of the last negative result immediately before "safe sex just fell apart." Since his last test, X had refused to be tested. As he put it, "I know I should; I am working up to it. I am terrified of what I might find."

He had never knowingly attempted suicide, nor had anyone in his family, nor was there a family history of psychiatric hospitalization. The patient met *DSM-IV* criteria for major depressive episode without psychotic symptoms. He had had one episode of hypomania in his late twenties following a job promotion. This was characterized by increased energy, altered sleep pattern from seven to five hours per night without residual fatigue, increased ambition, a feeling of elation, and modestly increased sexual desire. His sexual fantasy life and interpersonal sexual activity had remained unchanged but his self-masturbation increased from about five to ten times per week. The hypomanic episode had spontaneously subsided after three months.

He was a college graduate, had a stable, excellent work history, and long-standing close friendships.

Psychodynamically Relevant Past and Family History

The patient's fortieth birthday occurred at approximately the same time as his altered pattern of sexual experience and activity. In his late thirties he had noticed that it was more difficult to attract sexual partners than had previously been the case. Prior to that he would enter a gay bar, "do nothing in particular and leave with someone every time." To his chagrin, in recent years he found himself having to resort to patronizing prostitutes. He found the sexual activity pleasurable but considered the necessity to use this method of obtaining sexual release humiliating. He marked his fortieth birthday as signaling the passage from youth to middle age, which he dreaded. Nonetheless he considered the association between his altered sexuality and turning forty to be a "coincidence."

X was the youngest of several siblings and, to the best of his knowledge, the only gay one. He had had "crushes" on other boys from kindergarten age and dated the onset of clearly erotic desires to the third grade, when he was attracted to a teacher as well as a classmate. He knew that he was "different" from peers from about that age but did not fully realize that he was gay until his late teen years. He was identified within his family as having more girl-like than boylike interests, including theater and art, and was sometimes labeled "sissy" both within the family and by same-aged boys at school. Other than on two occasions, however—on Halloween and during a costume party—he did not cross-dress. He had never wished to be a girl or woman.

The family had pronounced heterosexist and homophobic values. His father, a blue-collar worker, and his mother, a homemaker, were openly contemptuous of men who seemed feminine in any way. Both parents were neglectful and abusive, especially to this particular child. For example, his father punished him with brutal beatings for minor infractions. His mother was publicly critical of his looks and often commented in front of his and family friends that his face could "be helped by cosmetic surgery." Others considered X attractive, however. On one occasion when he was eleven he had saved for a month to buy his mother a gift. She showed it to her friends in his presence with displeasure, saying, "This is all he could come up with." X, realizing that he was singled out especially by his mother for cruel treatment, decided that this was because she actually loved him the most. "She had to treat me badly in order not to show favoritism." Despite her hostility at times, his mother turned to him as her confidant. "She treated me at times like her girlfriend. We discussed interior decorating, clothing styles, and other girl-stuff."

When this man was twelve years old, more or less coincident with puberty, his mother developed breast cancer. At the onset of her illness she was forty years old, and her death, resulting from complications of metastatic disease, occurred thirteen years later. X vividly recalls his mother's fortieth birthday, which occurred while she was in the hospital recovering from a radical mastectomy. He remembers how "composed" both parents were about her illness. They prided themselves on responding to adversity "without emotion." Discussion of painful feelings was discouraged. Much more than his siblings, during his mother's decline from metastatic disease X had been involved with her. He had taken pride in "correcting" their previously difficult relationship prior to her death.

During the last years of her life a stressful event took place that had particular significance for him. One of X's brothers impregnated a girlfriend and her mother informed X's mother of her son's part in the behavior. X's parents were horrified. Observant Catholics, they belonged to "Right to Life" organizations and were deeply opposed to abortion. A few weeks later they attended an antiabortion fund-raising dinner of which their children were all informed.

When the patient's mother died fourteen years prior to the consultation, he had attended the funeral but had not experienced intense grief. Because of her intense disapproval of homosexuality, he had never "came out" to her. "She probably suspected, but we never spoke about it. For a man to love a man was simply unacceptable to her."

Approximately two months before the onset of his present problem, the patient's father died of a stroke. During his father's last years of life X had attempted to "build a relationship with him in order to correct the deficiencies" in his childhood relationship. He prided himself on his success in this venture. A few years before his father's demise X decided to come out to him. To his surprise, his father's attitude was accepting. "He told me that he had realized I was gay, and that he still loved me. We both cried." X was not only surprised that his father responded positively to his homosexuality but was also surprised at his father's admission of love. As had been the case with X's mother, he attended his father's funeral but did not experience intense grief.

Psychopathology and Psychodynamics

The patient's diagnoses were

> Axis I: Bipolar II Disorder
>
> Major Depressive Episode
>
> Cocaine and Alcohol Abuse
>
> Axis II: Mixed Personality Disorder with Narcissistic and Histrionic Features

Discussion

A psychodynamic perspective in addition to a descriptive one made possible a more specific model to inform psychotherapeutic strategy. The core part of the psychodynamic paradigm applied to this patient was provided by Freud in his classic essay, "Mourning and Melancholia" (Freud 1917). Freud observed that loss of an intensely ambivalent love relationship led to self-hatred via the defense mechanisms of repression and introjection. The hatred felt toward the lost object is repressed, and the object, with its associated affects, including unconscious affects, becomes part of the self-representation. Thus, instead of feeling angry at someone outside the self, the person experiences anger directed at the self. This produces depression and decreased self-esteem. Subsequent psychoanalysts applied Freud's model to losses other than death and elaborated upon his discussion of normal and abnormal aspects of grief (Bowlby 1980; Engel 1962).

Freud's ideas about pathological grief were supplemented with those of modern clinicians about internalized homophobia to shed light on this patient's narrative history (Malyon 1982; Friedman and Downey 1995; Downey and Friedman 1996; Isay 1989, 1996).

At the level of descriptive psychopathology it was observed that during the past seven months the patient had experienced a major depressive episode and that his symptoms were most severe on weekends, when he was lonely. This required psychopharmacological intervention, and antidepressants and mood stabilizing drugs were prescribed.

Most patients do not experience a change in the story line and imagery of their erotic fantasies associated with the onset of depression. In order to account for X's unusual reaction, a psychodynamic formulation was utilized. It was hypothesized that the patient was motivated by unconscious guilt as a result of pathological grief about the loss of both parents. The appearance of his bandaged mother celebrating her fortieth birthday in the hospital was indelibly etched on his mind, although he did not consciously realize its significance for his symptomatic reaction to his own birthday. Despite their reconciliation, X harbored unresolved unconscious anger toward her. Since she was overtly homophobic, he represented the cause of her abuse and neglect in his mind as a reaction to his homosexuality and activated a belief formed in his childhood but repressed and psychologically encapsulated: "She always hated me because I am homosexual." This understandably led him to feel angry. In a magical and irrational way he unconsciously concluded that her death had occurred because of the power of his rageful feelings. He formed a pathological identification with her, which influenced his sexual fantasies and activity. By participating in unsafe sex he could contract HIV at the same age that his mother contracted cancer and atone for his unacceptable (albeit unconscious) hostility. He thus experienced his mother's antihomosexual attitude as his own. The cognitive processes associated with this were unconscious, and all that the patient was aware of was depression and a desire to engage in receptive anal intercourse.

This psychodynamic reasoning was validated to some degree with data that emerged in his treatment. For example, he dreamed that he was a woman, lifting up her skirt to be vaginally penetrated by a "blue-collar type of guy." (The patient had on other occasions described his father and brothers as having a "blue-collar" style.) After beginning therapy X also revealed that shortly before his first consultation he had received treatment for an infection of his right nipple. He found himself "picking" at the nipple until he caused a bloody suppuration. The patient's mother's carcinoma involved her right breast, and X worried that he too might have breast cancer. He was successfully reassured about this by the physician who treated his infection.

An important aspect of psychodynamic reasoning involves the concept of condensation. Thus, although pathological identification with his mother contributed to the course of his disorder, other conflicts did as well—all having as a final end point self-hatred for being homosexual.

For example, another intrafamilial event that served as a symbolic nidus for symptom formation involved his parent's reaction to his brother's out-of-wedlock impregnation of a young woman. The fantasized elaboration of his memory of this provided a direct link to the patient's altered sexual fantasy life. It was conjectured that he constructed a narrative, "I wish to be the girl that my brother got pregnant." The imagery associated with this led to his intense sexual arousal in response to having a man ejaculate into his rectum—and also influenced his desire that the man not wear a condom. Also contained in this fantasy was repression of hostility toward the brother, for being favored over him, the sense of having been an innocent victim abused by the brother, and the wish that perhaps he would have been more loved if he had been a woman. Both parents had favored the female children over the males.

In addition to representing in a condensed way narratives about the patient's mother, and the girl his brother impregnated, it was hypothesized that the patient's unconscious guilt was exacerbated by the death of his father, which occurred shortly before the onset of his present problem. This too stimulated self-punitive activity in order to atone. Additional unconscious issues concerned the patient's conflicts about aging. He seemed to equate his perceived loss of sexual attractiveness as retribution, as if his mother's view of him when he was a child was valid. This fostered feelings of ugliness associated with his depression and hopelessness. Contracting a disease that would further shorten his life span spared him the necessity of imagining what he would be like as an elderly man.

Combined Psychodynamically Informed Psychotherapy and Pharmacotherapy

In the first session the patient agreed to a treatment plan consisting of psychotherapy and pharmacotherapy. Medication consisted of an SSRI antidepressant and a mood stabilizer. X elected to be seen once per week rather than more frequently and has subsequently appeared promptly for each appointment.

In the second session X's sexual activity was labeled as a suicide attempt equivalent. This was done in as concerned and nonjudgmental a fashion as possible. Verbatim notes were not taken during the session, but a reconstruction of the dialogue follows.

> DR. F: Are you aware of feeling so bad—so low—that you are actually trying to kill yourself?
>
> x: No, I want to live. I have lots of things I want to do with my life.
>
> DR. F: I get the sense that the "wanting to live" part of you is very deep and because of that part you are here after all. That part is not all of you though. We have to consider that the sexual activity you told me about expresses a desire not to live but to die—a kind of suicide attempt even though you don't experience it that way.

X appeared thoughtful when this was suggested and noted he had intense desires to die, and sometimes did imagine himself ending his life, but denied having a specific plan to do so.

The reason for not labeling his sexual behavior as suicidal in the first session was concern that he might not return for a second. Having established rapport, and in light of the dangerousness of the patient's behavior, the decision was made to intervene as soon as possible.

In the third session it was pointed out that the patient's mother had developed breast cancer at the age of forty. This was the same age as the onset of his self-destructive sexual activity. The patient agreed that this was "a coincidence." I commented that his mother had ultimately died of her illness and that HIV-related disease can be fatal as well.

During the first month of psychotherapy the patient continued his pathological sexual activity pattern on weekends. After our fourth session, however, he stopped and restricted his sexual activity to masturbation to the fantasy of receptive anal intercourse. The symptoms of his depression largely remitted and lability of mood, also a feature of his initial presentation, subsided. The patient is presently actively assessing the reasons for the limitations of intimacy in his previous sexual relationships and his hopes for future ones. Although not sexually active during the past two months, he hopes to become so in the future, but not in an impulsive way. He recognizes that the probability that he has become HIV+ are high, but describes himself as "not yet ready to be tested." He spontaneously stated that if he were to engage in sexual activity with someone he would wear a condom, behaving as if he were HIV+.

The major aspects of X's present problem have improved as a result of his treatment (which is ongoing). The improvement has been manifested by decreased depression and mood lability, increased impulse control, and cessation of unsafe sexual activity. The erotic fantasy of passive anal intercourse persists, however. X's improvement at present therefore cannot be considered stable, since the fantasy might motivate activity if impulse control decreases. This might occur for a number of reasons, the most likely of which would probably be psychosocial stress.

The case of X is unusual since his erotic fantasy life appeared to be influenced by unresolved unconscious conflicts that were activated by immediate life events. Although similar types of causal chains of events were hypothesized by psychoanalysts to influence behavior in the past, documentation of their influence on conscious erotic fantasy life has been sparse. Indeed, more frequently than not, psychoanalytically oriented psychotherapists have tended to blur the distinction between erotic and nonerotic fantasies. It might be that, as psychotherapists attend more explicitly to narrative material concerning the erotic domain, better understanding will emerge about the relationship between unconscious motivations and erotic experience and activity.

An important difference between the psychodynamic paradigm outlined here and that used by classical psychoanalysts of past generations is that the latter attempted to relate unconscious conflicts to the *etiology* of homosexuality. This line of speculation proved invalid and has been abandoned by most modern psychoanalysts (Friedman 1988; Isay 1989). There is no reason to think that the tendency toward maladaptive and destructive sexual activity is related to a specific type of sexual orientation.

Another difference between modern and classical psychoanalytic models of unconscious mental functioning concerns internalized homophobia. This construct has only been utilized in the dynamic psychotherapy literature since 1982 (Malyon) and subsequently in the psychoanalytic literature. In X's case internalized homophobia appears to have resulted from pathological internalizations of family members that occurred during critical periods of development. His peer relationships during childhood and adolescence were not pathological. In fact, close friends of both sexes have been a source of sustenance and security throughout his life. Sometimes this is not the case, however. Many gay patients are severely abused by peers during their juvenile and adolescent years (Herek 1995). Identification with the aggressor leads to internalized homophobia and post-traumatic stress reactions may be associated with other symptoms as well (Downey and Friedman 1996). Often such patients have experienced severe intrafamilial stress as well, and their developmental histories may be even more difficult than that of X.

Understanding and treating X illustrates the value of a combined descriptive and psychodynamic diagnostic assessment and a dual psychopharmacologic and psychotherapeutic treatment strategy. The treatment approach is based upon relating the erotic domain of X's experience and activity to the nonerotic domain. This type of construction of meaning—by therapist and patient together—necessarily extends beyond exclusive focus on ameliorating his depression.

The duration of X's psychotherapeutic treatment is difficult to predict because his goals after twelve sessions were different from his initial ones. Following psychotherapeutic exploration, he realized that the absence of an intimate passionate love relationship in his life did not occur by chance but rather was related to unconscious mechanisms of avoidance. He entered psychotherapy with the view that he had never loved anyone because he was unlucky. He now continues psychotherapy with the understanding that he avoided contact with potentially suitable partners because he was unconsciously fearful. He was thus able to set a new goal: enriching the depth of his sexual relationships. This occurs frequently in psychotherapy and is one reason why the psychotherapeutic process is complex.

Although the case of X raises many questions, it illustrates that assessment of psychotherapeutic outcome sometimes requires more than improvement in immediate symptoms. Fortunately for X, his treatment was paid for out of pocket and not by an insurance company. It is likely that many insurance plans would consider remission of depression as successful outcome and therefore refuse to subsidize additional treatment. In X's case, however, the persistence of his erotic fantasy is a warning signal that subsequent risky sexual activity might well occur. Hopefully this fantasy will subside as its root causes are explored in psychotherapy.

The case of X is also relevant from a public health perspective. Psychoeducational interventions for risky sexual behavior, although helpful, have not been universally successful. Thus many people who are fully aware of the dangerousness of particular types of sexual activities nonetheless engage in them. The reasons that particular individuals behave against their self-interest when aware of the dangers remain to be fully described.

11

Internalized Homophobia and Gender-Valued Self-Esteem in the Psychoanalysis of Gay Patients

This chapter discusses the relationship between self-condemnation for being gay and self-condemnation for feeling unmasculine. The patients who are its subjects are reasonably well-adjusted men, homosexual in erotic fantasy orientation, comfortable with gay identity and social role, integrated at a neurotic, nonborderline level (Kernberg 1975). Although they recall having been labeled "fag" or "sissy" as children, the most painful aspects of this taunting are now out of conscious awareness. They are usually integrated in the gay subculture and in conventional heterosexual society as well. During analysis, however, as often happens (Isay 1989), negative feelings about being homosexual come to the surface. Associated with these is intense shame about being unmasculine. As a general rule both the antihomosexual feelings and the shame about feeling unmasculine have been repressed and together constitute part of the patient's symptomatic "core"—the primary reasons for suffering and for the therapeutic intervention of psychoanalysis.

Although heterosexual men often experience low masculine self-esteem, gay patients are far more likely to fuse this feeling—or, more properly, this complex set of ideas, images, and feelings—with the *orientation* of their erotic fantasy life. For example, heterosexual patients who feel unmasculine are not likely to *attribute the cause of their unmasculinity to heterosexuality per se.* The gay patients discussed in this chapter unconsciously view their homosexual orientation as indissolubly intertwined with masculine inadequacy.

Internalized homophobia may follow upon early childhood abuse and neglect (Downey and Friedman 1995, 1996). In such instances patients tend to have *primary* psychopathology of various types—often masochistic-depressive—upon which internalized homophobia is superimposed *secondarily* later in childhood. Other individuals seem to reach late childhood without traumatic familial circumstances and without primary core psychopathology. In them internalized homophobia appears as a *primary* phenomenon, usually occurring as the result of interactions with family *and* nonfamily members, particularly peers. Both groups of patients, however, may *attribute* the exclusive cause of psychic suffering solely to negative attitudes about being homosexual. It remains for the analyst to help the patient understand the many developmental conflicts mobilized and symbolically represented in a condensed way as a reaction to homoerotic imagery (Friedman and Downey 1995; Downey and Friedman 1995, 1996).

Only some patients with internalized homophobia experience the type of gender-valued self-condemnation we discuss here. Since, to the best of our knowledge, we are the first to describe the phenomenon, its frequency is not known, although our clinical experience suggests that it is common.

Patients in this group generally *condense* diverse negative judgments about themselves with the specific negative judgment that is a reaction to "being homosexual." In the previous chapters we observed that most gay patients have had traumatic experiences with other males because of their gender-role behavior. During childhood they have been teased, threatened with physical violence, ostracized, and even assaulted by other boys (Herek 1996; Herek and Berrill 1992). Because of the psychological mechanism of identification with the aggressor, and for other reasons that vary from patient to patient, these traumatic interactions may result in a feeling of masculine inadequacy. Later in development, usually during adolescence, the sense of gender-role inadequacy may become attributed to erotic fantasies, whereas in actuality the erotic fantasies have become part of a negative self-valuation that began earlier. In order for the clinician to accurately formulate the psychodynamic aspects of the patient's internalized homophobia, he or she must understand the developmental psychodynamic significance of the patient's history of gender-identity/role experience and activity.

Brutal Abuse of One Boy by Another

Although there are no data indicating how frequently gentle, timid, or athletically awkward boys or those who enjoy stereotypic cross-gender activities are subject to such abuse, common sense and clinical experience suggest that it is common. The severity of mistreatment may be extreme, however, as evidenced by an illustration from the autobiography of Paul Monette, a gay author:

> It happened in the basement corridor just outside the boys' lavatory where the six grade had its lockers. Vinnie and a group of three or four others had somebody pinned in a corner. Vinnie was snarling and shoving.
>
> "Yea, you're a homo, ain't ya? Little fairy homo. Ain't that right?"
>
> Then he shot out a fist and slammed his victim's head against the wall. A bustle of students streamed past to their lockers, eyes front and pretending not to see. But my locker was just a few feet away; I couldn't help but hear it all if I wanted to get my lunch box. Besides, I was drawn to it now, as to a wreck on a freeway.
>
> "Homo, homo, homo," Vinnie kept repeating, accompanying each taunt with a savage rabbit punch. The victim pleaded, terrified, but trying not to cry. He vigorously denied the homo charge, choking it out between punches, which only made Vinnie angrier. He growled at two of his henchboys who pinned poor Austin's face to the wall. Vinnie made a hawking sound and spit a gob of phlegm on the brick besides Austin's face." "Come on homo, lick that off."   *(1992:35)*

Boys who are brutal such as Vinnie probably grow up to become sexist, rageful men, prone to violence. Perhaps some of these very same children commit hate crimes later in life (Herek and Berrill 1992). Their childhood behavior might be considered rehearsal for adult criminality.

Monette himself was not physically abused in this situation, but he identified with the victim whose *actual sexual orientation was in fact not known.* The boy was victimized not because of his sexuality but rather because of his gentle temperament and intellectual interests. Patients with childhood experience like those of the young Paul Monette, or the child whose assault he witnessed, are sadly not uncommon. Monette discusses other traumatizing experiences that did happen to him as a result of interactions with aggressive males later in his book.

Many gay men like Monette have had similar experiences as children. The patients we refer to here fall along a spectrum with regard to severity of abuse. Some were beaten, publicly humiliated, physically threatened; others were mocked and ostracized by boys like the little leaguers discussed earlier. In no instance, however, did the reactions leading to the type of negative self-assessment we discuss here result simply from fantasy.

Late childhood has unique phase-specific development tasks requiring mastery, one of which is the psychological movement away from the nuclear family and toward the world of peers (Engel 1962). During this time boys must maintain their sense of connection with nuclear family members and develop an additional network of connections with peers. Same-gender peer abuse and ostracism may lead to pervasive feelings of unworthiness and shame. Isolation from male peers may result either as a result of ostracism, anxious avoidance, or both (Friedman 1988).

The Representation of the Self as Inadequately Masculine: Theoretical Perspectives

We have thus far suggested that during late childhood or early adolescence some boys construct a fantasy about the self representing a fusion between negative attitudes and values about homoerotic imagery and a sense of masculine inadequacy.

These boys are probably only a minority of all those on a gay developmental track who have been abused by other boys during childhood. Such abuse is quite common (Saghir and Robins 1973; Herek and Berrill 1992) and there is no reason to think its effects are uniformly so pernicious. We believe that many men truly leave the consequences of their childhood traumata behind them, and integration into the gay subculture is instrumental in facilitating this felicitous pathway. Supportive relationships often have a therapeutic effect on trauma survivors, enhancing security, self-esteem, and buttressing the sense of identity (Gabriel 1996). This may be an important reason that so many gay people respond positively to "coming out." The complex processes involved in positive identity consolidation are fostered in the context of beneficent interpersonal interactions with other gay people.

The patients discussed here seem similar in much of their *manifest* behavior to those who appear to have put the worst consequences of trauma behind them. Only because of the exploratory uncovering work of dynamic psychotherapy or psychoanalysis does the repressed image of the damaged masculine self appear. This is not a research report but rather one focusing on psychological mechanisms. There is no way of knowing the descriptive characteristics that might distinguish patients discussed here from those that do not have a repressed self-representation of masculine inadequacy.

Case Example

A forty-five-year-old accountant is presently in his fourth year of psychoanalysis. He came for treatment because of depression stemming from difficulties in his relationship with his partner. The couple had been in a mutually monogamous relationship for many years, which was stable but, from the patient's perceptive, constricting. After much soul searching during the first year of treatment, A decided to end the relationship.

The issues that we discuss here, central in A's psychology, were not part of his initially identified reasons for seeking assistance. A had been openly gay for many years. There were no social or vocational circumstances in which his gay identity was not acknowledged. He was proud of being gay, socialized with both gay and heterosexual friends, gave money to gay charities, and marched in the annual Gay Pride parade. At an unconscious level, however, he continued to have negative feelings about being gay that exerted a subtle but important influence at work.

The major symptoms he experienced were intense shyness, severe anxiety when he had to speak up at committee meetings, aversion to conflict, and difficulty asserting himself when others behaved aggressively toward him. The traits sometimes impeded his functioning at the high executive level he had attained. A was ambitious and his excellent technical knowledge of his field was widely appreciated. His firm wished to move him even higher in its chain of command, but some were concerned that he had failed to demonstrate the type of executive performance necessitated by such a high level of corporate responsibility. .

In sessions A often found himself commenting on negative attributes of gay people shortly after discussing one of his own symptoms. In one session, for example, he remarked that he had felt "paralyzed with fear" when the (male) CEO of the company asked for his reactions to a report at a committee meeting. "I croaked out a few words but I felt like a fool." Later in the session he observed that one of his colleagues at work was a gay man with "effeminate mannerisms." "I hate that. It gives a bad message about all gays." Persistent questioning about the precise nature of the "bad" message led A to observe that "we are truly faggots. I don't want to be placed in the same category as those people." A's associations continued, and it became clear that when he used the label "those people," he meant all gay people. The therapist pointed out that he seemed to be inconsistent—A often expressed pride about being gay, was not in the closet, yet seemed to hold unconscious antihomosexual attitudes. A readily agreed. His feelings of disgust were in fact inconsistent, but they were real nonetheless. He seemed at a loss to understand their meaning.

Many sessions followed filled with dream imagery and stories in which A was condemned or mistreated by disapproving male and female authority figures. In these dreams he was usually a child, and the authority figures were adults who represented his parents. Rich associations followed and included memories of his father patiently playing catch with him, for days, weeks, and months of his childhood, but never able to teach him to "throw a ball like a boy. . . . Finally my father gave up and left me alone." A professed "relief" about this, but also experienced a sense of loss. "He seemed to lose interest in me when I couldn't do what he wanted." There were also dream narratives of his mother finding him doing something "horrible" and berating him. As might be expected, his associations were to masturbation. The sexually repressive atmosphere of his family was set by his domineering mother who never actually commented on the patient's masturbating, however. His self-condemnation derived entirely from his inner fantasy life. A began masturbating regularly at age thirteen. The imagery was always of male peers, and he always experienced shame and guilt associated with masturbatory activity. Interestingly, although his home was puritanical and unaffectionate, there was no evidence that it was antihomosexual. As far as A recalled, the topic of homosexuality was never discussed during his childhood.

Following much therapeutic work, A was able to have insight about the magical-irrational beliefs that led him to expect punishment for being gay. He unconsciously "believed" that his CEO had contempt for effeminate men and would ragefully attack him for being gay. This erroneous belief led him to experience severe anxiety when he had to address the CEO in a meeting. In reality, it seemed that the CEO was a brusque but unprejudiced man who focused on job performance in a nonheterosexist way.

It was only after three years of treatment that the patient's memories and associations of having been brutalized by male peers during late childhood fully emerged. He had previously alluded to many of the events, but in a bland way, as if they had been unimportant. Their full emergence followed transference interpretations. The specific material that led to such interpretation was a dream, occurring after a session discussing A's masturbation fantasies, in which a monster fell upon the patient as he was waiting to meet someone for an appointment and dismembered him. A awoke terrified and was unable to fall back asleep.

The dream led to increased understanding of A's projected fears and beliefs about the analyst, which were explored. He expected the analyst to condemn him as his mother had and/or reject him as his father had, and/or treat him with contempt the way the CEO would for being "a gay fag!" Once these fears and beliefs had been discussed, the material about his traumatic experiences as a boy emerged with full intensity. A had often been brutally abused by a gang of neighborhood bullies. He was taunted by being called "fag" and "homo." At that point in his life he had not identified himself as homosexual, and he was confused by these epithets. He felt that for some reason he deserved the abuse, and told no one about his many terrifying and humiliating experiences. One of the gang leaders took particular sadistic delight in tormenting A. He would not only call him "a girl" but would steal money from him as well. A tried to hide from this boy whenever possible. Years later he decided that the "masculine" thing to have done would have been to somehow stand up to the bullies, but he had never been able to. Secretly he decided that they were right—*he was* a fag and a homo.

These memories and associations were so traumatic that they were largely repressed and dissociated. They were not part of A's chief complaint and not identified as a reason for which he sought treatment. They were not even in full awareness until he had been in uncovering psychotherapy for years. They caused him to have a specific type of *gender-valued internalized homophobia,* however. These had many manifestations, but one particularly dramatic one occurred in vocational settings. A equated business meetings with confrontations with gangs of juvenile-aged sadistic bullies. His response to the actual trauma he experienced at their hands was to run and hide whenever he could. Now—in business situations—he could not actually hide. The best he could do was try not to take sides in a conflict, and to say as little as possible. However, he was sure that his CEO could see that he was behaving "unmanfully" and therefore that he was unacceptable: "Not executive material!"

A continues in analysis, but this symptom complex has greatly improved, as has his vocational functioning.

This is but a small segment of analysis meant to illustrate a few points about internalized homophobia. A's conflicts were largely unconscious and involved an equation in his mind between being gay and being unmasculine. The unmasculine self-image had its origins in different developmental phases of childhood. The phase that we emphasize particularly in this chapter is late childhood. His vocational performance was the result of symptomatic compromise formations. On the one hand, he was perfectionistic, intelligent, and ambitious, and strove to succeed. On the other hand, however, he did not wish to be the subject of attention of others in his corporation. He was irrationally terrified that corporate visibility would lead to attacks by other males, including his CEO. The reason for this abuse (in his unconscious mind) was that he was an "effete homosexual." Analysis of the symptom complex included separation of the different psychodynamic narratives that were folded into it in a condensed and disguised way. These included the disapproval of his father for his mild gender nonconformity as a child and of his mother because of his childhood sexual impulses and masturbatory activity. As is often the case, more primitive preoedipal conflicts were also exposed, in which preoedipal maternal representations physically attacked him in various ways. A core dynamic contributing to his symptoms involved his reaction to late childhood trauma by bullies. His identification with the aggressor contributed to the tenaciousness of his symptoms.

Additional Theoretical Issues

Early in the history of psychoanalysis unconscious fantasy was thought to consist primarily of forbidden wishes expressing primitive sexual and aggressive impulses. This model was in keeping with Freud's ideas about the primary and secondary process, the dual instinct theory, and the development of the reality principle (Fenichel 1945). Of subsequent contributors to the theory of unconscious fantasy, the most influential may have been Arlow, who extensively discussed unconscious fantasy from the perspective of structural theory (Arlow 1963, 1969a, b). Arlow pointed out that the creation of fantasy was an ever-present activity of the ego and that unconscious fantasies exerted a profound effect on behavior. He theorized that unconscious fantasies were best conceptualized as the products of intrapsychic conflict and that their analysis was based on the dissection of their components: each consisting of compromises between wishes and fears, id pressures, superego prohibitions, ego-syntonic functions and reality testing, and manifestly expressed in a disguised way. In a recent monograph on fantasy, Person summarized some of Arlow's contributions as follows:

> As already suggested, it has been recognized that many underlying wishes and motives operate in fantasy, including the need for the regulation of self-esteem, the need for a feeling of safety, the need for regulating affect and the need to master trauma.

> Moreover, in this recent view . . . fantasy encompasses not only the original wish but the defenses erected against it. All fantasies show the mark of the ego's synthesizing function and therefore, are more or less composites of wishes, defenses against them, superego directives, and reality consideration. *(Person 1995:63)*

In a review of psychoanalytic ideas about unconscious fantasy, Inderbetzin and Levy noted that although ego psychology marked an advance it also had limitations. It could not explain, for example, the persistence of certain core fantasies, their organization and their influence on present experience (Inderbetzin and Levy 1990). They summarized a different model of unconscious fantasy generation proposed by Slap and Saykin (1983) and Slap (1986). These authors applied the model of Piagetian schemata to the problems posed by psychoanalytic theory in this area. They suggested that repressed schemata consisting of memories, fantasies, and emotions organized in specific ways can become sequestered in the unconscious and exert powerful influences on behavior. In particular, Inderbetzin and Levy also summarized Sandler's idea that unconscious fantasy may exert a stabilizing adaptive function on mental functioning (Sandler and Sandler 1983; Sandler 1986).

All three models, Arlow's (1969a, b), Slap's (1986) and Slap and Saykin's (1983), and Sandler's (1986), appear to inform understanding of the clinical phenomena we discuss here. Thus the fantasy of the damaged masculine self has adaptive and stabilizing functions on psychological functioning as Sandler suggested. It functions as a neurotic symptom with many condensed overdetermined components in a way compatible with Arlow's theory. Understanding its origins and functions is also informed by a Piagetian type model in which the "schemata" that are repressed consist of fantasies of the self interacting with male peers. Condensed into these, or connected via associative pathways, are schemata from earlier phases of development.

Early, middle, and late childhood interactions are all frequently represented in what appears to be the same manifestly experienced fantasy construct. Not only are events from different developmental phases condensed with each other, but so are interactions that primarily involve females such as mother, other female authority figures, relatives, same-aged girls and interactions that primarily involve males including father, other male authority figures, relatives, and male peers. Our observations about this are in keeping with those made by Schafer about internalizations generally (Schafer 1968).

The question arises *why a negative view of the self as inadequately masculine functions as an organizing unconscious fantasy.* Why does the patient not abandon his negative self-representation unconsciously, when he discards it at the conscious level of mental functioning?

The answers to this may be found in the traumatic context in which a sense of self-defect originated. To date, the literature on trauma has stressed neglect, abuse, and/or the experience of diverse other catastrophes. The kind of trauma that is discussed here, gender-specific abuse of children by other children, has thus far not received attention in the psychoanalytic literature (Kardiner and Spiegel 1947; Krystal 1968, 1978; Burgress and Holmstrom 1974; Horowitz 1976; Lifton 1976; Green, Wilson, and Lindy 1985; Baum, O'Keefe, and Davidson 1990; Flannery 1990; Green 1990; Wolf and Mosnaims 1990; Walker 1991; Gerson and Carlier 1992; Ochberg 1995; Gabriel 1996). Severe trauma induces massive repression and dissociation—and its treatment involves the recovery of unconscious memories and fantasies.

The degree to which segments of the personality subsequently grow and develop may depend on preexisting primary psychopathology and/or innate vulnerability as well as the severity and duration of the trauma. Among the patients discussed here, although many parts of the personality were not subsequently impaired, others were. These individuals experienced difficulties in love and work and the capacity to experience pleasure for reasons they were unaware of.

The Construction of the Negative Self-Representation

The painfully negative self-representation is composed of layers upon layers of compromise formations. We conjecture that the juvenile-age unconscious fantasy self-representation functions almost as if it were part of the self-body image, or perhaps a new type of transitional object—providing a holding environment for the representation of the relational self that, while painful, fulfills important unconscious functions. Thus, the fantasies about the self during juvenile years seem to bridge *intrafamilial* relational fantasies and *peer* relational fantasies.

The body-self is represented as being physically defective, too fragile to fight a bully, too awkward to command respect for athletic prowess. The specific fantasy/memories of the body-self in action often consist of running away from a possible fight, being pushed and punched, physically hiding from a threatening group of boys, placating, or retreating. The fantasy of physically demonstrating subservience to dominant males, common in the patients we discuss here, is strikingly similar to behavior that is enacted in actuality by nonhuman primates and many other mammalian species (Ploog and MacLean 1963). A central component of the organizing fantasy, albeit disguised, is simultaneous identification with the abusive aggressors (A. Freud 1937). This is associated with sadistic impulses from earlier developmental phases. As is true of other types of abuse, a tie to an assaultive or condemning other is often experienced as preferable to no bond at all. The psychological pain stemming from the real and, later, the imagined relationship often functions as atonement for unacceptable sexual and aggressive impulses.

The experiences, memories, and fantasies upon which more adequate gender self-valuing is built tend to be organized at a more abstract level—in keeping with the more advanced age of the patient when positive gender self-valuing occurred. This stage of gender self-valuing is not organized around body image fantasies but rather around more general and abstract ideas about the relational self. As one patient put it, "When I got to college, I realized that all this macho male stuff was dumb! That's not what makes a real man! It's all posturing—and strutting—who needs it?"

Castration Anxiety and the Construction of the Unmasculine Self-Representation

A classical Freudian explanation for the phenomena discussed here would be castration anxiety. Freud considered the Oedipus complex to be biologically determined and castration anxiety also to be part of the "biological bedrock" (S. Freud 1937). Our model is different.

As explained elsewhere, we do not believe that the Oedipus complex is either universally experienced or biologically determined (Friedman and Downey 1994). We have suggested that the predisposition toward competitive/aggressive struggles with other males does appear to be influenced by prenatal androgens in humans as in other mammals (Friedman and Downey 1994). Boys often represent fantasized assault in somatic terms. Sometimes damage to self-integrity is symbolically represented as *bodily* integrity (in dreams or fantasy) simply because of an intrinsic attribute of mental functioning—to represent abstract concepts with concrete images. Often the fear symbolically represented is not sexual.

Therapeutic Considerations

The type of condensation outlined above is associated with symptoms that are often difficult to alleviate. There are no outcome studies indicating which clinical techniques are potentially most effective. Our approach is to examine the patient's memories and fantasies about specific interactions that appear to have been of importance in the construction of the negatively valued self-image. Once the psychological mechanisms involved in the process of self-devaluation are understood, their irrational unconscious determinants can be brought to light. It is not only the intellectual processes involved in understanding that lead to therapeutic improvement, of course. Mutual consideration of traumatic experiences by patient and analyst must be associated with empathic support. Rather than having to endure suffering alone as had been the case during childhood, the patient now has a bond with the analyst that exerts a healing effect.

Exploration of the meaning of these key interactions is often painful. Many sessions are usually required in order to help the patient better understand only a very small element in a complex internal narrative whose major theme is "I am an unworthy, inadequate, unmasculine man." The transference regressions occurring during the psychoanalytic process add to the complexity of the analytic work. Ultimately, if the work is successful, the end result is that the patient modifies his ego-ideal-supergo system, bringing his conscious and unconscious self-valuation into alignment with his *present beliefs* about gender-role behavior and his *present standards* for assessing masculine adequacy. This type of gender-role analysis must often be accomplished *in addition* to analysis of irrationally negative attitudes about erotic fantasy and activity per se. This was carried out in the treatment of A, the patient we discussed earlier. As a result, he was better able to distinguish between assertion and aggression and to become appropriately assertive in vocational situations.

Patients are diverse in the way in which they negatively code self-esteem in a gender-valued way. The particular mechanism emphasized in this chapter, and continuing a line of thought introduced earlier in the book, is identification with the aggressor during late childhood, contributing to an image of the self as unmasculine. In the patient A manifestations of trauma occurred largely in symptoms experienced around his vocational functioning. Other patients experience different types of symptoms as well as the manner in which the negative effects are experienced in other areas of functioning, such as love relationships, for example. Since this chapter focuses on a specific type of symptomatic constellation, other aspects of unconscious gender valuing could not be addressed. For example, both gay and heterosexual males may positively value aspects of the self that are seen as feminine. The positive aspects of the representation of the self as feminine in men may be experienced consciously and unconsciously.

12

Homophobic Parents

The parents of most lesbian/gay people are heterosexual and many harbor homophobic attitudes. They tend to seek assistance from mental health professionals for many reasons. The psychologist George Weinberg, who introduced the term *homophobia*, wondered how heterosexual people could be so horrified by homosexuality that otherwise apparently caring parents would actually consider it justification for rejecting their children (Weinberg 1972). Actually, parents who consult psychotherapists about their children's homosexuality are a select group in that they are usually motivated to preserve the child-parent bond. Hence they tend not to have the most extreme antihomosexual attitudes and beliefs of those found in the general population. People with such beliefs tend to reject their children and not to come to the attention of mental health professionals. Homophobic parents are diverse in every possible way and many different types of influence shape their attitudes. In order to be helpful to them, it is necessary to assess their cultural and religious beliefs, their level of education and general knowledge base (not only their knowledge of sexuality), and their life histories as well. This requires an initial working relationship.

Disclosure of Therapist's Sexual Orientation

Parents who are homophobic often avoid consultation with gay/lesbian therapists who they are likely to view as "biased" toward a gay affirmative agenda. The authors of this book, both heterosexual, are usually asked what their sexual orientation is at the outset of the consultation and immediately disclose it. (They adopt the same disclosure policy when seeing individual patients in consultation.) The parents with whom we have clinical experience, therefore, are different than those seen in gay affirmative mental health settings. Interestingly, in our experience, parents rarely ask whether we are "gay affirmative" but are usually interested in being understood and helped (no matter what their overt, manifest request is).

Countertransference Issues

Parents who seek consultation about homosexuality of their children are usually not formally identified as patients. Countertransference traps are common in work with them, since prejudicial attitudes may be difficult for therapists to tolerate, particularly if they are expressed with self-righteous anger and expectations that the therapist share the parental attitudes and behavioral ideals. Nonetheless, homophobic parents usually seek professional assistance with the goal of finding a way not to reject their children. In most situations it is possible to take an appropriately therapeutic stance and carry out an assessment of the reasons that the homophobic attitudes exist and the psychological functions that they serve. Although theoretically this might not always be possible, actually in the private office setting where consultation is voluntary, we have never seen patients to whom some type of help could not be offered and found useful.

In order to better understand parental homophobia, it is helpful to have an overview of what the parents of gay/lesbian patients are apt to be like.

Fathers

A consistent finding that has emerged across many independently conducted research studies and clinical reports is that the father-son relationship is likely to be problematic among gay youth (Friedman 1988; Isay 1989; Savin-Williams 1996). This is by no means invariably so, however, and both authors have had experience with warm supportive and loving relationships between gay patients and their dads. Nonetheless, problems are extremely common, particularly rejection—either overt or subtle—by the father. A speculation advanced by Isay is that such distancing may come about defensively because fathers sense their son's sexual attraction to them and anxiously withdraw (Isay 1989). This may sometimes happen. More commonly we feel that fathers experience the atypical gender role behavior/interests of their sons as extremely different from their own and feel alienated as a result. They need narcissistic gain from parent-child relationships in order to be involved parents and fail to find this in contact with a son who is obviously uninterested in what they are interested in. To them it is as if the son were saying, "I *don't* want to be like you when I grow up, Dad!" If sons are extremely gender-atypical, fathers may be embarrassed and angry, and reject them for psychodynamic reasons similar to those of juvenile boys whom we discussed earlier in this volume.

Another set of reasons for difficult father-son relationships may not be overt rejection by the father but rather poor fit between son and father. A son may require greater emotional contact than a father can supply for practical and/or emotional reasons. We have seen many gay youngsters, for example, who hunger for closeness to fathers who are well-intentioned and caring but work hard and long and are temperamentally not in touch with their feelings or expressive. Even though such a father may feel positively about his son, he still may be unable to meet his son's specific needs for parenting. The situation may be compounded when the son projects angry feelings onto his father and then experiences his father's withdrawal as motivated by hostility.

Relationships between gay young men and their mothers tend on average to be better. Are they comparable to relationships between heterosexual youth and their mothers? In a sense yes, and, as might be expected, in a sense no. Clinicians must keep in mind that mothers on average tend to be much more involved and accessible parents than fathers. Thus, if a child is suffering, lonely, and having difficulty with peers, which is likely to be the case with those gay youth who are in the clinical domain, the chances are greater that their mothers will be available to provide support than that their fathers will be. Gay youth are likely to have more interests in common with their mothers than their fathers as well, a circumstance that in itself fosters a closer relationship. Yet another issue must be kept in mind. All young people who have clinical difficulties are more likely to come from dysfunctional homes than those who never need help from mental health professionals. The relationship between the caretakers in the homes of such youth is likely to be fraught with tension. In such situations mothers often turn to children who are emotionally receptive to provide solace and support. Closeness between a gay son and a mother in this type of situation is quite common. When this is extreme, a triangular situation evolves, with the mother and son becoming allies and extruding the father. Even though such situations are often seen in practice, as a group they do not fit the model of a difficult, problematic, or troubled relationship between a gay young person and a parent. In fact, the mothers of gay male youth are often valued friends and supportive companions.

The parents of lesbians do not fall into a specific pattern, as might be expected, since lesbians as a group are more diverse in many ways than are gay males. Of course, individual families may be organized similarly to those of gay males. Mothers especially may experience disappointment if a daughter does not seem to be on a traditional heterosexual life track (Lasenza, Colucci, and Rothberg 1996). Clinical experience suggests that should similar familial-developmental problems exist, they are likely to involve childhood gender nonconformity, homophobia, and internalized homophobia.

The *New Yorker* Survey About Parental Homophobia

A recent informative survey about parental homophobia was carried out by the *New Yorker* magazine. The editors sought to compare attitudes about homosexuality (and other topics) between four hundred randomly selected ordinary people and those termed "elites," six hundred college graduates between ages thirty and sixty whose personal incomes exceeded $100,000 per year ("economic elite") and four hundred subscribers to the *New Yorker* ("cultural elite). Ordinary Americans were termed "Main Street," the economically advantaged were termed "Easy Street," and the *New Yorker* subscribers, "High Street" (Hertzberg 1998). When asked how they would react to a child who announced that he/she was homosexual, 36 percent of Main Street and 44 percent of Easy Street responded that they would be "totally accepting and supportive." Seventy-eight percent of *New Yorker* subscribers did as well. Twenty-eight percent of Main Street, 25 percent of Easy Street, and 6 percent of *New Yorker* subscribers responded that they would be upset and concerned and would communicate this to the child. A related question was, "Which would you prefer for your son or daughter: to be heterosexual, childless, and either unmarried or somewhat unhappily married; or to be homosexual, involved in a stable, happy relationship, and have children?" Fifty-six percent of Main Street, 44 percent of Easy Street, and 28 percent of *New Yorker* subscribers chose "Heterosexual, childless, and either unmarried or somewhat unhappily married." This latter finding indicates that many parents would prefer their children to suffer unhappy marriages, or not be parents, than be homosexual (Hertzberg 1998:29).

Clinical Issues

Not all homophobic attitudes/beliefs are psychodynamically motivated. The concept of psychodynamic motivation refers to experiences and acts that are the consequences of unconscious fears and irrational beliefs. Psychoanalysts are used to thinking about such phenomena as conversion symptoms and dissociative reactions as being primarily psychodynamically motivated. As Freud pointed out dramatically, so are many other things, including certain types of irrationally determined attitudes and beliefs about gay/lesbian people. As we have earlier observed, even when antihomosexual attitudes are primarily psychodynamically motivated, generally the resultant behavior tends to be more paranoid than phobic in the technical psychoanalytic sense.

There are many reasons outside the realm of psychodynamic motivations for having antihomosexual attitudes. Herek has stressed the importance of ignorance, magical thinking, antihomosexual religious beliefs, conformity with prejudicial norms (Herek 1984, 1991, 1996). Other commonly expressed and understandable concerns of parents are that 1. venereal disease and HIV are more prevalent among gay than heterosexual males, hence the gay lifestyle may be inherently dangerous (Friedman and Downey 1994); 2. lesbian/gay people are the targets of prejudice—sometimes violence—and the risk of abuse increases if they travel to unprotected areas, hence, progress against hate crimes notwithstanding, they are less able to live reasonably secure lives than heterosexual people (Herek and Berrill 1992); 3. stable relationships, particularly among gay males, seem more difficult to achieve than among heterosexual couples, hence the young gay male may be more prone to disappointment and trauma in love relationships; 4. child rearing is problematic if the parents are gay, and they may never become grandparents.

Homophobia is best understood as multidetermined, since people function at multiple levels of psychological organization that are parallel and concurrent. Although we discuss the psychodynamic determinants of homophobia here, we do not mean to suggest these are the only determinants, only that they are important and the people whose experience and behavior are influenced by them seem unaware of this influence. To such persons their manifestly experienced belief system appears perfectly reasonable and, often, the only "sensible" way to think.

Irrational Beliefs about Homosexuality

The manifest attitudes of homophobic parents are usually organized around myths about homosexuality that are common in society at large. There are many such myths, and the ways that they are used by homophobic parents are quite diverse, depending on the parents' psychiatric diagnoses (should such be present), developmental and psychosexual histories, psychodynamics, couple dynamics, and the relationship of the parent or parents to larger social systems of which the family is a part, such as religious, ethnic, and geographical systems. Of course, the parents themselves have not conceptualized any of this. From their perspective, the problem is the homosexuality of their child.

A common myth is that gay/lesbian people are sexually promiscuous. The concern about "sexual promiscuity" is generally associated with fears that the son or daughter will contract venereal disease or HIV infection or be emotionally damaged by uncaring and exploitative and even dangerous sexual partners. It is essential to establish exactly what the term *promiscuous* means to a particular set of parents. Most commonly they believe that the lesbian/gay person is prone to participate in sexual activity with strangers, to have sex for sex's sake (that is, for pleasure and not as part of loving relationships), and to get involved in impulsive/compulsive sexual activity. Regardless of their own religious beliefs, these parents tend to accept the late medieval-religious characterization of homosexual activity as lust-driven unnatural behavior that, because of its hedonistic quality, is immoral by Judeo-Christian standards. Whether or not the parents identify themselves as religiously observant, those who accept the "unnatural" argument generally believe that "natural law" is based on divine revelations that regulate sexual conduct, as expressed in Pauline theology.

Another type of myth involves the parents' ideas about normal sex-role behavior. For example, they may accept the stereotype that gay men are inherently feminine, e.g., "fairies" or "fags," and that lesbians are "dykes." They may believe this about their son or daughter even without indication from the social behavior of the offspring. As a general rule the reason this makes them anxious is that others may see them as well in gender-stereotypic devaluing terms, e.g., "If my son is a fairy, people might think that I, too, am a fairy."

223

Parents with this belief tend to associate homosexual activity with negatively valued cross-gender behavior. A gay son, in their view, may be prone to emotional instability, weakness, and lack of trustworthiness—"like a woman." A lesbian daughter might be assumed to be excessively confrontational, unmaternal, ungiving, and so on.

Yet another myth is that the parents somehow caused the homosexuality of their offspring as a result of familial interactions. They may believe that during childhood the mother was overinvolved and the father critical/detached. Parents with this belief thus adopt a frame of reference compatible with psychoanalytic beliefs about the etiology of homosexuality influential in the 1960s and perhaps 1970s (Bieber et al. 1962). Parents such as this are often conversant with the scientific literature about homosexuality. They may suggest that prenatal influences caused their child's homosexuality as well. Often parents condense this belief with the idea that they did something wrong to cause the son/daughter's homosexuality—e.g., "We fought during the pregnancy, causing stress which led to her homosexuality." Here homosexuality in the child is perceived as punishment for parental misdeeds. Yet another myth is that the child has voluntarily chosen to be homosexual. Here the child is conceptualized as willful and immoral, desiring revenge against high-minded parents. These are by no means the only myth beliefs parents bring with them when they consult therapists about homosexuality in their children.

Responding to Simple Ignorance with Psychoeducation

The easiest type of situation to deal with therapeutically is that in which parents are more or less psychologically intact, but have anxieties and erroneous beliefs about homosexuality that stem from simple ignorance. The erroneous beliefs may be prejudicial in content, without being motivated by prejudicial feelings against homosexual people. They may simply be believed as factually true—in the same way that many false beliefs are—because they were learned during the parents' formative years from idealized authority figures. It is helpful for clinicians, after establishing rapport, to answer questions about homosexual behavior from parents like this as directly as possible. For example, people are sometimes surprised to learn that the sexual behavior of lesbians is closer to that of heterosexual women than gay men and that lesbians are not at heightened risk of HIV infection. Generally, even well-informed and well-educated lay people are not aware that research on national samples of gay

men representative of the general population reveals that the number of lifetime sexual partners of most is the same as the number of lifetime sexual partners of most heterosexual men. It is true that some gay men have had so many
partners that they are essentially "off the curve" for heterosexual men, but this
applies only to a small minority (Friedman and Downey 1994; Coleman and
Simon-Rosser 1996).

One helpful way of illustrating how the myth of promiscuity in gay men
is prejudicial is to explain the way in which prejudiced ideas are created: a
quality of some members of a group is attributed to all members of that
group. If one doesn't know a particular person in the group who is the target
of prejudice, one nonetheless believes that he or she must possess or behaviorally express that negative attribute. An example of an antisocial, negatively
valued social behavior, for example, is sexual violence. We often point out
that rape of women carried out by heterosexual men does not mean that all
heterosexual men are potential rapists. Recently, heterosexual rape has been
used as an instrument of political coercion, torture, and revenge—in Bosnia,
for example—yet there was no intimation in the press or popular culture of
such sentiments as "Of course, the Yugoslavian women were raped. Heterosexual men are like that. What else could a captive population expect? American heterosexual men are all potential rapists as well. The solution to this terrible social problem is to influence men not to be heterosexual." The reason
the conduct of some gay men is taken to be representative of all but the conduct of some heterosexual rapists is taken to be deviant behavior is that prejudicial feelings against gay men influence beliefs about them.

In challenging parental concerns that gay relationships are inherently
unloving, we point out that durable, successful, loving relationships are difficult to achieve in heterosexual couples as well. Despite many barriers, some
gay and heterosexual couples do establish them, however (McWhirter and
Mattison 1984, 1996; Klinger 1996). Most of our patients, regardless of their
sexual orientations, want to find a loving partner with whom to share their
lives. Gay men and lesbians differ in many of their attitudes about sexuality
and love, however. Gay men tend to be more similar to heterosexual men and
lesbians to heterosexual women than to each other. Although gay couples
achieve loving committed relationships, gay men are less likely to be monogamous than heterosexual men (Klinger 1996). Of course, one reason for this
is that women tend to endorse monogamy more frequently than men do, and
some heterosexual men are probably monogamous out of consideration for
their partners' feelings. Certainly, a robust market for heterosexual prostitu-

tion exists worldwide and is not usually taken as evidence that a heterosexual lifestyle makes true love difficult to attain.

Among parents who erroneously believe that they "caused" homosexuality in their children—and in whom this belief is not adhered to for psychodynamic/pathological reasons—discussions of the origins of sexual orientation can be enlightening. Our experience is that even parents who lack knowledge of biology can become reasonably sophisticated consumers of scientific information in this area. Review of the genetic, neuroendocrine, and historical issues discussed earlier in this book is often quite helpful.

In response to the question "Did my child choose homosexuality?" we feel it helpful to discuss sex differences in sexual orientation. Boys do not choose their sexual fantasies, nor do their sexual feelings and motivations follow upon political beliefs or deep emotional relationships they make during adolescence or adulthood. Homophobic parents are sometimes concerned that their son has been "seduced" into homosexuality. A time of particularly high stress for families occurs when a teenaged child leaves home to go to college or to pursue some other path on his own. Parents who are worried that the increased freedom will lead to homosexuality or who are reacting to the fact that their child has "come out" after leaving home are sometimes astonished to learn that boys, theirs included, usually had sexual desires long before that. In those destined to become gay adults, the object of their sexual desires is often male beginning as early as age eight or nine (Herdt and McClintock 2000).

Girls are much more diverse than boys, but some experience the same type of sexual development as boys do: being sexually attracted to members of the same sex from childhood or adolescence. Other girls, however, experience homosexual desire much later when they are fully grown women. Sometimes women during adolescence or adulthood do seem to *choose* homosexuality, usually for political reasons. Although their initial decisions may be based on political/social values, they are unlikely to persist in homosexual relationships unless their sexual feelings follow suit (see chapter 8, this volume).

The issue of cross-gender behavior in a child is a particularly complex one, since a common prejudicial stereotype is that gay/lesbian people have pathologically disturbed gender/role behavior. The most common way in which this type of homophobic anxiety is expressed, in our experience, is that a parent has identified cross-gender behavior in a child and requests treatment for the child to prevent homosexuality. This is, of course, a "chief complaint" that is more complex than it seems. On the one hand, the parents may have a prejudicial stereotype about gay/lesbian people. On the other hand, however, the cross-gender behavior they have identified may in fact be more common among those on a lesbian/gay developmental track than heterosexuals. Furthermore, while cross-gender behavior in itself is not inherently pathological, some types of cross-gender behavior, particularly toward the extreme part of the spectrum and in younger children, can signal psychological disturbance in itself—apart from a possible relationship to homosexuality (Zucker and Bradley 1995). We suggest that when cross-gender behavior in a child is the parent's chief complaint, the clinician must be especially aware that assessment is the initial task. The therapist must assess not only the child but the meaning of two domains to each parent—cross-gender behavior and homosexuality. Only following careful assessment and establishment of a working alliance with them can psychoeducation be helpful.

Sexual Orientation Conversion

Often clinicians are confronted by caretakers who wish them to convert their child from homosexual to heterosexual. Here the therapist is viewed analogously to a surgeon and the homosexuality of the offspring to a tumor. The parents turn to the therapist for rescue and generally lack insight into the nature of the dilemma they need rescuing from (that is, themselves), instead attributing all their family's problems to the offspring's homosexuality. The *function of the wish* in the family system must be assessed. The clinician should not simply respond to this request as a manifest reality but should ask himself, "What are the psychodynamic reasons that this is expressed as an urgent need?" Often this request hides a difficulty between the caretakers, and attention is diverted from this to a teenager who is scapegoated. For example, it may be easier for the parents to focus on the sexual orientation of a teenager than on communication and sexual difficulties they have with each other.

Some parents who initially request assistance from clinicians in converting their offspring from homosexual to heterosexual may be responsive to psychoeducation. Topics for psychoeducation include all aspects of homosexuality, the causes and treatments of depression, adolescent sexuality, and other areas as well. Most such parents, however, probably need some type of psychotherapeutic intervention. A key area that they may have trouble understanding and accepting concerns the sexual rights of adolescents. It may well be that the parental request for sexual reorientation of their child is the first contact a dysfunctional family system has with mental health professionals.

Many different issues are usually conflated in the request by parents to get the consulting therapist to collaborate with them in encouraging their gay adolescent to change his or her sexual orientation. On the other hand, if people request information about sexual orientation change, we try to answer their questions as directly as possible. The topic of sexual orientation conversion is a controversial and complex one. We discuss it in chapter 15 of this book and defer further elaboration until then.

Coming Out As a Family Issue

The psychological processes involved in coming out as part of gay/lesbian development have been discussed by others (Broido 2000; Reynolds and Hanjorgiris 2000; Cass 1996; Brown 1995; Gonsiorek 1995; Savin-Williams 1996). Many heterosexual parents struggle with the problems involved in the public recognition of their child's homosexuality by others who are not in the family. Not infrequently, parents live in suburban or rural communities with conventional attitudes and values. For them socializing with a child who is openly gay, even one who is fully adult and has long left the family home, involves a "coming out" of the family. Unlike their offspring, however, they may have no desire to "come out" to their neighbors and friends. They feel conflicted between a desire to accept their child and a desire to conform to the conventional, heterosexist values they endorse. These parents may feel that they fully accept their child as long as her homosexuality is kept discretely out of view when visits home occur.

From a clinical perspective familial relationships may be made more problematic by the fact that the offspring may or may not be prone to trying to find some sort of middle ground with her or his troubled parents. Understandably, many lesbian/gay people feel that their sexuality is an authentic part of themselves and that their partners must be respected and accepted, as would be the case if they were of the opposite sex. They consider their parents' shame their parents' problem. Particularly with younger gay/lesbian patients, some might rebelliously flaunt the very types of behavior their parents object to. Parents and children in these situations become involved in power struggles that are common between younger patients and their parents in areas other than sexual orientation. The range of problems and coping strategies is great, and clinicians may find it distressingly difficult to make therapeutic alliances, and keep lines of communication open so that therapeutic work can proceed.

Parents with Psychological Disturbances

Mild Psychopathology

Some parents, while not necessarily suffering from an Axis I or II disorder, nonetheless have unconscious conflicts that are projected and displaced onto their child, the person who is identified as a patient. The son or daughter may symbolically represent a parent's sibling or childhood friend, or the parents may have a rigid and irrational need for a child to live out parental fantasies that are heterosexist or reparative for other reasons. For example, unhappily married parents might unconsciously or even consciously wish their children to achieve happiness in a conventional marriage that they themselves could not. Often, the unconscious fantasies of such parents involve, either in actuality or in fantasy, their relationship to their own parents.

In making an assessment of possible psychodynamic influences on parental attitudes toward their child's sexual orientation, it is necessary to take a sexual history from the parents. In order to carry this out, it is necessary to interview people individually as well as in the presence of their partners. Extremely common is the finding of some "trouble spot" or abnormality in the history of one or both parents and/or in their present sexual relationship. In these instances the lesbian/gay child is scapegoated to divert attention from the sexual and interpersonal difficulties of the parents themselves.

Often a consultation may be helpful to patients, even when from the clinician's perspective it is incomplete, as in the case vignette described here:

A fifty-six-year-old professional woman requested consultation because her twenty-five-year-old daughter had just come out to her. The mother became distraught and queried her gynecologist who referred her for consultation.

Early in the initial meeting it was established that this daughter, an only child and graduate student, not only had not informed her father about her sexual orientation but had sworn her mother to secrecy. The mother had supported this secrecy, both women agreeing that the father would never be able to tolerate this unwelcome news.

229

This woman was seen in two consultation sessions. The father, who remained unaware not only of his daughter's sexual orientation but also of his wife's appointment with a psychiatrist, was never interviewed.

The parents had long been living in a dysfunctional marital relationship. The mother, raised in an observant Roman Catholic family, had become much less religious in her later years. Her husband, also Catholic, was quite observant. Both parents were opposed to divorce, held conservative views about politics and family values, and were involved in "Right to Life" antiabortion activities.

Regarding the sexual adaptation of the couple, all that could be established was that their relationship had been asexual for more than ten years. The mother had not experienced sexual desire or sexual fantasies for many years and indicated that the sexual part of her life was over. Although she did not report missing sexuality (despite having been fully sexually responsive as a younger women), she did admit that she missed romance and often wished that a man would show interest in her. She ruefully described herself as being of an age when a woman becomes "invisible" to men, although she was in fact slender, well-groomed, and attractive.

These facts were established in the initial interview as well as one important additional piece of information, namely, that the mother-daughter relationship in this family had been extremely close until the daughter became a teenager. After that the bond had remained intense but became rebellious. The mother admitted that at that time she had felt as if she had lost her "best friend."

The therapist answered a few questions about homosexuality at the end of this interview and arranged a second meeting. On this occasion she focused on the mother's homophobia. Without even putting a label on her attitude, it was possible to frame discussion of it in such a way as to direct the mother's attention to the psychological functions served by her attitudes in her own adaptation. Obviously, without having a relationship with her in which she was identified as a patient, true interpretative work was not possible. However, it was possible to point out that by investing her daughter's sexual orientation in such a negatively intense manner she had found a focus for complaint outside her own frustrating relationship with her husband.

This woman did not have major overt symptoms of Axis I or II disorders. Even consultation with a mental health professional—something that only "crazy people did"—was not part of her worldview. She elected not to return for more visits. However, she was able to discuss the history of family "secrets," which, in this instance, went back to the previous generation. In addition, she discussed the meaning of the fact that she and her daughter now shared an important secret from which the father in the family had been excluded. She was also able to consider the fact that the daughter in this family had sexual values that were radically different from her parents.

This type of consultation is common and illustrates the complexities of the "naturalistic" clinical situations one encounters in the practice of psychiatry. The "patient," if you will, (the mother) was disabused of erroneous beliefs about homosexuality, and the psychodynamic roots of some of her antihomosexual attitudes were framed. More was left unsaid and undone, of course. The clinical impression was that the consultation would in fact help her establish a better relationship with her daughter. She would be less judgmental and fearful about her daughter's homosexual orientation. However, she was unlikely to alter her marital or sexual-romantic adaptation.

More Severe Psychopathology

We now come to parents who have pronouncedly antihomosexual attitudes that are heavily psychodynamically influenced and in whom one or both has a psychiatric disorder according to *DSM* criteria (American Psychiatric Association 1994).

Interview of both members of the couple together and separately is necessary in order to establish diagnoses and also to acquire appropriate historical information.

Stone, Kernberg, and Friedman have all emphasized the benefit of assessing an individual not only for the presence or absence of Axis I and II disorders but also for a descriptive and psychoanalytic perspective on the type of personality defenses employed and the level of personality integration present (Kernberg 1975; Stone 1980; Friedman 1988). It is really not possible to understand marital interactions between people who have mental disorders without doing this. Even though the person who is identified initially as the subject of the consultant's attention is the couple's child, nonetheless, the parents and their marital interaction usually becomes the primary focus.

Once the diagnostic and dynamic framework is established, a formulation must be made about the function of the child in the family system. This is always done from a historical perspective. Particularly salient is the question "What function did this child serve in the family before the child's sexual orientation was known?"

From the child's perspective, coming out marks a major transitional point in the establishment of her or his identity. From the perspective of the types of parents we are considering here, however, the child's coming out is a threat to the equilibrium of a fragile shared defensive structure. That structure is the fantasized identity/role of the child in the family, which serves reparative functions in one or both parents.

The clinician must ask: Why should these particular parents have needed (a) to have made in the first place this construction involving their child's role in the family? (b) to have extended and elaborated this construction over time? (c) and, finally, to be invested in a new concern—the sexual orientation of their child—at this particular time in each of their individual histories, in the history of their couple relationship, and in the history of the entire family structure of which they and their lesbian/gay child are a part?

This clinical approach most frequently reveals difficulties in multiple areas.

From the diagnostic perspective, regarding the individuals in the family system, each parent often carries one or more psychiatric diagnoses. Commonly enough the mother is depressed, often with recurrent major depressive episodes alternating with dysthymia. She may abuse alcohol or other substances. The father might also have some type of depression and, in addition, an Axis II diagnosis with prominent narcissistic and paranoid features. The maternal pedigree might reveal many women with depression and men with antisocial behavior. The paternal pedigree might reveal the same or perhaps a number of relatives with bipolar disorder. Scattered throughout the family of mother and father may be gay/lesbian people, some of whom have special meaning to the parents and, often, special meaning to the parents of the parents as well.

The sexual histories of each parent may have been problematic throughout their lives. The mother, for example, may have had unwanted pregnancies for which she received medical terminations. Her feelings about these may have remained conflicted. Not rarely, she has been in love with someone before the father. It had gone badly—she had been rejected or perhaps abused in the relationship or relationships. The father may have his version of a similar history of disappointments and failures. Of particular importance is that either or both may have had difficulties with their personal sexual orientation during their lives. Commonly enough, bisexual fantasy has been experienced and unwanted in these homophobic people and has stimulated intense guilt. It is not unusual for homosexual activity to have occurred.

The religious value systems of the parents and their gay/lesbian child may be in conflict as well. The conflict may, in fact, involve specific religious attitudes toward homosexuality.

All of this may be present in addition to the more or less routine but serious life stresses that are so common as to be expected but that may be coped with maladaptively in this family system. Routine life stresses include such events as job loss or change and the death or serious illness of siblings, friends, or parents of the parents, menopause, difficulties with functioning of the reproductive organs such as breast or prostate cancer.

Moreover, there is the specific nature of the parental psychopathology. One or both parents may use extreme rigid denial and projection or be integrated at a low borderline level. The way in which their specific character defenses function is obviously crucial.

This vast canvas has to be at least sketched in before the manifest issues about sexual orientation can be appropriately conceptualized, let alone responded to. It is particularly important to appreciate that simple psychoeducation is likely to fall on deaf ears in cases like these unless the parents' dynamics and psychopathology are appropriately met clinically.

For the sake of simplicity, we have limited the discussion to situations in which the consulting individuals were married and the biological parents of a gay/lesbian person. Obviously, the consultant's clinical terrain may be even more complex than discussed here, since the persons requesting consultation may be divorced, separated, widowed, and may be without a sexual partner (her- or himself) or may be living with someone who is not the parent of the gay/lesbian child.

Whether or not parents realize it prior to the first session, an important underlying reason for consultation with a mental health professional is nearly always to find a way to preserve the bond with their child. Rather quickly in the initial interview, the therapist/consultant must assess the degree of parental psychopathology with a view toward establishing the type of therapeutic alliance that would support some kind of ongoing education/therapeutic work with the parents. If this can be successfully accomplished, the parents gradually become receptive to learning more about the functions served by their beliefs and fears about their child's homosexuality in the family system and for each of them as individuals. Although only a small number of such parents will want ongoing, long-term treatment for themselves, many can be helped to a better understanding of themselves and their adolescent or adult offspring. This offers in turn the chance for development of more accepting and mutually supportive attitudes between the family members. The worst fears of the parents, that the child's homosexuality signifies the loss of the parental-child relationship and the death of the family, can be assuaged.

13

Psychopathology, Suicidality, and Homosexuality: New Developments

In the 1950s Evelyn Hooker, a psychologist, carried out an important psychodynamically informed investigation (Hooker 1957). Hooker reasoned that the large psychoanalytic literature on the etiology of homosexuality might be biased toward global psychopathology and therefore not be valid. Psychoanalytic patients understandably seek assistance because of psychological distress and impairment in functioning. It was therefore risky for psychoanalysts to generalize about all homosexual people from a patient sample. Through word of mouth, Hooker recruited highly functional, socially well-integrated homosexual men. She matched these with a heterosexual control group and administered Rorschach tests to all the subjects. Their written records were blindly rated for psychodynamic features that were thought to be characteristic of homosexual men—after mention of sexual orientation was edited out of the record. The results were astonishing—and contrary to what would be expected if psychoanalytic theories about the etiology of homosexuality were accurate. The judges were unable, on the basis of Rorschach responses, to predict sexual orientation! Hooker's meticulously designed research provided evidence that ultimately supported the decision to delete homosexuality as a psychiatric diagnosis from the *Diagnostic and Statistical Manual* of the American Psychiatric Association (American Psychiatric Association 1980; Bayer 1981).

Following these investigations, descriptive studies failed to find differences of various forms of psychopathology among nonclinical samples of homosexual compared to heterosexual people (Gonsiorek and Weinrich 1991). Reports by psychoanalytic clinicians emphasized similarity in functioning between homosexual and heterosexual individuals (Isay 1989). Studies testing the hypothesis that homosexual people have phobic anxiety about heterosexuality had negative results (Freund et al. 1974). Research on specific disorders such as sexual abuse of children did not reveal an increased frequency of homosexual perpetrators (Groth and Birnbaum 1978). Critical review of the psychoanalytic literature revealed that certain ideas, then popular among psychoanalysts, were not solidly supported. These included the theories that homosexuality was intrinsically related to narcissism and/or masochism and/or paranoia (Freud's discussion of the Schreber case notwithstanding) (Freud 1911; Friedman 1988, 1999).

Recent Population-Based Studies Report Increased Psychopathology Among Gay Men and Lesbians

Although descriptive studies finding similarity in psychopathology between nonclinical homosexual and heterosexual samples had been reported, the number of subjects investigated was small and the studies were not of randomly selected members of the general population (Saghir and Robins 1973; Siegelman 1974). The more recent research we report on below corrected these limitations. Four studies were carried out by epidemiologist/public health investigators, each agreeing with the others. The results of these investigations indicate that gay men and lesbians are indeed more likely to experience certain psychological difficulties than are heterosexuals. We discuss the new extra-analytic research and its relevance for clinical work with gay and lesbian patients. There has also been recent descriptive research on youth suicide, which we consider in the second part of this chapter.

Herrel and colleagues (1999) utilized a twin registry created during the Vietnam era to study the lifetime history of suicidality in relation to homosexuality-heterosexuality in middle-aged men. The comparison groups in this investigation were those who were exclusively heterosexual compared to those who had participated in sexual activity with same-sexed partners during adulthood. The latter group, consisting of 2 percent of a sample numbering several thousand, had been clearly more suicidal during the course of their lives. Most twins were each heterosexual, and, of more than 6,000 individuals, 15.3 percent reported suicidal ideation and 2.2 percent had attempted suicide. In contrast, 16 pairs of twins each reported homosexual activity (32 men). In this group 56.3 percent had experienced suicidal ideation and 18.8 percent had attempted suicide. There were 103 pairs in whom one twin had male sexual partners during his adulthood and the other had been exclusively heterosexual, 25.2 percent of the heterosexuals reported suicidal ideation and 3.9 percent had attempted suicide, 55.3 percent of twins who had sex with male partners reported suicidal ideation and 14.7 percent had attempted suicide.

The increased suicidality of those men who had homosexual experience compared to those who had been exclusively heterosexual is striking. The fact that the control group in this investigation were co-twins was a particularly strong feature of this study. This research did not study men from the perspective of developmental psychodynamics, however. Thus the relationship between the many dimensions of sexual orientation and suicidality were not included in the investigation. The timeline relating the feelings of the subjects about their homosexual orientation, and the intricate psychological processes involved in establishing a homosexual identity, were all omitted from investigation. The research did not investigate homophobia experienced by the patient during his life or internalized homophobia. Nonetheless the finding about suicidality is important from both a research and a clinical frame of reference.

Cochran and Mays reported on lifetime prevalence of suicide symptoms and affective disorders among 3,648 randomly selected men, representative of the general population, between seventeen and thirty-nine years of age (Cochran and Mays 2000a). Fourteen of these had only male sexual partners during their lifetime, 94 had male and female partners, and the rest of the group was exclusively heterosexual in activity. Of those who had same-sexed partners 19.3 percent had attempted suicide during their lives compared to 3.6 percent of the heterosexuals. Suicidal thoughts and wishes were also elevated among those with male sexual partners. Although differences in prevalence of depression did not attain statistical significance, there was a trend for those with male sexual partners to have increased prevalence of recurrent depression during their lives.

The same investigators carried out a separate study, using a different data base, of randomly selected men and women representative of the general population (Cochran and Mays 2000b). Out of 9,908 subjects participating, all reported at least one sexual partner during the preceding year (2,479 subjects who were contacted had no sexual partners during the preceding year and were not part of this study), 1.6 percent of the sexually active sample reported same-gender sexual partners, 57 percent of this group was male, and one-third had engaged in sexual activity with partners of both sexes.

Men with same-sexed partners were at greater risk for the diagnosis of major depression and panic attacks than those with exclusively opposite-sexed partners. Women with same-sexed partners were at greater risk for the diagnoses of drug and alcohol dependency than women with exclusively opposite sexed partners. Both men and women with same-sexed partners used mental health services more frequently than those who were exclusively heterosexual (Cochran and Mays 2000b).

The findings in the above studies were compatible with results obtained from a population-based study carried out in the Netherlands. Sandfort and colleagues (1999) examined differences between exclusively heterosexual and nonheterosexual subjects in lifetime and twelve-month prevalence rates of mood, anxiety, and substance use disorders in a representative sample of the Dutch population aged eighteen to sixty-four. The population studied consisted of 5,998 people who had been sexually active during the preceding year: 2.8 percent of 2,878 men and 1.4 percent of 3,120 women had same-sex partners. Of the men, 82 had sex only with males, and 6 with men and women. Of the women, 43 had sex only with women, and 6 with men and women. Both homosexual men and women were found to have at least one *DSM-III-R* psychiatric diagnosis more frequently than heterosexuals (American Psychiatric Association 1987). Homosexual men had increased present and lifetime rates of major depression and anxiety disorders. Lifetime prevalence of alcohol abuse was higher in heterosexual than homosexual men. During the past year homosexual women had higher prevalence of alcohol and drug dependence than heterosexual women. They also had higher lifetime prevalence of major depression and alcohol and drug dependence.

Neither Cochran and Mays (2000a, b) nor Sandfort et al. (1999) carried out research that was psychodynamically informed. Neither group studied homophobia, internalized homophobia, coming out, or many other developmentally meaningful events. These limitations notwithstanding, although the methods were slightly different, their findings are compatible with each other. These studies came from the public health/epidemiology sector and utilized definitions of assignment into "homosexual" or "heterosexual" groups on the basis of sexual activity only. People who had sex with males and females were grouped with exclusively homosexual individuals for the purpose of data analysis.

Psychoanalysis, Homosexuality, and Psychopathology

Despite their limitations, taken together these investigations indicate that certain types of psychopathology are in fact increased among people whose sexual partners are not exclusively of the opposite sex. This should not be taken to mean that homosexuality is intrinsically pathological, however. It is important to emphasize this because some psychoanalysts (a minority) in North America—and many more in other parts of the world—still adhere to the view that homosexuality itself is inherently pathological. In the epidemiological/public health studies discussed above, most people who had sex with same-sexed partners did not manifest symptoms of psychiatric disorder, including suicidal or depressive symptoms (Cochran and Mays 2000a, b). Not only are many gay/lesbian people unusually creative and productive, as Freud pointed out in his letter to the mother of a homosexual (1935; reproduced in chapter 16), there have never been any studies suggesting that sexual orientation influences the capacity of people to function at the highest psychological levels according to any standard chosen.

Lesbian Mothers

An additional domain of information is available about the functioning of homosexual women—their effectiveness as parents. Millions of lesbian women are mothers, and there has been progressive interest in their parenting capacities from the judicial system, child welfare institutions, and mental health systems. If the prevalent older psychoanalytic theories were valid, it stands to reason that lesbians would be inadequate mothers.

Studies of diverse design have compared the psychological adjustment of lesbian mothers to heterosexual mothers and found no differences. Nor have lesbian mothers been shown to adhere to sex-role stereotypes in any unusual fashion. For example, they do not tend to encourage girls to be "masculine" (in keeping with stereotypic paradigms of masculinity) or boys to be "feminine." Independent investigators have compared divorced heterosexual and lesbian mothers' attitudes and behavior toward contact with the father of their children and found no differences. Research on gender identity development, sexual orientation, and psychological adjustment of children of lesbian mothers compared to heterosexual mothers has revealed no differences (Patterson 1995, 1996).

Although the studies reviewed above are nonpsychoanalytic (i.e., not of psychoanalytic patients), some were carried out by psychoanalytically informed investigators (Kirkpatrick 1987). The number of studies of lesbian parenting and their diversity of design suggest that the assumptions of the classical psychoanalytic literature about the inherent association between lesbianism and psychopathology are invalid.

The Influence of Homophobia

Although there have been no direct studies to date indicating that increased prevalence of psychological disturbances among nonheterosexuals is due to homophobia, this is certainly a credible hypothesis. Whereas progress has been made toward tolerance and acceptance of people of all sexual orientations, much homophobia persists not only in the general society but even among mental health professionals (GAP 2000).

The influence of homophobia would certainly explain why psychological symptoms are more common among lesbian/gay people than heterosexuals (Meyer 1995). Their specific symptom profile, however, raises additional intriguing questions. It is notable that gay men have a tendency to develop increased depression and anxiety symptoms—symptoms usually more common among women, and lesbians who also manifest increased lifetime depression in some reports also have a tendency to develop increased substance abuse—symptoms usually more common among men. This raises the question whether common factors influence both childhood gender atypicality in lesbian/gay people and a tendency for those predisposed toward psychological disturbances to manifest these in a "gender-atypical way" as well (Bailey 1999).

Additional Clinical Issues in Adults

The fact that gay/lesbian/bisexual people may be more predisposed to certain types of symptoms/disorders than heterosexuals is an important one for therapists to be aware of. It is helpful to know—from a purely descriptive perspective—that lesbians might be more prone to alcohol and drug abuse than heterosexual women. Similarly, therapists might ask a gay depressed man about suicidal thoughts with particular thoroughness.

In clinical situations therapists are faced with the complex task of trying to determine to what degree the person's problems are a function of a specific psychiatric disorder, such as major depression, for example, and to what degree they are a function of his/her unique attributes of self, including the way he/she experiences being gay or lesbian. Both dimensions of functioning are important, and therapists must approach the diagnostic/assessment initial interviews with both frameworks in mind. For example, a middle-aged gay man might seek help because of feelings of ugliness. Living alone and without a sexual partner, he doubts that he can attract one. Both his social/sexual isolation and his impaired self-regard might be consequences of depression. On the other hand, his depression may be a reaction to his existential circumstances. Usually both are true. People become depressed because they are isolated, and they become more isolated because they are depressed. The therapist who works with such a patient must be conversant with the aspects of his difficulties that are clearly related to *psychopathology* in the sense conceptualized by the descriptive psychiatrists who constructed the recent versions of the *DSM*. The assessment of his present problem must include his specific symptoms of depression, particularly those such as hopelessness that are associated with suicidality, and other symptoms that may be associated with his depression, such as alcohol or substance abuse, for example, or symptoms of personality disorder(s), duration of the present problem, and impact on his adaptation. Particularly in light of research indicating that socially isolated males are at risk for suicide, and that this might be even more true of gay males, the patient's degree of social interaction would be carefully assessed. The descriptive part of the assessment should also include a family history, with particular care paid to mood disorders, suicidal behaviors, alcohol and substance abuse, and a history of developmental trauma.

A different but overlapping behavioral dimension has to do with the patient being a middle-aged gay man. The therapist must be familiar with pathways of gay male development. Among many factors to be considered are the history of self-awareness of being gay and the complex processes of coming out. To what degree are conflicts about coming out, for example, still present, or reactivated as a function of the man's depression? As is true of all patients, it is necessary to ascertain this man's sexual history. We have earlier discussed the way in which male self-esteem is integrally related to sexual functioning and to feelings of attractiveness. Here the therapist must be aware not only of male sexual behavior but specifically of patterns of sexual behavior common among gay males. What types of sexual relationships has this man participated in during his life? How recently? Does he masturbate? What are his fantasies? With regard to his future sexual behavior, what does he hope for? How sexually attractive does he feel?

Another area concerns exposure to sexually transmitted diseases, particularly HIV. Virtually every gay man knows people who have died of HIV-related illnesses, and most have lost loved ones. To what degree has this man participated in risky sexual behavior? What is his HIV status? (Friedman and Downey 1994; Hayes et al. 1997).

Yet another area concerns the history of his exposure to overt heterosexism and homophobia. Here the issue of revelation of the therapist's sexual orientation is a topic to be considered. Many gay/lesbian patients have been traumatized by heterosexual people during their lives, and some have had either traumatic or unsuccessful experiences with heterosexual therapists who were uninformed about homosexual behavior. This being the case, many understandably seek to learn the sexual orientation of the therapist in the initial sessions. Although a classical psychoanalytic position about this would be not to reveal the therapist's sexual orientation, we do believe that revelation is often indicated in light of the enormous social turbulence still current around homosexuality. Our clinical experience has been that such revelation does, of course, influence the initial transference—just as knowledge of a therapist's gender does. As psychoanalysis or uncovering therapy progresses, however, unconscious issues shape the clinical process to a greater and greater extent, and the initial revelation becomes much less salient.

The same guidelines about descriptive psychopathology and homophobia apply to lesbians as well as gay men. Certain existential aspects of life are similar between gay men and lesbians as well. Both, if without partners, tend to yearn for loving, romantic/sexual connections as heterosexuals do. Both have to cope with living and working in a largely heterosexual and heterosexist world. In addition, however, the clinician must be aware of how the patient/client feels about herself as a woman and what her sexual orientation means to her. If she is in a committed relationship, does she feel sexually alive, or has the relationship succumbed to the loss of sexual vitality that seems to occur more in lesbian than gay male partnerships (Herbert 1996)? Does she feel that she and her partner are able to be mutually supportive yet each retain her sense of individuality? Is there a way in which she feels overwhelmed and lost in a type of intimacy that has fewer boundaries than she would like? Is she lonely in the company of her partner? What is the woman's life history of sexual partnerships? Has she always been lesbian or has she come to that realization later in life? Is she a mother? If so, how are her concerns about parenting influenced by her lesbianism? If not, does she wish to be? How does her partner feel about this? Does the couple plan to adopt a child, or conceive a child with or without the new reproductive technologies?

These issues may be an integral part of a given person's successful coping strategy or may be the source of conflicts and symptom formation. When the latter occurs, the research studies reviewed above suggest the need for clinicians to be especially sensitive to the possibility of mood disorders, substance abuse, and alcohol being present even if not necessarily part of the chief complaint.

Youth Suicide

Another area in which descriptive research has been carried out is that of suicidal behavior in gay/lesbian and bisexual adolescents and young adults. Youth suicide is a major public health problem, and it is helpful to identify high-risk groups so that appropriate therapeutic interventions can be offered them. Clinical guidelines for treating suicidal young people are somewhat different than for adults. In this section of the chapter we first discuss the recent research on attempted and completed suicide and then clinical issues.

Emerging recent data suggested that attempted suicide, and the psychiatric difficulties associated with it, is a problem deserving of particular attention in gay and bisexual adolescents and young adults.

For example, a twenty-one-year longitudinal study of 1,265 children was recently carried out in New Zealand (Fergusson, Horwood, Beautrais 1999). Subjects were asked about their sexual orientation (heterosexual, gay or lesbian, bisexual) and their sexual relationships since age sixteen. Nine men and eleven women identified themselves as gay/lesbian/bisexual. These individuals were at increased risk for major depression, generalized anxiety disorder, conduct disorder, nicotine dependence, substance/abuse/dependence, suicidal ideation and suicide attempts. Compared to 28.0 percent of the heterosexual youth, 67.9 percent had experienced suicidal ideation, and 32.1 percent had attempted suicide compared to 7.1 percent of the heterosexuals.

The number of gay/lesbian/bisexual subjects in the study cited above was small, but the outcome was compatible with larger population-based studies carried out in the United States. A sample, randomly selected in 1987, of 36,254 seventh to twelfth grade students in Minnesota provided data for a large study of adolescent health. Students who described themselves as homosexual (81 males and 38 females) and bisexual (131 males and 144 female subjects) were compared with regard to suicidal ideation and attempts to heterosexual groups (Remafedi et al. 1998). Among women there were no statistically significant differences in suicidal behavior. Suicidal ideation was more frequent among the homosexual/bisexual males than the heterosexual males, however. Of the homosexual/bisexual youth, 28.1 percent had attempted suicide compared to 4.2 percent of the heterosexual youth.

Faulkner and Cranston (1998) obtained data from a random sample of high school students in Massachusetts in 1993. In this study participants were classified according to whether they had sexual experience confined to the opposite sex (1,563 subjects), the same sex, or both. Because of the small sample size, data for individuals who engaged in exclusively homosexual behavior and those who were bisexual were pooled for analysis, as were data for males and females (105 subjects). Equal numbers of males and females reported at least some same-sex experience. The homosexual/bisexual students reported suicidal ideation more frequently than the heterosexual students. Twelve percent had attempted suicide in comparison to 2.3 percent of heterosexuals; 7.3 percent had attempted suicide four or more times in comparison to 1 percent of heterosexuals; 7.7 percent of those reporting sexual experience with the same gender had made a suicidal attempt requiring medical attention in the twelve months prior to data collection in comparison to 1.3 percent of the heterosexual youth. The homosexual/bisexual youth were also more likely to have experienced alcohol and drug dependence or abuse, to have been threatened or victimized at school, and to have avoided going to school because they felt unsafe.

Garofalo and colleagues (1999) reported on data collected from a representative population-based sample of Massachusetts high school students in 1995. Responding to both a sexual orientation and a suicide attempt question were 3,365 students. Students were assigned to a category on the basis of self-identification—gay, lesbian, bisexual, or not sure of their sexual orientation. The males were 6.5 times more likely to report a suicide attempt than the heterosexual males, and the females twice as likely compared to their heterosexual female peers. Statistical analysis revealed that among the females other variables may have influenced the outcome, so that sexual orientation was an indirect influence. Homosexual or bisexual orientation was clearly predictive of reported suicide attempts for the males, however. In another report Garofalo and colleagues (1998) noted that gay/lesbian/bisexual youth from the same data base were more likely than heterosexuals to engage in multiple drug abuse, high-risk sexual behavior, and other high-risk behaviors.

These investigations were compatible with many other studies of gay/lesbian youth in which samples were not randomly selected but recruited in other ways. When compared with heterosexual youth, frequency of attempted suicide was consistently elevated (Muehrer 1995; Remafedi 1999). Other studies of adults indicate that if suicidal history was positive, attempts were most likely to have been carried out during adolescence (Bell, Weinberg, and Hammersmith 1981; Saghir and Robbins 1973). Some research has indicated that attempted suicide was not only more frequent but also of greater potential lethality—a variable associated with completed suicide (Remafedi et al. 1991).

A different type of study, of completed suicides in the New York City area, was carried out by Shaffer et al. (1995). Earlier, an uncontrolled study carried out in San Diego County in the 1980s had revealed that 10 percent of suicides occurred in gay men and none in lesbians (Rich et al. 1986). Data were collected about 120 of 170 suicides occurring in individuals under age twenty. These subjects were matched to controls by age, sex, and ethnicity. Trained interviewers obtained information from people in the deceased individuals' social network about whether the person had had homosexual experiences or had declared that he had a homosexual orientation. Three males who had successfully committed suicide fit these criteria. All had been suffering from severe depression, and two had chronic substance abuse as well. The difference in prevalence of homosexual orientation between suicides and controls was not significant. The investigators concluded that their study had failed to uncover a relationship between death by suicide and homosexual orientation.

Nonetheless, this research raised questions about such an association. For example, five of the control subjects revealed that they had been teased for being gay/effeminate in school; in no instance, however, did their parents report any abnormal gender role behavior to have been present! This illustrates that next of kin, interviewed about details of an adolescent's personal life, may not be well informed. Moreover, common sense suggests that if shame and guilt about unacceptable homosexual wishes influenced a young person to commit suicide, he would be likely to remained in the closet until his death. In this instance, the negative findings of the postmortem study must be assessed along with the accumulating positive findings about suicide attempts and psychopathology. In general, female adolescents and young adults are more likely to attempt suicide than males, but males are more likely to die as a result of suicide. We believe that enough research has been done to warrant the conclusion that homosexual/bisexual *male* youth are at increased risk for attempted suicide, and possibly completed suicide, than comparable heterosexual youth.

Male Peer Brutality: A Particular Problem for Gay Youth

A theme that we have stressed throughout this book is that males are much less tolerant of atypical gender-role behavior than females, and that this intolerance appears to be even stronger among teenagers and young adults than those who are older. Life can be a misery for boys, from juvenile age on, who are tormented by their peers because of feminine interests and/or behavior. A reason for this abuse, and one not usually discussed by dynamically oriented psychotherapists, is that some boys are innately brutal and sadistic.

Although gender role abuse during childhood has not yet attracted widespread attention from mental health professionals, bullying has (Nansel et al. 2001). Aggressive abuse of children by other children has been identified as a major problem during middle anad late childhood and adolescence (Haynie et al. 2001; Hanish and Guerra 2000; Gibbs and Sinclair 2000; Mynard et al. 2000; Glover et al. 2000; Carney 2000; Berthhold and Hoover 2000). Bullying is widespread, and has been reported in many different countries including the Netherlands (Limper 2000), Spain (Ortega and Lera 2000), Ireland (Omoor 2000), England (Cowie 2000), Finland (Olafsen and Viemeroe 2000), Greece (Andreou 2000), Italy (Smorti and Ciucci 2000; Baldry and Farrington 1999), Australia (Peterson and Rigby 1999), Malta (Borg 1999). In keeping with what common sense suggests, the cost paid in suffering of victims is often high, and the deleterious effects persistent (Gibbs and Sinclair 2000; Salmon et al. 2000; Mynard and Alexander 2000).

Boys who torment those with atypical gender-role behavior have not, to the best of our knowledge, been studied by behavioral scientists. Generally the abuse is not severe enough for the perpetrators to enter the criminal justice system, nor do they tend to be in the mental health delivery service system. We suspect that when they are studied, many will have come from dysfunctional families and/or have themselves experienced abuse. We believe that boys such as these are in the minority, but they may exert leadership roles in peer groups. In that regard, a recent study of bullying on the school playground was instructive. The subjects were 120 first through sixth graders who were videotaped at play. When bullying occurred, an average of 4 peers passively watched it happen. Many boys were found to model the behavior of bullies and/or join with them in abusing victims (O'Connell, Pepler, and Craig 1999). Therapists of victims often have to work on environmental change, providing sanctuary for their patients by helping them find protected settings. We believe that experiencing brutality from male peers is a crucial reason that attempted suicide is so prevalent among gay male youth. Other stresses influencing suicidal behavior have been identified as well, as might be expected, including early awareness of homosexuality, dropping out of school, suicide attempts by friends and relatives, and lack of social support (Remafedi 1999; Rotheram-Borus and Hunter 1994).

Clinical Issues

The more suicidal the patient, the more likely hospitalization will be necessary to avert the risk of suicide. We do not discuss the indications for hospitalization or hospital treatment in this chapter. Our emphasis is not on suicidal emergencies but rather underlying psychodynamic-psychopathological clinical issues that are helpful in understanding suicidal gay, lesbian, and bisexual young people.

As with adults, psychopathology must be diagnosed according to the descriptive criteria of the *Diagnostic and Statistical Manual* of the American Psychiatric Association (*DSM*). Particular attention should be devoted to the likelihood that multiple diagnoses are present. Patients are likely to suffer from some type of mood disorder and personality disorder. Substance and alcohol abuse may be present as well (Lock and Steiner 1999).

Certain topics should be the topic of particularly careful clinical inquiry. Risky sexual behavior must be assessed, and HIV status determined. During adulthood HIV risk is increased among gay men and not lesbians. Gay male adolescents with serious psychopathology are, of course, also at risk for HIV. Homosexually active adolescent women may well have had male sex partners with whom they have engaged in unsafe sexual activity.

Atypical gender role behavior is more likely in young men than young women to be associated with suicidality (Harry 1983). This does not mean that individual women are immune from gender role abuse, however. The combination of severe psychopathology in the patient and deviance from conventional gender role behavior may well lead a young woman to be the target of abuse similar to that so commonly experienced by young men.

For both sexes the therapist needs to create a psychodynamic developmental timeline. The history of psychopathology must be temporally correlated with the patient's history of gender role and sexual experience and activity. For example, consider a suicidal-depressed gay fifteen-year-old patient. The clinician should carry out a detailed assessment of suicidal intent and immediate suicide risk. In addition, the following areas should be explored:

THE PAST HISTORY AND TYPE OF DEPRESSION. Is the depression unipolar, bipolar, or mixed? Is the patient chronically depressed, with major depressive episodes (MDE) superimposed on chronic underlying depression? When was the earliest severe depression? How does the history of depression relate to the history of suicidal fantasies and past acts (if present)?

THE HISTORY OF HOMOSEXUAL FANTASIES. How old was the patient when he/she first realized he/she was sexually and romantically attracted to the same sex? How did he/she feel about these sexual desires? What is the temporal relationship between his/her depression and the recognition of sexual desire? Did the person become depressed (or more depressed) because of homosexual urges? Is masturbation associated with guilt and shame?

THE HISTORY OF SEXUAL ACTIVITY. Has the patient been sexually active? If so, is the suicidal crisis related to difficulties in a sexual/romantic relationship?

PAST HISTORY OF GENDER NONCONFORMITY. To what degree has the patient experienced gender role nonconformity? Has this been associated with difficulties with peers or parents? What are the patient's peer relationships like? Is the suicidal depression a reaction to having been the victim of gender role abuse?

GAY IDENTITY AND COMING OUT. The psychological processes involved in establishing a gay identity have been extensively described, as have those associated with coming out (Cass 1996). Where is the patient in regard to these processes? Is identity confusion/diffusion present? Is this associated with confusion about the establishment of gay identity?

HOMOPHOBIA AND INTERNALIZED HOMOPHOBIA. Is the suicidal depression a reaction to having been the victim of overt homophobia? Does the patient berate herself or himself for homosexual desires?

The Family System

In addition to understanding the timeline of the patient's difficulties, it is also necessary to understand the environment in which she or he has been raised. Certain types of deleterious effects on development may be likened to nuclear explosions and derail all children, no matter what their personality or sexual orientation profiles are. Severe abuse, neglect, and violent trauma, such as occurs in war or devastating poverty, would be examples of this. In such circumstances, attachment bonds may be torn apart and physical security may be threatened.

These situations are unfortunately common. Often, however, the difficulties that patients experience, although painful, are not as extreme as these. The problems of most gay/lesbian and bisexual suicidal young people emerge in some type of family setting. As we have discussed in the last chapter, the vast majority of gay/lesbian adolescents have heterosexual parents, and many of these have negative attitudes about homosexuality. This is one reason there is frequently a delay of years between the time someone realizes that he/she is gay and tells others about it, e.g., "comes out" (Herdt 1989; Stein 1993; American Academy of Pediatrics Committee on Adolescence 1993). During these years, teenagers are apt to live with what they feel is a dreadful secret and harbor the conviction that they would be rejected by their families if this emerged.

The younger the patient, the more necessary it is to assess the parents independently. Such assessment is often best carried out by another therapist-colleague, but there are many situations in which this is simply not practical, and the primary therapist of the young person must assess the family environment as well. In carrying out such assessment, the therapist should not simply accept his patient's view of what the caretakers are actually like. Simply because a teenager is lesbian/gay doesn't mean that she/he is less likely to project and distort than other young people. Therapists are sometimes surprised to learn that parents who have difficulty accepting their child's sexual orientation may not be as homophobic as expected.

A pedigree of the family must be made that goes beyond attitudes about sexual orientation and gender. The presence of heritable psychiatric disorders must be determined, and a timeline for major familial traumata constructed. For example, in families of divorce, when partners left and new partners came into the family setting, and what all participants were like, is crucial to determine. It is important to ascertain not only their attitudes about homosexuality but about many other things as well. How did they feel and act with regard to male-female role behavior? How related, caretaking, and involved were they? Did they have psychiatric difficulties such as depression or substance abuse? Were they abusive or neglectful toward the other caretaker?

In assessing suicidal gay youth, the clinician should have a paradigm of development that includes the concept of *cumulative stress*. Thus the parent(s) and patient may attribute the patient's difficulties entirely to conflicts about homosexual orientation. In fact, the effects of prolonged intrafamilial stress, loss, and other early trauma may have produced depression, anxiety, and other symptoms throughout the patient's childhood. Conflicts both conscious and unconscious about many painful developmental nodal points may be "packaged," as it were, in the manifest "problem" experienced by the patient ("I am gay") or by the parent(s) ("My son/daughter is gay"). Exploration of the patient's presented complaint usually reveals conflicted unconscious internalizations with significant others occurring at different phases of childhood, contributing to a final common pathway leading to his/her present difficulties.

Need for Future Research

In this chapter we have emphasized how important it is for psychodynamically informed clinicians to be aware of descriptive and epidemiological/public health studies of psychopathology in gay/lesbian and bisexual people. It is also important to be cognizant of the unique areas of knowledge that clinicians can contribute to further knowledge in this area. For example, there are no studies that have documented the specific ways in which an interpersonal environment of suicidal young people is homophobic, how the homophobia was expressed and by whom, and its impact upon suicidality. Studies comparing homophobia in parents between gay/lesbian suicide attemptors and nonattemptors have not yet been undertaken. Pedigree studies comparing familial history of depression and suicidality between gay suicide and nonsuicide attempts have yet to be done. There are presently no data indicating that fathers of suicidal gay youth are more unaccepting or uninvolved with them than are fathers of suicidal heterosexual youth.

There is also need for detailed, psychoanalytically informed discussion of the relationship between self-esteem, suicidality, internalizations, and the psychotherapeutic process in gay/lesbian people. Are there particular patterns during the kind of regressions that occur in psychotherapy when gay/lesbian youth are particularly prone to suicidal activities? What can be said about the influence of the transference on such behavior(s)?

The problem of youth suicide is one of unusual urgency and widespread public health importance. In this area the type of knowledge available to psychodynamically oriented therapists of the intimate lives of their patients seems uniquely important. Common sense indicates that shame, guilt, and conflict foster suicidality. Successful interventions depend on knowledge of the specific details. Throughout the world there is all too frequently a split between psychoanalysts and psychodynamically oriented clinicians, on the one hand, and nonpsychoanalytically oriented behavioral scientists, on the other. It is particularly important that, in the future, interdisciplinary teams include psychoanalytically informed clinicians working to shed light on this area.

14

Coming Out at Eighty-Four:
The Psychotherapeutic Treatment of
Internalized Homophobia in a Lesbian Patient

Since the depathologization of homosexuality, substantial attention has been devoted to the psychological functioning of gay and lesbian people throughout the life cycle, including development during old age (Cabaj and Stein 1996). Older gay men have been discussed in the literature, somewhat more than lesbians, and the psychodynamically informed literature on older lesbians remains sparse (Berger and Kelly 1996; Raphael and Robinson 1980). One dimension of healthy development in gay and lesbian people involves the complex psychological processes that together have been termed coming out (Troiden 1979; Coleman 1982; Cass 1989, 1996). Investigators tend to agree on the broad psychological patterns but differ somewhat on the particular stages involved. Mattison and McWhirter have recently described five steps of coming out: self-recognition as gay, disclosure to others, socialization with other gay people, positive self-identification, and integration and acceptance in the larger community (Mattison and McWhirter 1995).

In this chapter we discuss the beneficent effects of coming out in an older lesbian patient who sought psychotherapy for depression, but not for any conflicts that she identified as being related to her homosexual orientation. In the narrative presentation of the treatment by JID, we focus on psychotherapeutic techniques that assisted the patient in achieving her therapeutic aims.

The patient, JE, a seventy-six-year-old Protestant, white retired literature professor, began treatment a year and a half after her female lover of fifty years had died. Although she thought that her suffering was simply due to the loss of a loved one, her problems were actually exacerbated by the social isolation she experienced as a women with a lifelong, secret homosexual orientation.

None of her social circle was gay or lesbian, and none knew about her sexual orientation. Deeply honest and idealistic, JE experienced chronic shame and guilt as a result of having to cloak her lesbian self in a heterosexual disguise. Her sense of painful detachment was amplified after the death of her beloved partner. In sharing their separateness from the outside heterosexual world, the two had provided consensual validation and ongoing support to each other.

At first meeting, JE was a well-groomed, slender, white-haired woman whose face resembled a mask of grief. Her symptoms were those of a major depressive episode without suicidal ideation or psychotic symptoms. Complaining of the loss of meaning and purpose in her life, she was preoccupied with guilty ruminations about her dead lover—how she should have been nicer to her during their lengthy relationship and the many times (in her own mind) that she had failed her. JE was anhedonic, and the immediate precipitant of the consultation session was that her suffering had become so severe she was unable to function at the full-time volunteer activities she had pursued since retiring from academia.

It is not possible to describe a fifty-year-long love relationship adequately in a clinical paper or even to communicate a sense of what it was really like. Respecting this limitation, we emphasize certain aspects of the partnership in keeping with the main themes of this report—the effect of internalized homophobia on JE's capacity to participate in a loving sexual relationship, its influence on her depression after the loss of her lover, and its subsequent psychotherapeutic treatment.

JE had met M at a summer school for teachers in the 1930s, and mutual feelings of admiration, romantic attraction, and passionate desire soon emerged. At that time JE was in her late twenties and had never experienced interpersonal sexual activity with anyone. All of her early attractions and crushes had been on girls her age or on slightly older women such as teachers. Her romantic/sexual desires were at odds with her attitudes and beliefs about homosexuality. In many ways she was a conventional person—albeit an intellectual—and endorsed many traditional values. She longed to be accepted by "normal" (that is, heterosexual) society and felt pained by the split between public and private personae necessitated by her sexual orientation.

M came from a staid but sophisticated upper-middle-class family, had exquisite manners, and had received education at the best private schools. She was devoutly Christian and particularly knowledgeable about the Bible. By comparison JE felt herself crude, untutored, with rougher manners, a public school education, and a much less sanguine religious faith. A quality that JE loved about M was her self-possession and confidence. M felt JE was too self-effacing and unassertive. She was much less homophobic than JE and believed that a loving relationship between two women could include sexual expression; God would not disapprove of such a union. With M's encouragement and support the painfully guilt-ridden JE yielded to her desires, and they developed a sexual relationship.

During their first fifteen years together, JE and M each lived with her mother and traveled in Europe on summer vacations. On their trips they shared a bedroom and a bed. They presented their relationship to their mothers as a close friendship. JE was not aware of feeling guilty about misleading her mother, who she was sure would not approve of her relationship with M. JE's father had abandoned the family when she was an infant. Throughout her childhood her mother had emphasized that men were not to be trusted and that male-female sexual relationships were dangerous and should be avoided. Although her mother was antisexual, she did not verbally condemn homosexuality. During the years of JE's childhood, the topic of homosexuality was simply not discussed in most families, including her own. Later, as an adult, JE had no doubt that her mother's attitude about homosexuality was strongly negative.

The relationship between JE and M was characterized by deep happiness over shared values, intellectual and career pursuits, travel, friendships, and life goals. Although JE was romantically and sexually attracted to M, she was also ashamed and guilty about having sexual desires. She was able, however, to participate in sexual activity without dysfunction.

After about ten years of being involved with M but totally closeted, JE experienced an identity crisis about whether she was truly homosexual. L, a male friend of many years, made a romantic overture and proposed marriage to her. No passionate or sexual relationship developed, but JE felt that fate had provided a chance to adopt a conventional heterosexual lifestyle—given her age, another might not be forthcoming. Although she was in her late thirties, she was not aware of desires for motherhood, nor were such uncovered during subsequent psychotherapy. In an agony of guilt, JE told M of her decision to marry L. The relationship between the two women continued, however; M was reproachful but restrained and not rejecting. Both JE and L were conflicted about the marriage, and, after a brief interval, it was he who finally broke the relationship off. At this point JE became depressed, full of self-rebuke for her willingness, even temporary, to leave M in the hopes of a heterosexual future. JE's depression became so painful that she sought psychotherapy. Her female therapist supported her homosexual identity. Thus this therapy was directed at neutralizing JE's irrational self-hatred and giving her the sense that her life was enhanced, not hurt, by the relationship with M. After about a year JE's depression had resolved and the psychotherapy was terminated by mutual decision.

While her mother was alive, JE maintained a consciously ambivalent tie to her. The women were extremely close, and JE's mother confided in her about everything. JE was by far the more competent person and from adolescence was the caretaker and emotional provider in the relationship. During adulthood she was the financial provider as well. JE introduced her mother to all of her friends, including M (of whom she approved). Her mother seemed to accept the summers that JE spent with M without resentment, but was greatly appreciative when JE returned home.

At the time of her mother's death, JE did not experience a clinical depression but rather a sense of relief. M's mother had died at about the same time, and JE and M were now able to live together.

JE's mother's death seemed, however, to influence her sexual relationship with M. The nonsexual aspects of the relationship flourished and each partner thrived on the intimacy, friendship, and mutual support. However, JE became even more preoccupied with guilt about sexual expression and found it necessary to avoid M's sexual overtures. Without much discussion, M seemed to accommodate to this. JE remembers this lengthy period (fifteen years) after they first moved in together, when the couple was rarely sexual together but shared deep feelings of intimacy and friendship, as the happiest time she experienced in the relationship.

It was after this period of abstinence that JE experienced a crush on a younger woman. This time she did not share her feelings with M. The feelings passed, but JE was so preoccupied with guilt for having mentally "left M" (although no physical infidelity had occurred) that she resumed sexual activity with her as a way of repairing the bridge. With this return to some sexual activity, for reasons she was unaware of, JE began to experience guilty ruminations about her mother. Despite the fact that her mother was deceased, JE thought of many ways in which she had not been a good enough daughter. These ruminations were not about her sexual behavior, however. Simultaneously, she became aware of a sense of emotional distance between M and herself. Although this occurred coincident with the return to sexual intimacies between the women, JE did not consciously connect the two, nor was she able to verbalize her sense that something had changed.

Despite these vicissitudes, the two women continued devoted partners until, in their seventies, M began to experience a deterioration in her physical health. JE took over more and more executive tasks as M's eyesight diminished and she developed circulatory problems. M was seventy-five years old when she died of a stroke in the hospital. JE had left her side only a few hours earlier to go home and rest.

During the first year after M's death, JE focused on the tasks that needed completion—first the funeral, then sorting M's belongings and giving them to members of her family. As she sorted books and papers, she came across notes to her, written by M, to be read after M's death. For example, JE would reread poetry she and M had enjoyed together and find a note in the margin indicating that M had suspected that JE might read this after she had died and that JE should notice a particular passage or that now M felt different about something they had previously discussed. These notes provoked feelings of pain but also facilitated the mourning process and were experienced as simultaneously comforting.

JE became more aware of the full extent of her loss after about a year. Her grief worsened, and she developed symptoms of a major depressive episode. She became preoccupied with her lack of religious faith and worried that if she did not become as religious as M had been, they would not be able to be reunited in the hereafter. Fantasies of having a heterosexual relationship returned and increased her feelings of guilt toward M. She also felt despair that, because she was now so old, another relationship—hetero- or homosexual—seemed impossible. It was at this point—seeing no reason to go on living (though not suicidal), anhedonic, and with many somatic symptoms of depression—that JE sought psychiatric treatment with the therapist (JID). With antidepressant medication and psychotherapy the most severe symptoms of depression remitted after a few months, and after two years her sad preoccupation with M had greatly diminished. JE reestablished vital contacts with colleagues and friends, and a sense of purpose returned to her life. She did not seek another romantic/sexual partner, however (and has been unpartnered since).

Psychotherapeutic Treatment

The goal of the first two years of psychotherapy was to mitigate the patient's self-hatred as much as possible. The initial phase of the treatment was char-

acterized by JE's grudging compliance with the requirement of the fundamental rule that she say whatever came to mind. Doing so made her embarrassed. Resentful and grumbling, she nevertheless made the effort, communi-
cating to the therapist that she did so not because the process interested her
but because the therapist believed it was necessary.

She dreamed profusely and hated it. She found the same troublesome
topics emerging: she had to abandon her activities and run back to save an
elderly woman (associated usually with her mother, sometimes with M); she
was attracted to some young woman who was not M and wanted to have a
sexual relationship with her but didn't because she was afraid or disgusted; she
was being punished, imprisoned, or killed for terrible misdeeds.

The initial transference was to the therapist as an exacting maternal figure. For instance, in a dream from this phase of the treatment, which was unusual in that it depicted the therapist undisguised, the therapist admonished
her not to "do anything lewd." Then the patient noticed (in a dream) that the
therapist had an electroshock machine. Her associations were that the therapist was like her mother in wanting her to avoid sex. The electroshock machine was the treatment JE would receive if the talking cure didn't work. The
patient's grief and depression were seen as punishments for unacceptable sexual desires. Because they caused her to require therapeutic attention, the requirement that she attend sessions was seen as additional punishment—a humiliating discipline that other (heterosexual) people did not require because
they were "normal."

Psychotherapeutic interventions designed to mitigate the constant on-
slaught of the patient's harsh superego for having sexual feelings at all, and
homosexual desires in particular, were helpful. Toward the end of the second
year of treatment, JE took a trip during which she wrote her long decreased
mother a letter criticizing her for child-rearing mistakes but offering forgive-
ness. Also during the second year of treatment, she experienced grief for never
having attempted to lead a conventionally heterosexual life.

The Lesbian Writers Project

At this point JE was no longer grief-stricken and was somewhat less ashamed
of her sexuality. She was still quite isolated, however, since she was unwilling
to confide in anyone about her sexual orientation. In fact, she harbored a
"dread fear," which was to be recognized as a lesbian. The only sign that there

was any means of access to the prison of guilt and shame she still occupied was that she had opened the closet door wide enough to admit the therapist.

A problem in therapeutic strategy now emerged. The traditional psychotherapeutic techniques, confrontation, clarification, interpretation about JE's internalized homophobia, were followed by increased self-hatred. This negative reaction to intervention appeared to be specific and not part of a more global psychopathological process such as a negative therapeutic reaction, for example (Freud 1923; see chapter 9). A technique was called for that resulted in strengthening the therapeutic alliance and the patient's ego defenses while at the same time diminishing the self-hatred resulting from internalized homophobia. The therapist decided to attempt a supportive enactment. A great source of pride for JE throughout her life was teaching about writers; reading continued to provide her with great satisfaction and to be a major source of security and self-esteem. Aware of this, the therapist mentioned to JE that she thought it might be enlightening to read fiction authored by homosexual women. Did JE have any suggestions about whom to read?

JE responded with delight and a long list of authors and books. JE and the therapist began to read the works of these women and to discuss them during the sessions. The treatment became less painful for JE partly because the therapist was now with her mentally on a daily basis, since engaged in the same activities, and partly because reading with M had been a treasured activity. JE's affect became considerably brighter. She linked this to the knowledge of the many illustrious women including Willa Cather, Simone de Beauvoir, Colette, and Virginia Woolf who had entered her closet. Thus, although JE had not "come out," she had let a number of others "come in" to her mental world, and her sense of isolation was much reduced. While the process of reading together had comforted her in ways both nonverbal and verbal, the content of the reading had detoxified the condition of her homosexuality to some extent.

The introduction of lesbian writers into the treatment was followed by another change in the structure of the treatment situation.

A Heart Attack

JE suffered a heart attack and was hospitalized. The therapist learned of this from JE's neighbor, who called to explain why JE would not be at her routine appointment. Seeking to contact the patient, the therapist learned that she was in a room without a phone. The therapist spoke with the nursing staff and asked them to convey the message that she would like to visit if permitted. JE agreed. At the bedside, the therapist found JE in a mood of intense denial of her need for others, including (and perhaps particularly) the therapist. JE explained that she had declined a phone because of the expense that would be added to her medical bill. Finding JE to be rigidly insistent—beyond reason about this matter—the therapist decided upon an intervention. Explaining that it was customary for hospitalized patients to receive get-well gifts, she had decided to provide the patient with one. She offered JE a choice—flowers or a bedside phone.

This was in fact more of a pseudo choice than an actual one. JE prided herself on her physical sturdiness and stoical coping style. The therapist suspected that the possibility of receiving flowers as a get-well gift would not be well received. Thus the patient would really be left with only one possibility—a pathway out of her imposed isolation. JE was reluctant to accept any gift at all, but the therapist was adamant. Finally, JE agreed, and the therapist arranged for a phone to be installed, which she paid for. She was thus able to maintain contact until JE was discharged.

JE returned to regular office sessions three or four weeks later. In the early sessions that followed her release from the hospital she elaborated her fantasy that the analyst was Mother Thérèse who had picked JE up out of the gutter and restored her to health through faith and love. She expressed feelings of love for the therapist as well.

Her attitude toward her illness was stoical; indeed she stated calmly that "I know I could die at anytime and that's all right, but I seem not ready to go yet." Shortly after resuming the psychotherapy, however, and without antecedent discussion, JE began to reveal that she was a lesbian to selected people in her social network. This act of self-revelation, undertaken at the age of eighty-four, was the first time JE had ever told anyone except psychiatrists and her partner about her homosexuality. JE's decision occurred without preceding exploration of her closeted situation. Of course, some assessment of this had occurred at the beginning phases of therapy. After that, however, the therapist followed the patient's lead in the sequence of the themes explored as therapy unfolded.

JE's emergence from the closet was fashioned in a personal way, appropriate for someone of her age and station in life. A dignified, deliberate person, she chose to proceed with coming out in small steps, as she approached other tasks. She revealed her sexual orientation only to people whom she knew well and whom she judged not likely to be homophobic. (None expressed any surprise or disapproval at the news.) She also began to donate small sums of money to gay/lesbian charities and to subscribe to gay/lesbian magazines. At the beginning of the coming out process, JE experienced increased depressive self-hate, the major symptom of her internalized homophobia. This was analyzed and the symptom resolved. Her depressive mood was gradually replaced by a sense of increased self-worth, security, and pride. A profoundly honest person who believed it was important to live a moral life, she felt relieved to discard the trappings of a false self.

At the same time, she has not felt inclined to join gay/lesbian groups of any type, but rather to present herself to the world as a professor, one of whose attributes is that of being lesbian. This change in her social presentation of self was associated with an identity change as well. Rather than having her personality dominated by conflicts about being homosexual, her sense of herself as a lesbian was now progressively integrated into other aspects of her personality. The quality of her life was enhanced because of her capacity to tap dimensions of meaning and pleasure that had been impossible because of the rigid internal focus on conflicts about homosexuality. This plateau having been achieved in psychotherapy, other areas of growth that are outside the scope of this report could then occur.

Discussion

JE is now ninety-two years old. It has been eight years since she came out of the closet, and therapeutic sessions continue at a frequency of every few weeks. The effect of coming out on her psychological adaptation has been dramatic, and persistent improvement in her sense of self-authenticity and self-regard has occurred. As a person with a highly developed conscience, the sense of having to live duplicitously had made her feel chronically anxious and ashamed in a way familiar to lesbian and gay people. There is no experience that is analogous for a heterosexual person. Since then, pride has replaced the shame associated with deception. The positive effects of coming out on JE's adaptation are compatible with those described by researchers (Meyer 1995). Her circumstances were unusual, however, since she endured the stresses of being in the closet for more than fifty years. We can find no other instances in the literature in which a patient made this type of self-transformation at age eighty-four and had its positive effects documented on sustained follow-up.

The immediate therapeutic interventions that facilitated coming out involved two enactments: the lesbian writers project and the therapist's visit to the hospital and gift of the phone. Interestingly, there was virtually no discussion of being in the closet prior to JE's abandonment of it—and very little in preceding years. Thus nonverbal processes of communication proved to be crucial in JE's treatment in addition to the traditional verbal processes of psychotherapy.

The Therapeutic Enactments

We use the term *enactments* here to refer to an experience (or experiences) between patient and therapist in which both participated in activities whose goal was to increase the patient's level of adaptation. During these activities the therapist gave up the role of observer and commentator and instead adopted the role of participant (Panel 1989; Chused 1991; Roughton 1995). Despite this, at no point did the therapist forsake the therapeutic role. In the interactive experience of the enactment the patient's needs and the progress of the therapeutic process were primary, not the therapist's gratification.

The first enactment occurred because the patient had apparently reached a treatment plateau. Substantial symptomatic improvement in her depression had occurred, yet she still felt empty and devoid of purpose. The therapist decided that this was primarily due to traditional psychotherapeutic maneuvers. How to proceed? Many possible treatment strategies were considered and rejected (including the possibility of formal psychoanalysis). The therapist finally decided that JE came most alive in sessions when discussing literature— her lifelong love. As it happened, the therapist, too, loved literature and in fact had seriously entertained the notion of becoming a literature professor before she became a psychiatrist-psychoanalyst. By chance, at this point in her career the therapist had also become particularly interested in lesbian writers. The mutual interest was associated with increased awareness on the therapist's part of her capacity to identify with JE. She realized that not only did JE become more vital when discussing literature during sessions but she herself did as well. JE's harsh superego had battered both of them; respite was needed.

The discussion of lesbian writers marked the first stage of JE's coming out. Although she had revealed her sexual orientation to the therapist at their very first meeting, exploration of the meaning of being a lesbian had been only possible in part before this stage had been reached. Perhaps this was because JE needed to identify with other women who were similar to her in more dimensions than sexual orientation. The intellectuals she met in her literary explorations seemed more real, and certainly less threatening, than any with whom she might have come in contact in her social life. In fact, at this point in her treatment, no one other than the therapist knew that she was lesbian.

The Heart Attack

JE's heart attack raised a host of questions about psychotherapeutic strategy. What should an appropriate therapeutic stance be when a patient becomes seriously ill? Should the therapist wait for the patient to call or actively reach out? If contact is made, should it be limited to brief telephone chats, primarily to set up and direct attention toward subsequent therapeutic work to be carried out in the office setting?

In this case the therapist, finding herself unable to contact JE by phone, was determined to visit her if possible. Many factors were weighed before making this decision, including JE's existential circumstances (especially her social isolation), her tendency to be self-denying and to become more isolated when stressed, and the danger of exacerbation of depression. At a conscious level the therapist was not especially aware that her own anxiety about JE's health led to a need to establish contact with someone she greatly cared about. Subsequently, however, she realized that this contributed to her decision as well. She obtained JE's permission for the visit, however, in keeping with her understanding of her patient and generally accepted ethical guidelines.

The therapist had no idea that the gift of the phone would ultimately have an impact on the patient coming out of her closet. Rather, she intuitively realized that she and the patient's powerful and malevolent superego were engaged in a struggle. One sought isolation, withdrawal, and probably the patient's death—the other, contact, communication, and renewal. After years of therapeutic work, the therapist realized that the patient would probably accept the phone and, in fact, she did.

Love, Guilt, and Shame

From a psychodynamic perspective the myocardial infarction threatened to actualize a dread fear of the patient's—that she had been punished, perhaps fatally, for being lesbian. Her withdrawal from interpersonal contact was a tacit sign that she had lost her struggle to enter the mainstream of humanity. The therapeutic enactment not only communicated her therapist's determined refusal to accept her patient's symptomatic stance but was also clearly an act of love. Love itself is not an instrument of cure in psychotherapy, however, and its expression is fraught with the many dangers that are associated with boundary violations. The therapist, in deciding to act in this fashion, felt confident that her loving feelings (of which she was aware) were not leading her to make a countertransference error. The psychotherapeutic process, as subsequently revealed, has supported this judgment.

Supportive Versus Insight Psychotherapy

JE's treatment consisted of a mixture of supportive and insight therapy, but more the former than the latter. Her symptoms, life circumstances, and coincident stresses called for interventions that tended to support ego defenses and immediate adaptive capacities (Ursano, Sonnenberg, and Lazar 1998). There were lengthy intervals, however, during which more exploratory work was carried out. As is always the case in the psychotherapeutic treatment of patients with internalized homophobia, it was necessary to separate out the many narratives condensed into a single negative self-label: "I hate myself because I am homosexual." The patient was able to make major gains in understanding the way in which these narratives adversely influenced her sense of security, self-esteem, and tendency toward social isolation. The area of sexuality itself proved to be difficult to explore, however. JE was almost eighty years old by the time she felt able to move psychologically beyond her partner's death. She felt unmotivated to engage in a sexual partnership with anyone else—and had essentially retired from the sexual arena. The therapist followed JE's lead in exploring sexuality, largely limiting interventions to efforts to ward off superego attacks for not having been more sexually active when M was alive. There is no way of knowing whether JE would have been able to overcome the sexual inhibitions stemming from internalized homophobia, had she participated in exploratory psychotherapy when she was younger. Unfortunately, during the years when this might have been possible, most psychoanalytically trained psychotherapists would probably have tried to motivate her to become heterosexual. Notably, the one therapist she saw many years before beginning her present treatment did the reverse and supported her relationship with M. The psychotherapeutic work carried out at that time was, however, not exploratory, and the concept of internalized homophobia was as yet unknown.

The Sexual Orientation of the Therapist

JE was referred to the therapist because of depression, not for issues of her sexual orientation. At the beginning of treatment JE did not ask the therapist to disclose her sexual orientation. During their many years of work together, however, it emerged that the therapist was heterosexual. As the treatment revealed, this proved no obstacle to therapy, as is often the case. Although the patient-therapist match is sometimes best when concrete facets of their personae are identical, such as sexual orientation, gender, race, religion, this is often not necessary (Marmor 1996). Of course, certain aspects of JE's and the therapist's psychological profiles were the same, including the fact that both were women professors who loved literature. The crucial aspect of the therapeutic relationship, however, was that JE was able to feel recognized and understood and to feel trusting of the therapist. They shared a common humanity.

This chapter has not been a complete case discussion in the traditional sense. Rather, we have focused on a specific narrative line: the treatment of internalized homophobia and the positive effects of coming out of the closet. However, these central aspects of the treatment process were not part of JE's chief complaint. She was only partially aware of the way in which her feelings about being lesbian had caused her to suffer during the course of her life. JE had no expectation that her unconsciously irrational feelings of self-hatred for being lesbian could be ameliorated by psychotherapy.

In recent years much attention has been devoted to the negative consequences of internalized homophobia (Meyer 1995) and the positive effects of coming out. Most of the literature in these areas has focused on patients much younger than the one discussed here. In addition to discussing psychotherapeutic techniques involved in treating internalized homophobia, we have tried to convey a sense that psychotherapy involves a relationship between two people. Unpredictable events often occur during the process that require flexibility and even ingenuity on the parts of both participants.

15

Sexual Orientation and Psychoanalysis: Current Problems and Controversies

Psychoanalytic developmental and clinical theory is presently incomplete in many areas, and clinicians often find it difficult to anchor their techniques in ideas that are generally accepted throughout the world. Absence of empirical validation of key concepts has provided a context for turbulent disagreement and polarized debate. We have selected three topics to discuss in the field of sexual orientation/gender psychology that are especially fraught with conflict. The first of these is bisexuality.

Constitutional Bisexuality

The notion of a universal, basic bisexual disposition in human beings was close to Freud's heart from the very beginning of his explorations. In 1899 he wrote Fliess: "But bisexuality! You are certainly right about it. I am accustoming myself to regarding every sexual act as process in which four individuals are involved" (Masson 1985). In *The Three Essays on the Theory of Sexuality* Freud commented:

> Psycho-analytic research is most decidedly opposed to any attempt at separating off homosexuals from the rest of mankind as a group of a special character. By studying sexual excitations other than those that are manifestly displayed, it has been found that all human beings are capable of making a homosexual object-choice and have in fact made one in their unconscious.
>
> *(Freud 1915 [1905])*

Arguably the most important psychoanalytic text that attempted to present Freud's views in a systematic matter was Fenichel's *The Psychoanalytic Theory of the Neuroses* (1945). Fenichel, whose encyclopedic work informed an entire generation of psychoanalysts, commented: "Initially, everyone is able to develop sexual feelings indiscriminately. . . . A certain amount of sexual feeling toward one's own sex remains in everyone as a residue of the original freedom of choice" (Fenichel 1945).

In 1990 an updated edition of a glossary of psychoanalytic terms and concepts was conjointly published by the American Psychoanalytic Association and Yale University Press (Moore and Fine 1990). The entry on bisexuality states:

> Through identification with both parental objects, every human being has the potential to a greater or lesser degree, to invest libidinally in both sexes. By adulthood one component tends to be largely unconscious and a relatively exclusive hetero- or homo-sexual orientation has evolved. Bisexual men and women do not deal with sexual anxieties by repression, and so alternate hetero- and homosexual behavior. Although the frequency of each type of sexual contact may vary, homosexual eroticism is often predominant.   *(1990:33)*

Our perspectives about bisexuality are quite different than these.

Freud's (and Fenichel's) views, based on libido theory, were expressed prior to the development of the research discussed in the first part of this book. The psychoanalytic glossary treated Freud's observations, understandable at the time they were made, as being as valid in 1990 as they were in 1915.

Freud also assumed that there is a universally experienced homosexual infantile developmental phase. This idea has long been abandoned, however, both within and outside of psychoanalysis (Friedman 1988). Had there been such a developmental phase, one might credibly posit persistence of repressed unconscious homosexual desires in those without manifest homosexual fantasy. Since there is no such phase, the assumption of persistent unconscious homosexual desire in all people lacks support. This is not to suggest that all people do not form identifications with males and females. Psychoanalysts routinely hear of dreams in which men are pregnant and women have penises, for example. There are two points to emphasize about such cross-gendered identifications. The first is that they generally do not influence gender identity. No patient has ever left an analyst's office believing she/he was of the opposite gender after having been put in touch with their opposite-sexed identifications. Second, homosexual imagery in adults does not generally appear to be a response to unconscious cross-gendered identification. With regard to the relation between sexual anxiety and repressions, in bisexual patients either the homo- or heterosexual component of erotic imagery may be repressed for varying periods of time. We return to this topic at the end of the section of this chapter dealing with sexual orientation change during treatment.

We restrict further discussion of bisexuality here to bisexual fantasy that meets the criteria for erotic fantasy we discussed in earlier chapters. There is actually no empirical evidence that this is a universal experience or that even the potential to become erotically aroused by partners of both sexes is universal. As we noted in chapter 1, the majority of men and women have never experienced sexual desire for the same sex as well as the opposite sex during their lives, but many have. From the clinical perspective, the topic of bisexual fantasy becomes the source of considerable complexity because of its relationship to ego identity (Erikson 1959). On the one hand, there is no evidence that the history of bisexual fantasy is symptomatic, and we do not believe that it should be thought of in a medical or pathological context. On the other hand, patients who have identity difficulties for one reason or another, and who happen to experience bisexual fantasies, often find their capacity to experience homo- and heterosexual desire anxiety provoking. Such patients often try to attribute significance to their erotic fantasies for their sense of identity. Thus the question "Am I homosexual or heterosexual?" assumes great significance for them. Many vignettes of patients in this category have previously been discussed, and we refer interested readers to Friedman (1988:126–143).

In summary we suggest that the theory of constitutional bisexuality was credible when it was proposed but has outlived its usefulness. Most of the phenomena it sought to explain are now best understood in terms of attachment theory (Goldberg, Muir, and Kerr 1995; Carter, Lederhendler, and Kirkpatrick 1997) and gender psychology (Maccoby 1990, 1998; Tyson and Tyson 1990; Tyson 1994; Fagot 1995; Geer and Manguono-Mire 1996). Other ideas deriving from the theory, such as the notion that all people have unconscious homo- and heteroerotic objects, lack empirical validation, although all have probably identified with people of both sexes.

Sexual Orientation Conversion Therapy

The topic of sexual orientation conversion therapy is one of the most controversial in modern psychiatry, and discussion of it invariably evokes anxiety and anger in different groups and for different reasons. Our emphasis here will be to frame the issues in ways that are especially relevant for psychoanalysts and psychoanalytically oriented psychotherapists.

Reparative Therapy

We find it helpful to keep in mind the relationship between politics and psychotherapy in thinking about sexual orientation conversion. This is especially so because antihomosexual bias is a serious problem in contemporary America and the idea that lesbian/gay people can and should be "converted" to the heterosexual mainstream has been used by some to further discrimination and prejudice.

Psychoanalytic ideas influential in the 1950s and 1960s were expressed in somewhat simplified form by Dr. Joseph Nicolosi, in a book entitled *Reparative Therapy of Male Homosexuality: A New Clinical Approach* (1991). Nicolosi, a clinical psychologist, is not psychoanalytically trained, and although his book utilized theories originally published by psychoanalysts, he did not discuss them in a therapeutically neutral context, as a psychoanalyst would. Rather, he focused on concepts he believed would assist patients who sought to replace homosexual with heterosexual desires and behavior. The most important of these is that male homoerotic desire is rooted in a sense of masculine self-defect. Certain types of nonsexual relationships with men can enhance a man's sense of masculinity, and along with supportive heteroerotic experience, can lead to sexual orientation change. In addition to his speculation about how sexual reorientation might be achieved, Dr. Nicolosi's volume contains prejudicial antihomosexual stereotypes. For instance, he wrote:

> The inherent unsuitablity of same-sex relationships is seen in the form of fault-finding, irritability, feeling smothered; power struggles, possessiveness, and dominance; boredom, disillusionment, emotional withdrawal, and unfaithfulness. Although he desires men, the homosexual is afraid of them. As a result of this binding ambivalence, his same-sex relationships lack authentic intimacy. Gay couplings are characteristically brief and

very volatile, with much fighting, arguing, making-up again, and contin-
ual disappointments. *(1991:110)*

The outspoken political advocacy by some psychotherapists whose ideas
echo those expressed in Nicolosi's book to legitimize antihomosexual views
led the major mental health organizations to publish position statements out-
lining a modern approach to the sexual reorientation issue. The statement
from the American Psychoanalytic Association may be found at the end of
this section of chapter 15, and the statement from the American Psychiatric
Association in an appendix to the chapter.

Politics and Psychotherapy

The boundary between psychoanalytic psychology and political ideology has
not been breached only by reparative therapists. On the other side of the political spectrum, some psychoanalytically oriented gay psychotherapists have
introduced political ideology into discussions nominally about psychoanalytic
theory and practice. This has most commonly occurred not only with respect
to conversion therapy but in regard to the relationship between childhood gender nonconformity and adult homosexual orientation as well (Drescher 1998).
In order not to lead the discussion astray, we refer interested readers to discussions of this in the literature (Friedman 2000, 2001; Drescher 2001). Our point
here is that the confounding of politics, psychology, and therapeutics has been
committed because of antihomosexual bias in some cases and gay activism in
others. In both instances distortion of facts and theories by anti- or pro-ho-
mosexual political groups has occurred, and the ideas expressed do not appear
to be representative of beliefs held by most therapists.

Patients/Clients Who Seek Conversion Therapy

The needs of patients/clients that seek sexual orientation conversion seem out
of step with the attitudes of many contemporary clinicians. The erotic fantasy programming of these people is predominantly homosexual, but their value
systems interdict homosexual activity or membership in the gay subculture.
They seek to become "heterosexual" to whatever degree this is possible. Some
such individuals are, of course, predominantly motivated by irrational un-

conscious antihomosexual beliefs. Their desires to avoid homosexuality are best thought of as being symptomatic. In many other instances, however, this cannot be considered to be the case. Whether because of religious convictions or diverse other reasons, such people are unable to positively sanction homo-sexual activity or participation in a gay lifestyle. They may accept gay and les-bian people but, even so, are unable to tolerate a gay role for themselves.

The Facts About Sexual Orientation Conversion

In order to place the clinical issues in an empirically grounded perspective, we summarize the major facts and open questions about sexual orientation con-version as best as we can. Many of the problems in this area were anticipated and discussed by Lief and Mayerson (1965) andd Lief and Kaplan (1986). There have been a number of more recent reviews of studies of conversion, and we refer interested readers to those (Haldeman 1991, 1994). As reviewers have correctly noted, there are no adequately designed studies that demon-strate that "reparative" therapies are therapeutically efficacious as a general rule. Because of the paucity of research, however, it has also not been empir-ically proven that these reparative therapies are never helpful. Two addition-al studies of conversion therapy are presently being carried out. Dr. Robert Spitzer, at the New York State Psychiatric Institute in New York City, has re-cruited subjects who claim that they have been helped by conversion therapy (Bialer 2001). He has developed a detailed sexual history questionnaire and is systematically assessing their claims. Also in New York City two psycholo-gists, Drs. Shidlow and Schroeder (Bialer 2001), have recruited subjects who have undergone conversion therapy. Unlike Spitzer, who limited his sample to those who claimed a positive result, Shidlow and Schroeder describe both positive and negative results, such as loss of self-esteem, financial resources, lack of change of sexual orientation, and other negative consequences of the intervention. The results of these studies were not available at the time this manuscript was completed. Preliminary data from the Spitzer investigation suggest that among subjects selected on the basis of a belief that reparative therapy had helped them, many did indeed state that their sexual arousal pat-tern and activity had changed in a meaningful manner from predominantly homosexual to predominantly heterosexual. Another finding of this study was that some of these subjects believed that their homosexual desire was rooted in a sense of masculine self-defect. It is important to stress that the research strategy used by Spitzer was not a point-of-entry study. In other words, he did not assess all patients from the time they began therapy in order to determine therapeutic efficacy. Since patients who were not helped were omitted from investigation, Spitzer was not able to study the very important issue of complications of treatment. To use an analogy, a given drug might have a desired therapeutic effect, only to cause damaging side effects in most people who used it. Relatively few may have obtained a desired result without having serious side effects. For them, the treatment was helpful. For most, however, it was not, or may even have been harmful. Other patients who were not harmed may not have been helped. Spitzer's ex-patient group is disproportionately weighted toward people with strong religious beliefs that negatively sanction homosexuality.

Reparative Therapy Is Not Dynamic Psychotherapy

Although based on ideas originally contributed to the literature from the psychoanalytic sector (Socarides 1978), reparative therapy should not properly be considered a form of psychodynamic psychotherapy. It is basically a behaviorally oriented type of intervention, but lacks the systematic structure of manual-based therapies such as cognitive behavioral therapy of depression or dialectical behavioral therapy of the borderline syndromes. There is no manual for sexual reorientation therapy. Its basic principles seem to be applied by a diverse group of counselors and therapists from the mental health and religious sectors.

Sexual Orientation Change During Psychotherapy

One way of thinking about sexual orientation change is to ask, What kinds of data are presently available to provide clinicians information about such change? We briefly alluded in chapter 2 to plasticity versus rigidity of sexual fantasy. How much do psychoanalytically oriented therapists actually know about sexual fantasy changes during or as a consequence of dynamic psychotherapy? (This question is a more general one than simply whether patients can be "converted" from homosexual to heterosexual fantasies.) There is astonishingly little information to provide clinicians with a data base in this area. For example, it would be helpful to have verbatim transcripts of a patient in which erotic fantasies are verbalized during psychoanalysis or psychotherapy. Longitudinal assessment and ratings by independent judges could determine the extent to which fantasies had changed during treatment. Follow-up assessment could assess whether such change has persisted. No such study has ever been undertaken.

A different strategy might be to have an independent investigator longitudinally assess sexual fantasy (and perhaps activity) at periodic intervals during the course of psychotherapeutic treatment. This could be achieved through questionnaires or structured interviews. Unfortunately, this, too, has not been done.

Our clinical impression, as we noted in chapter 2, is that for most men and some women the limits of potential sexual fantasy change during psychotherapy or psychoanalysis are rigid and the range of possible change is small. For many women and some men, however, more plasticity appears to be possible. There are no published data that might assist clinicians to form an initial impression about possible change in the case of individual patients. Since psychoanalytic patients may come from different groups—one in which significant and meaningful change in erotic fantasy is possible, and one in which it is probably not—the reporting of individual cases provides no basis for a sound general guideline to therapists.

The Special Problem of Bisexuality

We return to the subject of bisexuality here because it has special significance for understanding sexual orientation change (Friedman and Downey 1999).

There is no generally acceptable bisexual social niche. Accordingly, many people with bisexual fantasies label themselves as heterosexual or gay/lesbian. During dynamic psychotherapy or psychoanalysis, they may experience a change in consciously perceived balance of heterosexual/homosexual fantasy desires. Either component may be repressed or experienced with heightened intensity for many reasons. This in turn may lead people to participate in sexual activity that is immediately motivated by such fantasies. We suspect that many cases of "sexual fantasy change" reported as a result of psychotherapy or psychoanalysis actually fall into this category. Both patient and therapist believe that sexual fantasies of one type—usually homosexual—have been replaced by those of another type—usually heterosexual—hence that the patient has changed his/her sexual orientation as a result of treatment. Neither systematic sexual history reporting nor detailed follow-up data are available to confirm the claim that such change has actually occurred, however, or whether (if it has) it is persistent. Among men we have failed to find a single published case in which adequate documentation has been provided that sexual fantasy that was totally homosexual has been replaced by sexual fantasy that is completely heterosexual as a result of psychoanalysis or dynamic psychotherapy. On the other hand, meaningful movement toward heterosexual fantasy has occurred in some men, associated with pleasureful and meaningful heterosexual activity, and, when in keeping with their therapeutic goals, has greatly improved the quality of their lives. When this has occurred, however, some homosexual fantasy has usually persisted.

The published literature on sexual fantasy/activity in women during or following psychoanalysis or dynamic psychotherapy is too sparse and diverse to discuss here.

In the discussion above our emphasis has been on people who are predominantly homosexual and who seek to be predominantly heterosexual. In keeping with the substantial emphasis on heterosexuality and heterosexism throughout American society, this is, among men, the most common profile that therapists tend to see. We have seen occasional gay patients who have been disturbed by ego-dystonic heterosexual desires, however. In the instances in which this has occurred the heterosexual fantasies appear to have been maladaptive responses to unconscious irrational fears and to have subsided with appropriate psychotherapy.

Countertransference Issues

The issue of change in sexual fantasies during psychotherapy is fertile field for countertransference problems. In our view the soundest guidelines for clinical practice are those that inform psychotherapists who practice dynamic psychotherapy generally. Psychotherapists should not impose their value systems on patients but rather try to form professionally appropriate relationships with them and understand them as well as possible. The perspective is also expressed in the resolution recently adopted by the American Psychoanalytic Association, originally sponsored by the Committee on Gay and Lesbian Issues. It states:

The American Psychoanalytic Association has officially adopted the position statement initiated by The Committee on Gay and Lesbian Issues:

1. Same-gender sexual orientation cannot be assumed to represent a deficit in personality development or the expression of psychopathology.

2. As with any societal prejudice, anti-homosexual bias negatively affects mental health, contributing to an enduring sense of stigma, and pervasive self-criticism in people of same-gender orientation through the internalization of such prejudice.

3. As in all psychoanalytic treatment the goal of analysis with homosexual patients is understanding. Psychoanalytic technique does not encompass purposeful efforts to "convert" or "repair" an individual's sexual orientation. Such directed efforts are against fundamental principles of psychoanalytic treatment and often result in substantial psychological pain by reinforcing damaging internalized homophobic attitudes.

(American Psychoanalyst 2000)

Childhood Gender Identity Disorder

One of the most common aspects of discrimination against gay and lesbian people is the use of disparaging gender role epithets such as *fag* or *sissy*. Because many gay men and lesbians have suffered gender role abuse as children, some psychotherapists have argued that the diagnosis of gender identity disorder (GID) in children should be removed from the *Diagnostic and Statistical Manual of Mental Disorders* (American Psychiatric Association 1994; Richardson 1996; Isay 1997). They believe that this will diminish anti-homosexual discrimination in the same way that removal of the diagnosis of homosexuality from the *DSM* did. Our position is different (Friedman 1998).

The disorder begins early in childhood, often at age three or four or even earlier, and usually affects boys. Follow-up studies indicate that most children with GID grow up to become gay adults. Most gay adults, however, have not had childhood GID. Therapists who specialize in treating these children do not believe that it is usually possible to predict the sexual orientation that evolves later in development. Clinicians are responsible to all children with GID, not just those who grow up to become gay men.

The introduction of *DSM-III* ushered in a way of diagnosing psychiatric disorders that was radically different from previous editions of *DSM*. *DSM-*

III was based on the idea that groups of symptoms and traits covary to form disorders. A number of specific behaviors had to be simultaneously present for a psychiatric diagnosis to be made. Isolated symptoms or traits usually have no specificity.

Thus even though many gay men were the targets of prejudice when they were children because of some behaviors that are criteria for the diagnosis of childhood GID, these isolated behaviors do not constitute a disorder. Nor do they discriminate between gay and nongay men. For example, many adult cross-dressers are actually heterosexual (McConaghy 1993).

In considering whether a particular diagnostic category should be in *DSM*, psychiatrists should rely on published studies in addition to the experiences of clinicians. Review of empirical findings about a particular subject is a process analogous to peer review of a journal article. Conclusions must not be based on the opinions of authorities or the advocacy of particular groups.

Most clinicians who have experience working with these children agree that the reason for the psychopathology is not simple social discrimination because the boys are feminized. There is disagreement among experts about what the criteria for the disorder presently called GID should be. There is consensus, however, that the children are psychiatrically disturbed. Elimination of the diagnosis would mean that patients now in this category would not be able to have their psychiatric treatment expenses reimbursed by insurance companies.

Social discrimination is unfortunately directed against people in many groups, some psychiatrically disturbed, some not. Psychiatrists, while being sensitive to the consequences of discrimination, should not delete psychiatric disorders from *DSM* simply because of such abuse (Zucker 1999).

We have selected three areas to discuss in this chapter because of their topical interest. Controversies are very much a product of their times, whether in psychoanalysis or in other fields. The first subject we discussed, bisexuality, is controversial because some psychoanalysts believe that Freud's observations about psychosexual development, including the libido theory and the theory of constitutional bisexuality, are in fact valid. Some also disagree with the idea that extrapsychoanalytic knowledge has much to offer psychoanalysis. For them data obtained from the psychoanalytic situation are unique. The notion that such data can be compared to data from other fields is controversial, even unacceptable.

Opposite and incompatible views about conversion therapy have emerged only recently in the history of psychoanalysis. The notion that patients should experience a change in sexual object as a result of psychoanalysis seemed uncontroversial to most psychoanalysts in the 1960s. The proposition recently accepted by the American Psychoanalytic Association about the goals and purposes of psychoanalysis seems uncontroversial today (*American Psychoanalyst* 2000). The application of simplified psychoanalytic ideas in the general mental health community, and by political and religious groups, has produced much turbulence and misunderstanding. The basic controversy in the general mental health community appears to center on whether sexual orientation conversion therapy should ever be practiced. We note that many patients presently receive such therapy. Most are probably religiously observant and their therapists apparently come from diverse disciplines. Given that this type of intervention is available to mental health consumers in the community, it should be carefully studied by objective investigators.

The debate about childhood gender identity disorder seems to be about the basic procedures presently utilized by the psychiatric community to label specific forms of behavior as being mental disorders. The issues are quite different than were those involved in the debate about whether homosexuality should be considered a mental disorder. Although that discussion occurred simultaneously with the early phase of the gay rights movement, the decision to delete the diagnosis of homosexuality was not based on the discrimination endured by lesbian/gay people but rather on whether they met the criteria adopted by the psychiatric profession for mental disorder. Many behavioral scientists at that time felt that they did not. Some prominent psychoanalysts and psychiatrists, such as Judd Marmor, for example, vigorously supported depathologization of homosexuality (Marmor 1980; Bayer 1981). The major impetus to depathologize childhood gender identity disorder seems to come not from clinicians and behavioral scientists with expertise about children but rather from others who argue that the diagnosis fosters discrimination, particularly against gay/lesbian people. We believe that the basic, time-honored mechanisms used by the American Psychiatric Association to arrive at decisions of nomenclature should continue to be used in this instance. Presumably, the opinions of experienced clinicians and behavioral scientists who have studied children with gender identity disorder will provide the most important input to the profession in reaching conclusions about this matter.

American Psychiatric Association Position Statement on Therapies Focused on Attempts to Change Sexual Orientation (Reparative or Conversion Therapies)

This statement was proposed by the Commission on Psychotherapy by Psychiatrists. It was approved by the Board of Trustees in March 2000 and by the Assembly in May 2000.

Background

In December of 1998, the Board of Trustees of the American Psychiatric Association (APA) issued a position statement (1) that APA opposes any psychiatric treatment, such as "reparative" or conversion therapy, that is based on the assumption that homosexuality per se is a mental disorder or is based on the a priori assumption that a patient should change his or her homosexual orientation (Appendix 1). In doing so, APA joined many other professional organizations that either oppose or are critical of "reparative" therapies, including the American Academy of Pediatrics, the American Medical Association, the American Psychological Association, the American Counseling Association, and the National Association of Social Workers (2).

The following position statement expands and elaborates on the earlier APA statement in order to further address public and professional concerns about therapies designed to change a patient's sexual orientation or sexual identity. It augments rather than replaces the 1998 statement.

Overview

In the past, defining homosexuality as an illness buttressed society's moral opprobrium of same-sex relationships (3). In the current social climate, claiming homosexuality is a mental disorder stems from efforts to discredit the growing social acceptance of homosexuality as a normal variant of human sexuality. Consequently, the issue of changing sexual orientation has become highly politicized. The integration of gays and lesbians into the mainstream of American society is opposed by those who believe that such an integration is morally wrong and harmful to the social fabric. The political and moral debates surrounding this issue have obscured the scientific data by calling into question the motives and even the character of individuals on both sides of the issue. This document attempts to shed some light on this heated issue.

The validity, efficacy, and ethics of clinical attempts to change an individual's sexual orientation have been challenged (4–7). To date, there have been no scientifically rigorous outcome studies to determine either the actual efficacy or harm of "reparative" treatments. There are sparse scientific data about selection criteria, risks versus benefits of the treatment, and long-term outcomes of "reparative" therapies. The literature consists of anecdotal reports of individuals who claim to have changed, people who claim that attempts to change were harmful to them, and others who claimed to have changed and then later recanted those claims (8–10).

Although there are few scientific data about the patients who have undergone these treatments, it is still possible to evaluate the theories that rationalize the conduct of "reparative" or conversion therapies. First, they are at odds with the scientific position of APA, which has maintained, since 1973, that homosexuality per se is not a mental disorder. The theories of "reparative" therapists define homosexuality as a developmental arrest, a severe form of psychopathology, or some combination of both (11–16). In recent years, noted practitioners of "reparative" therapy have openly integrated older psychoanalytic theories that pathologize homosexuality with traditional religious beliefs condemning homosexuality (17–19).

The earliest scientific criticisms of the early theories and religious beliefs informing "reparative" or conversion therapies came primarily from sexology researchers (20–28). Later, criticisms emerged from psychoanalytic sources as well (29–40). There has also been an increasing body of religious thought arguing against traditional, biblical interpretations that condemn homosexuality and that underlie religious types of "reparative" therapy (41–47).

Recommendations

1. APA affirms its 1973 position that homosexuality per se is not a diagnosable mental disorder. Recent publicized efforts to re-pathologize homosexuality by claiming that it can be cured are often guided not by rigorous scientific or psychiatric research, but sometimes by religious and political forces opposed to full civil rights for gay men and lesbians. APA recommends that APA respond quickly and appropriately as a scientific organization when claims that homosexuality is a curable illness are made by political or religious groups.

2. As a general principle, a therapist should not determine the goal of treatment either coercively or through subtle influence. Psychotherapeutic modalities purporting to convert or "repair" homosexuality are based on developmental theories whose scientific validity is questionable. Furthermore, anecdotal reports of "cures" are counterbalanced by anecdotal claims of psychological harm. In the last four decades, "reparative" therapists have not produced any rigorous scientific research to substantiate their claims of "cure." Until such research is available, APA recommends that ethical practitioners refrain from attempts to change individuals' sexual orientation, keeping in mind the medical dictum to "First, do no harm."

3. The "reparative" therapy literature uses theories that make it difficult to formulate scientific selection criteria for this treatment modality. This literature not only ignores the impact of social stigma in motivating efforts to change homosexuality, it is a literature that actively stigmatizes homosexuality as well. The "reparative" therapy literature also tends to overstate the treatments' accomplishments while neglecting any potential risks to patients. APA encourages and supports research by the National Institute of Mental Health and the academic research community to further determine "reparative" therapy's risks versus its benefits.

Appendix 1. APA Position Statement on Psychiatric Treatment and Sexual Orientation (approved Dec. 11, 1998) (1)

The Board of Trustees of the American Psychiatric Association (APA) removed homosexuality from the Diagnostic and Statistical Manual of Mental Disorders (DSM) in 1973 after reviewing evidence that it was not a mental disorder. In 1987 ego-dystonic homosexuality was not included in the revised third edition of DSM (DSM-III-R) after a similar review.

APA does not currently have a formal position statement on treatments that attempt to change a person's sexual orientation, also known as "reparative therapy" or "conversion therapy." In 1997 APA produced a fact sheet on homosexual and bisexual issues, which states that "there is no published scientific evidence supporting the efficacy of 'reparative therapy' as a treatment to change one's sexual orientation."

The potential risks of "reparative therapy" are great and include depression, anxiety, and self-destructive behavior, since therapist alignment with societal prejudices against homosexuality may reinforce self-hatred already experienced by the patient. Many patients who have undergone "reparative therapy" relate that they were inaccurately told that homosexuals are lonely, unhappy individuals who never achieve acceptance or satisfaction. The possibility that the person might achieve happiness and satisfying interpersonal relationships as a gay man or lesbian are not presented, nor are alternative approaches to dealing with the effects of societal stigmatization discussed. APA recognizes that in the course of ongoing psychiatric treatment, there may be appropriate clinical indications for attempting to change sexual behaviors.

Several major professional organizations, including the American Psychological Association, the National Association of Social Workers, and the American Academy of Pediatrics, have made statements against "reparative therapy" because of concerns for the harm caused to patients. The American Psychiatric Assocation has already taken clear stands against discrimination, prejudice, and unethical treatment on a variety of issues, including discrimination on the basis of sexual orientation.

Therefore, APA opposes any psychiatric treatment, such as "reparative" or "conversion" therapy, that is based on the assumption that homosexuality per se is a mental disorder or is based on the a priori assumption that the patient should change his or her homosexual orientation.

References

The statement was drafted and submitted to the commission by Jack Drescher, M.D., deputy representative of the Lesbian, Gay, and Bisexual Psychiatrists in the Assembly. At the time of writing, the members of the Commission on Psychotherapy by Psychiatrists were Norman Clemens, M.D. (chairperson and Board liaison), Glen Gabbard, M.D. (vice-chairperson), Barton Blinder, M.D., Ph.D., Jerald Kay, M.D., Susan Gaber Lazar, M.D., Julia Holman, M.D., Jesse Wright III, M.D., Bernard Beitman, M.D. (consultant), K. Roy MacKenzie, M.D. (consultant), John Markowitz, M.D. (consultant), William Sledge, M.D. (consultant), Eva Szigethy, M.D. (consultant), Michael Thase, M.D. (consultant), Marcia Goin, M.D., Ph.D. (Board liaison), Robert Kimmich, M.D. (Assembly liaison), William Bebchuk, M.D. (liaison with the Canadian Psychiatric Association), Michael Hughes, M.D. (corresponding member), David Reiss, M.D. (corresponding member), Andrew Siegel, M.D. (corresponding member and Assembly liaison), Bradley Strong, M.D. (APA/GlaxoWellcome Fellow), Michele Baker, M.D. (APA/Bristol-Myers Squibb Fellow), and Khanh-Trang Nguyen, M.D. (APA/Zeneca Fellow).

1. American Psychiatric Association: Position statement on psychiatric treatment and sexual orientation. Am J Psychiatry 1999; 156:1131

2. National Association for Research and Treatment of Homosexuality: American Counseling Association passes resolution to oppose reparative therapy. http://www.narth.com/docs/acaresolution.html

3. Bayer R: Homosexuality and American Psychiatry: The Politics of Diagnosis. New York, Basic Books, 1981

4. Haldeman D: Sexual orientation conversion therapy for gay men and lesbians: a scientific examination, in Homosexuality: Research Implications for Public Policy. Edited by Gonsiorek JC, Weinrich JD. Newbury Park, Calif, Sage Publications, 1991, pp 149–161

5. Haldeman DC: The practice and ethics of sexual orientation conversion therapy. J Consult Clin Psychol 1994; 62:221–227

6. Brown LS: Ethical concerns with sexual minority patients, in Textbook of Homosexuality and Mental Health. Edited by Cabaj R, Stein T. Washington, DC, American Psychiatric Press, 1996, pp 897–916

7. Drescher J. What needs changing? some questions raised by reparative therapy practices. New York State Psychiatric Society Bulletin 1997; 40(1):8–10

8. Duberman M: Cures: A Gay Man's Odyssey. New York, Dutton, 1991

9. White M: Stranger at the Gate: To Be Gay and Christian in America. New York, Simon & Schuster, 1994

10. Isay R: Becoming Gay: The Journey of Self Acceptance. New York, Pantheon, 1996

11. Freud S: Three essays on the theory of sexuality (1905), in Complete Psychological Works, standard ed, vol 7. London, Hogarth Press, 1953, pp 125–243

12. Rado S: A critical examination of the concept of bisexuality. Psychosom Med 1940; 2:459–467. Reprinted in Sexual Inversion: The Multiple Roots of Homosexuality. Edited by Marmor J. New York, Basic Books, 1965, pp 175–189

13. Bieber I, Dain H, Dince P, Drellich M, Grand H, Gundlach R, Kremer M, Rifkin A, Wilbur C, Bieber T: Homosexuality: A Psychoanalytic Study. New York, Basic Books, 1962

14. Socarides C: The Overt Homosexual. New York, Grune & Stratton, 1968

15. Ovesey L: Homosexuality and Pseudohomosexuality. New York, Science House, 1969

16. Hatterer L: Changing Homosexuality in the Male. New York, McGraw-Hill, 1970

17. Moberly E: Homosexuality: A New Christian Ethic. Cambridge, UK, James Clarke, 1983

18. Harvey J: The Homosexual Person: New Thinking in Pastoral Care. San Francisco, Ignatius, 1987

19. Nicolosi J: Reparative Therapy of Male Homosexuality: A New Clinical Approach. Northvale, NJ, Jason Aronson, 1991

20. Kinsey A, Pomeroy W, Martin C: Sexual Behavior in the Human Male. Philadelphia, WB Saunders, 1948

21. Kinsey A, Pomeroy W, Martin C, Gebhard P: Sexual Behavior in the Human Female. Philadelphia, WB Saunders, 1953

22. Ford C, Beach F: Patterns of Sexual Behavior. New York, Harper, 1951

23. Hooker E: The adjustment of the male overt homosexual. J Pers Assess 1957; 21:18–31. Reprinted in Homosexuality and Psychology, Psychiatry, and Counseling: Studies in Homosexuality, vol 11. Edited by Dynes WR, Donaldson S. New York, Garland Publishing, 1992, pp 142–155

24. Bell A, Weinberg M: Homosexualities: A Study of Diversity Among Men and Women. New York, Simon & Schuster, 1978

25. Bell A, Weinberg M, Hammersmith S: Sexual Preference: Its Development in Men and Women. Bloomington, Indiana University Press, 1981

26. LeVay S: A difference in hypothalamic structure between heterosexual and homosexual men. Science 1991; 253:1034–1037

27. Hamer D, Hu S, Magnuson V, Hu N, Pattatucci A: A linkage between DNA markers on the X-chromosome and male sexual orientation. Science 1993; 261:321–327

28. Bern D: Exotic becomes erotic: a developmental theory of sexual orientation. Psychol Rev 1996; 103:320–335

29. Marmor J (ed): Sexual Inversion: The Multiple Roots of Homosexuality. New York, Basic Books, 1965

30. Mitchell S: Psychodynamics, homosexuality, and the question of pathology. Psychiatry 1978; 41:254–263

31. Marmor J (ed): Homosexual Behavior: A Modern Reappraisal. New York, Basic Books, 1981

32. Mitchell SA: The psychoanalytic treatment of homosexuality: some technical considerations. Int Rev Psychoanal 1981; 8:63–80

33. Morgenthaler F: Homsosexuality, Heterosexuality, Perversion (1984). Translated by Aebi A, edited by Moor P. Hillsdale, NJ, Analytic Press, 1988

34. Lewes K: The Psychoanalytic Theory of Male Homosexuality. New York, Simon & Schuster, 1988. Reissued as Psychoanalysis and Male Homosexuality. Northvale, NJ, Jason Aronson, 1995

35. Friedman RC: Male Homosexuality: A Contemporary Psychoanalytic Perspective. New Haven, Conn, Yale University Press, 1988

36. Isay R: Being Homosexual: Gay Men and Their Development. New York, Farrar, Straus & Giroux, 1989

37. O'Connor N, Ryan J: Wild Desires and Mistaken Identities: Lesbianism and Psychoanalysis. New York, Columbia University, 1993

38. Domenici T, Lesser R (eds): Disorienting Sexuality: Psychoanalytic Reappraisals of Sexual Identities. New York, Routledge, 1995

39. Magee M, Miller D: Lesbian Lives: Psychoanalytic Narratives Old and New. Hillsdale, NJ, Analytic Press, 1997

40. Drescher J: Psychoanalytic Therapy and the Gay Man. Hillsdale, NJ, Analytic Press, 1998

41. Boswell J: Christianity, Social Tolerance and Homosexuality. Chicago, University of Chicago Press, 1980

42. McNeil J: The Church and the Homosexual, 4th ed. Boston, Beacon Press, 1993

43. Pronk P: Against Nature: Types of Moral Argumentation Regarding Homosexuality. Grand Rapids, Mich, William B. Eerdmans, 1993

44. Boswell J: Same-Sex Unions in Premodern Europe. New York, Villard, 1994

45. Helminiak D: What the Bible Really Says About Homosexuality. San Francisco, Alamo Press, 1994

46. Gomes PJ: The Good Book: Reading the Bible With Mind and Heart. New York, Avon, 1996

47. Carrol W: On being gay and an American Baptist minister. The In-Spiriter, Spring 1997, pp 6–7, 11, Appendix 1

Chapter 16

Origins of the Model of
Homosexuality as Psychopathology

In the United States organized psychoanalysis has rejected the pathological model of homosexuality. This was the result of a paradigm change that had occurred, so far-reaching that younger therapists entering the field today often ask why homosexual orientation was once considered, in itself, to be evidence of profound psychological disturbance. The historical roots of this belief, almost universal among psychoanalysts for about four decades, are discussed below. By way of introduction, however, it is helpful to review selected contributions of psychoanalysts and scholars who helped change what appeared to be a view of sexual orientation that was solidly anchored in psychoanalytic culture.

In the early 1980s the psychoanalytic community was wary of the decision made by the American Psychiatric Association to pathologize homosexuality. There was widespread concern that psychiatrists may have been subject to political pressure in a way that many psychoanalysts found troubling.

The chairman of the Program Committee of the American Psychoanalytic Association at that time was Richard Isay. He organized a panel sponsored by the American Psychoanalytic Association in 1983, "Toward the Further Understanding of Homosexual Men." Isay, Stanley Leavy, Robert Stoller, and Richard C. Friedman delivered papers that, although different in content, were similar in their criticisms of the older, traditional models that had been universally accepted just a few years earlier (Panel 1983). Isay soon became a leader in a struggle to liberalize thinking about homosexuality within the American Psychoanalytic Association. He shocked the membership by coming out at a meeting and used his own experience as a gay man to challenge invalid assumptions common among psychoanalysts at that time about the pathological personality structure of gay men. Isay further spoke out against the prevailing belief system generally accepted in the early 1980s by delivering many lectures and leading discussions at psychoanalytic institutes. For a number of years he was the only openly gay psychoanalyst at the American Psychoanalytic Association. Isay went on to write more than one book, but his first, *Being Homosexual* (1989), was the most influential in fostering paradigm change. At the turn of the century such influential behavioral scientists as Havelock Ellis (1938) and Magnus Hirschfeld (1914) had pointed out that homosexual men were similar to heterosexual men in every respect save for the erotic object. This point had been largely ignored in the psychoanalytic literature until the contributions of Isay. By discussing the psychoanalytic treatment of men from the healthier part of the spectrum, Isay demonstrated that most psychoanalytic writing about homosexuality was biased toward sicker patients. He argued that homosexual orientation was directly due to primary biological determinants, but did not elaborate upon this theory.

Kenneth Lewes's book, *The Psychoanalytic Theory of Male Homosexuality*, also influential, was a critical discussion of the history of psychoanalytic ideas about male homosexuality from Freud to the recent past (Lewes 1988). The book stopped just prior to the 1983 panel held at the winter meeting of the American Psychoanalytic Association. He pointed out that the concept of constitutional predisposition, originally stressed by Freud, had been replaced in the traditional psychoanalytic literature by a model stating that early developmental trauma caused homosexuality. We discuss this in greater detail later in this chapter. Lewes observed that after Freud's publication of the Schreber case in 1911, psychoanalytic writings about homosexuality tended to move toward considering it psychopathological per se. This drift occurred even though the Schreber case was primarily about paranoia and not manifest homosexuality. Lewes also critically assessed the prejudicially antihomosexual publications of Edmund Bergler (Bergler 1944, 1951, 1956, 1958). Lewes noted that gynecophobic and homophobic attitudes colored many psychoanalytic articles during the post–World War II years. He pointed out that sexist attitudes in psychoanalytic thought were vigorously challenged from the outset by women analysts; however, negative attitudes toward homosexuals were not similarly challenged by homosexual analysts. A woman analyst could appeal to common sense and use her own psychobiography as data for argument against prevailing theories, yet no psychoanalyst could publicly declare that he was homosexual and then make the same type of introspective argument against prevailing psychoanalytic theories. If he had done so, he would have imperiled his career and his standing in the community. We agree and note that, even when Richard Isay did this, in the 1980s, he mobilized considerable resistance and even outrage. Lewes also observed that the first article in the psychoanalytic literature on countertransference reactions in the treatment of homosexual patients was written as recently as 1980 (Kwar 1980; Lewes 1988). Lewes's historical perspective provided additional scholarly evidence to help alter the pathological model.

Friedman's book, also published in the late 1980s, *Male Homosexuality: A Contemporary Psychoanalytic Perspective,* preferred additional reasons for dispensing with the pathological model (Friedman 1988). Friedman integrated research in neurobiology, sexology, and developmental psychology with psychoanalytic developmental theory. He suggested that homosexual orientation be conceptualized in terms of four major dimensions of psychological functioning: erotic fantasy, erotic activity, ego identity, and social role.

Friedman observed that the psychoanalytic literature made no distinction between homosexual patients who suffered from major psychopathology, such as schizophrenia, severe depression, the borderline syndromes, and those who did not. All symptoms were usually attributed to homosexuality, itself thought to be due to early life emotional stress. Psychoanalysts at that time tended to believe that there was an association between homosexuality, narcissism, and masochism and that, despite some psychoanalytic scholarship to the contrary (MacAlpine and Hunter 1953; Blum 1980; Lothane 1992), paranoid delusions were a defensive reaction to unconscious homosexual wishes. In a critical discussion of the psychoanalytic literature, Friedman pointed out that these assumptions were not adequately supported and in fact that there was no inherent association between homosexual orientation and any psychopathological syndrome. Emphasizing that it was inappropriate to make generalizations about all homosexual people from data obtained from the psychoanalytic situation, Friedman proposed a way in which the observations of sex researchers such as Kinsey could be integrated with psychoanalytic theory and practice (Kinsey, Pomeroy, and Martin 1948, 1953).

Friedman suggested that, in gay men, the homoerotic image should be considered autonomous, and not motivated by unconscious anxiety. The psychoanalyst who treats such patients during adulthood might reconstruct a childhood history of trauma preceding the (remembered) origins of the homoerotic image. Even so, however, the homosexual image during adulthood, operating autonomously and in a fixed way, and delinked from unconscious conflict, would not be expected to alter as a result of psychoanalytic intervention. Moreover, personality development was not arrested or otherwise impaired in such men.

The contributions of Isay, Lewes, and Friedman were complementary to each other. Whereas Isay and Lewes were themselves gay, Friedman was not. His work followed a pathway outlined earlier by psychoanalysts who developed the biopsychosocial model (Engel 1962) and Judd Marmor, who had objected to the pathological model of homosexuality during the post–World War II years (Marmor 1980).

Psychoanalysis and Homosexuality: Recent Contributions

Richard Isay continued his earlier line of thought in a number of publications. He provided insights about the development of sexual identity in homosexual men, garnered from his psychoanalytic experience (Isay 1991a). Issues pertaining to disclosure of sexual orientation and to transference and countertransference were also discussed in articles on the homosexual analyst (Isay 1991b, 1993). Isay also emphasized that it is usually not possible to change a man's sexual orientation in psychoanalysis or psychoanalytically oriented therapy and that attempts to do so are often harmful (Isay 1996). He discussed the psychodynamics and treatment of gay men married to women, pointing out that they appeared to marry for neurotic reasons. Psychoanalytic intervention helped them accept their homosexual orientation (Isay 1998). In these articles and in many lectures, Isay directed the attention of the therapeutic community to the widespread and deleterious influence of heterosexism on psychoanalytic attitudes and practices in the treatment of gay men. Psychoanalysts, in recent books, have elaborated on these issues and discussed additional topics as well. A lesbian-feminist perspective has been presented by Magee and Miller (Magee and Miller 1997), an interpersonal-relational view by Drescher (Drescher 1998), and a self-psychology framework by Cohler and Galatzer-Levy (Cohler and Galatzer-Levy 2000).

We now turn our attention to consider the origins of the pathological model of homosexuality in psychoanalysis.

As the founder of psychoanalysis, Freud entertained complex and inconsistent views about homosexuality. In a famous letter to the mother of a homosexual, he stated that homosexuality is neither a vice nor an illness. He spoke out against persecution of homosexual people and pointed out that many great men, among them Plato, Michelangelo and Leonardo da Vinci were homosexual. He also observed that it was generally not possible to change sexual orientation with psychoanalysis:

Dear Mrs. . . .

I gather from your letter that your son is a homosexual. I am most impressed by the fact that you do not mention this term yourself in your information about him. May I question you, why you avoid it? Homosexuality is assuredly no advantage, but it is nothing to be ashamed of, no vice, no degradation, it cannot be classified as an illness; we consider it to be a variation of the sexual function produced by a certain arrest of sexual development. Many highly respectable individuals of ancient and modern times have been homosexuals, several of the greatest men among them (Plato, Michelangelo, Leonardo da Vinci, etc.). It is a great injustice to persecute homosexuality as a crime, and cruelty too. If you do not believe me, read the books of Havelock Ellis.

By asking me if I can help, you mean, I suppose, if I can abolish homosexuality and make normal heterosexuality take its place. The answer is, in a general way, we cannot promise to achieve it. In a certain number of cases we succeed in developing the blighted germs of heterosexual tendencies which are present in every homosexual, in the majority of cases it is no more possible. It is a question of the quality and the age of the individual. The result of treatment cannot be predicted.

What analysis can do for your son runs in a different line. If he is un-happy, neurotic, torn by conflicts, inhibited in his social life, analysis may bring him harmony, peace of mind, full efficiency whether he remains a homosexual or gets changed. . . .

Sincerely yours with kind wishes,
Freud (Freud 1935)

In a letter to Ernest Jones Freud affirmed the right of homosexual people to become psychoanalysts (Freud 1921). In other writings, however, he took a different stance, which critics have suggested stemmed from a number of biases (Friedman 1988; Lewes 1988; Fisher and Greenberg 1985; Domenici and Lesser 1995). In considering these it is important to have a historical perspective. We are now more than forty years past the Stonewall riots—the uprising at the Stonewall Bar in New York City by gay people who resisted arrest because of their homosexuality. This is generally considered the beginning of the gay rights movement (Duberman 1991, 1993), which challenged prejudicial views of gay and lesbian people throughout society, including those held by psychiatrists. Some of Freud's ideas, and many of those in the first generations of his followers, appear to have been influenced by historical and cultural prejudices, and perhaps some of the anger expressed at Stonewall was directed against these. We have learned much since then, and psychoanalysis is certainly less biased against gay/lesbian individuals. We no doubt have other prejudices that are difficult for us to see because of the limitations of perspective imposed by our historical and cultural circumstances.

Freud suggested a number of theories about the *etiology* of homosexuality. These included castration terror stimulated by the sight of the mother's genitals and the alteration of the sexual object from the mother to a female with a penis, prolonged and excessive early closeness to the mother leading to pathological identification with her and therefore the wish to love others who are like oneself, the so-called negative Oedipus complex in which, for a number of possible reasons, the child identifies with the opposite-sexed rather than same-sexed parent, and the turning of rage toward same-sexed siblings—and presumably father—into homosexual love via the defense of reaction formation (Freud 1905, 1910, 1918, 1922; Lewes 1988; Wiedemann 1962, 1974, 1995).

Homosexuality As Psychopathology

In the United States during World War II and the postwar years, most psychoanalytic writings about homosexuality utilized Freud's drive theory and his model of childhood development. The emphasis in the literature was to put forth a model directed at explaining the etiology of homosexuality and relating this to specific types of psychopathology in homosexual patients (Bayer 1981; Lewes 1988). Psychodynamically oriented practitioners were offered no way of conceptualizing homosexuality except in the framework of developmental derailment, character pathology, and sexual pathology. These psychoanalytic models of homosexuality were accepted not only by psychoanalysis and psychiatry but by the other mental health professions as well.

Continued Influence of the Pathological Model

The pathological model of homosexuality has long been abandoned by psychoanalysts in the United States. The theoretical beliefs of some psychoanalysts about homosexuality are inconsistent, however, and older ideas about psychopathology are adhered to despite the fact that new ones are also endorsed. A recent study of such beliefs of eighty-two psychoanalysts was recently carried out (Lilling and Friedman 1995; Friedman and Lilling 1996). Most analysts strongly disagreed with the idea that homosexuality is a mental illness, or that heterosexuality is the only normal outcome of psychosexual development, or that a primary goal of treatment should be to convert homosexuals to heterosexuals or to establish heterosexual behavior. As a part of this study, thirteen individuals were selected who most strongly equated homosexuality with psychological health. Even so, they were found to hold some theoretical ideas that were incompatible with those beliefs. For example, none strongly disagreed with the idea that sexual activity between men unconsciously maintains the symbiotic tie to the mother and that the unconscious sense of the maternal connection protects the ego from disintegration during sex. Another idea that the analysts did not reject was that aversion to the female genitalia is an intrinsic aspect of male homosexual motivation (Friedman and Lilling 1996).

Our impression is that many psychoanalysts throughout the world presently hold mutually contradictory beliefs about homosexuality. This presumably has an influence on clinical practice. We turn now to consider how the idea that homosexuality is inherently pathological came to be influential in organized psychoanalysis. Scholarly commentary has suggested that this occurred because of antihomosexual bias (Lewes 1988; Young-Bruehl 1996; GAP 2000). We agree but note that a biased attitude toward homosexual individuals was only one example of a widespread belief system that influenced psychoanalytic attitudes toward all of behavior at that time. We comment below on a number of specific psychoanalytic attitudes and assumptions that, acting in concert, contributed to bias against homosexual people in particular. We discuss this from a historical perspective beginning with the relationship between American psychiatry and psychoanalysis in the 1940s.

Psychoanalysis and World War II

Psychiatric disturbances of combat soldiers were a significant problem during the Second World War. In major campaigns more than 20 percent of all casualties were primarily behavioral reactions to combat (Hale 1995).

At the beginning of the war American psychiatrists were divided into two groups: organically oriented and psychoanalytic. The former tended to be institutionally based and to specialize in the treatment of the severe psychoses with electric convulsive therapy (ECT), insulin coma therapy, and sedation, and, rarely, psychosurgery (Redlich and Freedman 1966). To the degree that they counseled their patients, they tended to be directive and advice giving. In contrast, the psychoanalytically oriented psychiatrists were younger and conveyed the enthusiasm of intellectual explorers. They were convinced that they were at the "cutting edge" of modern advances in the behavioral sciences. A few had been psychoanalyzed by Freud, and others had studied with other pioneer psychoanalysts. The psychoanalytically oriented psychiatrists emphasized outpatient more than inpatient treatment and, unlike the other psychiatrists, were convinced that their approach was directed not only at symptom relief but at correcting the underlying causes of mental illness.

When the war came the organic psychiatrists had relatively little to offer, either by way of understanding etiology or delivering effective treatment to traumatized combat troops. The psychoanalytically oriented psychiatrists did, however. Training programs were set up in the armed forces and in civilian psychoanalytically oriented psychiatric centers temporarily working for the military.

The type of psychodynamic approach that was actually utilized so effectively with soldiers during World War II was not, in fact, strictly "psychoanalytic"—as the term came to be defined in the postwar years. Major psychoanalytic ideas were accepted—such as that of the role of unconscious conflict in symptom formation and the significance of early childhood in shaping adult motivation. Psychoanalytic jargon and technical concepts were avoided. Psychiatrists working with combat soldiers applied therapeutic methods that were practical, flexible, and driven by the necessities of war. Hypnosis, abreaction, and catharsis were widely used, as were mixtures of organic and psychodynamic therapies—such as, for example, the use of pentathol to assist in recovering repressed memories (Grinker and Spiegel 1945). In the military time-limited therapy was the rule, not the exception, and psychoanalysis as a treatment technique was obviously impractical. The willingness of the wartime psychoanalytically oriented psychiatrists to choose approaches to treatment based on their effectiveness and to apply psychoanalytic wisdom to pressing immediate problems led to respect for psychoanalysis throughout the armed forces and American society. Psychoanalysts achieved high status and became role models for most younger physicians who aspired to become psychiatrists.

By the 1960s a majority of professorial positions in the most respected departments of psychiatry in the United States were held by psychoanalysts and/or candidates at psychoanalytic institutes. A psychoanalytic perspective about normality and psychopathology (including homosexuality) was taught to medical students and psychiatric residents at the nation's premier medical schools (GAP 1962).

The American Psychoanalytic Association was responsible for setting and enforcing standards for the training of psychoanalysts at psychoanalytic institutes throughout the United States. Skepticism about the validity of ideas accepted by organized psychoanalysis was discouraged. This phase of psychoanalytic history exactly coincided with the publications of most of the influential psychoanalytic articles on the pathological model of homosexuality. Charles Socarides, for example, is the most outspoken American psychoanalyst still advocating the general validity of the pathological model. The first papers on homosexuality that he published in the *Journal of the American Psychoanalytic Association* and the *International Journal of Psycho-Analysis* appeared in 1963—on female homosexuality—and in 1968—on male homosexuality (Socarides 1963, 1968). In these articles, in keeping with the conventions of the day, he used his clinical experience with patients as the exclusive data base to support generalizations about all homosexual people.

Teachers at psychoanalytic institutes were almost always full-time psychoanalytic practitioners who taught at and administered the psychoanalytic institutes on a part-time basis. Despite contributions by a few eminent women, the psychoanalytic institutes tended to be run by middle-aged and elderly men in private psychoanalytic practice (Hale 1995).

During this period there was increasing emphasis on what today would be termed classical Freudian psychoanalysis as opposed to psychodynamically oriented psychotherapy. This led in turn to a narrowing of the patient base appropriate for treatment. The technical dimensions of the psychoanalytic treatment led to a selection bias—toward reasonably functional middle- or upper-class people—and away from those with severe psychiatric illnesses. The patient was required to have adequate "observing ego" to be able to participate in the psychoanalytic process and simultaneously learn to understand him or herself. Patients with psychoses, impulse disorders, addictions, and/or severe identity problems were usually deemed "unanalyzable," although not necessarily without the capacity to profit from less intensive psychotherapy. This occurred despite the ongoing interest of some psychoanalysts, such as Harold Searles, for example, in working with such patients (Searles 1965).

This approach to behavior was different than that which had been found useful to assist soldiers in combat. It also signified a radically different attitude toward patients. Military psychodynamically oriented psychiatrists were interested in helping all who needed assistance. The postwar psychoanalysts, however, became primarily committed to helping patients who could be treated with a specific technique: classical psychoanalysis.

Historians have speculated that the extreme conservatism of psychoanalysis during the 1950s and 1960s may well have been a reaction to the intense struggles occurring throughout American society over such issues as communism, the cold war, segregation, and the war in Vietnam. It is understandable that an organization whose roots were in prewar Europe, many of whose leaders were émigrés who fled Nazi persecution, might have wanted to construct an oasis of stability—an island of reason and professional expertise in an unstable, unexpectedly threatening environment. Even psychoanalytic leaders who were not émigrés were aware of the hostile reactions to Freud's work experienced by early psychoanalysts. Perhaps they wished to protect psychoanalysis by cloaking it in a conservative uniform. The institutional structures that psychoanalysis created in the United States and the intellectual isolation these engendered eventually led to diminished influence of psychoanalysis on psychiatry and academic medicine in general.

A great deal of attention has been devoted to the defects of organized psychoanalysis in the 1950s, 1960s, and even later (Fisher and Greenberg 1977; Grunbaum 1984, 1998; Edelson 1984). One that we feel requires particular emphasis, even more than has already been expressed, was the mistrust of the scientific method by the institutes of the American Psychoanalytic Association.

Psychoanalysis and Science

Although the American psychoanalysts were, by and large, physicians, their psychoanalytic institute training heavily emphasized the *clinical case method*. Psychoanalysis was the only medical specialty whose therapeutic endeavors were not rooted in science. The scientific method was ignored—even frequently proclaimed irrelevant—by many psychoanalytic educators.

As a result of the scientific method, empirical knowledge has rapidly grown in chemistry, physics, and biology. Modern medicine and surgery are based on such knowledge. For example, the treatment of diabetes mellitus is informed by understanding the relationship between glucose metabolism and insulin secretion. The treatment does not rest entirely on the cumulative insights of clinicians—no matter how penetrating—about the utility of insulin.

During the post–World War II years this was not the case with psychoanalysis. The theory of treatment was based entirely on ideas about psychology derived from the treatment of patients (or observations about sociocultural behavior) made primarily by Freud and, to a much lesser extent, by his followers.

If inferences are made on the basis of the clinical case method, they must be tested via application of the scientific method before general principles can be assumed to be true. The clinical case method is basically illustrative—not demonstrative. Thus the clinical case method cannot in itself be the basis for general principles of either human motivation or treatment of psychological disorders. In rejecting the scientific method, the psychoanalytic institutes became more and more peripheralized in the world of medicine and isolated from the general intellectual community.

Although the psychoanalytic institutes carried out little research, scientists in allied fields did. It was largely because of their efforts that psychoanalysis radically modified its ideas about the psychological development and functioning of women. For example, Freud's theory about vaginal-clitoral relationships in development and in sexual functioning was not abandoned because of progress within psychoanalysis but, rather, because of the psychophysiological observations of William Masters, a gynecologist, and his associate, Virginia Johnson (Masters and Johnson 1966; Fisher and Greenberg 1977). The sexologists demonstrated that there was no physiological difference between vaginal and clitoral orgasms and that the most common sensory source of erotic stimulation was the clitoris.

Freud's theories about women had been earlier challenged from within the psychoanalytic movement, most notably by Karen Horney (1939). Neither she nor her followers influenced the psychoanalytic mainstream to modify its view of women, however.

Modern psychoanalytic ideas about the psychological development of girls and women were also influenced by research on sexual differentiation and gender identity carried out by many nonpsychoanalytic investigators (Money and Ehrhardt 1972; McEwen 1983). These basic scientists made it possible for the psychoanalyst Robert Stoller (1968) and others to propose alternative models for the development of gender identity than those suggested by Freud.

These two examples illustrate that the most far-reaching paradigm changes that organized psychoanalysis made in the 1950s, 1960s, and 1970s came from work done by nonpsychoanalysts whose discoveries were based on the scientific method.

This is not to suggest that all psychoanalysts were antiscientific. Important investigations were carried out by psychoanalytically trained investigators at many academic medical centers and universities. Psychoanalysts carried out systematic research in psychobiology and psychosomatic medicine, sleep and dreaming, child development, diverse psychiatric disorders, outcome of treatment, and in other areas (Benedek and Rubenstein 1942; Engel 1962; Kernberg et al. 1972; Holzman 1976; Wallerstein 1986). Much of this research, in fact, did not take place at psychoanalytic institutes. When it did, it tended to be peripheralized and not given high status. Rare exceptions to this general trend did occur. Benedek and Rubenstein's study demonstrating cyclic changes in fantasy associated with the hormonal changes of the menstrual cycle, at the Chicago Institute, achieved immediate acclaim, locally and nationally. Nonetheless, this research has not been widely cited in the more recent psychoanalytic literature. The need for psychoanalytic institutes to more adequately integrate research into their culture was recognized by many scholars (Holzman 1976; Holt 1989). Yet the cultural shift never adequately occurred.

Attitudes of Psychoanalytic Institutes

In the psychoanalytic institutes candidates were expected to conform to the attitudes, values, and expectations of their teachers. Clinical process was valued but not objective assessment of outcome, critical analysis of basic assumptions, or experimental testing of hypotheses. The institutes were therefore not protected by procedural methods from systematic error. Such error occurred in their generally accepted psychoanalytic theories of homosexuality. Thus theories about the psychodynamics and psychopathology of homosexuality were accepted because they were approved by psychoanalytic authorities, not because they were based on validated research studies.

We have stressed the general intellectual climate of American psychoanalysis in the 1950s and 1960s because it was during those years that the influential articles on the pathological model of homosexuality were published. Although we have taken a critical stance, we do not seek to convey the impression that psychoanalytic education was entirely arid. In fact, inspiring teachers discussed Freud's work and the subsequent psychoanalytic literature in institute classrooms. Many patients were helped by psychoanalysis. The insights of their analysts proved helpful and the cumulative wisdom of the field was usefully applied to ameliorate their suffering. Others, however, were misunderstood because of biases of which the field of psychoanalysis as a whole seemed unaware. The reason that we have stressed the negative dimension of the psychoanalytic institutes to such a degree is that the rigidity with which the pathological model of homosexuality was believed and the tenacity with which it was defended when under attack in the 1970s were anchored in an overall zeitgeist, as it were: that of the authoritarian, clinically focused psychoanalytic institute.

Let us now return to consider the area of homosexuality itself.

Sandor Rado's Theory of Sexual Orientation

Of the distinguished émigré psychoanalysts, the most important with regard to psychoanalytic ideas about homosexuality during the postwar years was Sandor Rado.

Rado was brought from Berlin to become the first director of the New York Psychoanalytic Institute in 1931. Following psychoanalysis by Karl Abraham, Rado had become director of training of the Berlin Psychoanalytic Institute. Initially enamored of Freud, by the time Rado came to New York he had become critical of the sycophancy, intolerance of criticism, and grandiosity that flawed the psychoanalytic movement. He was committed to building bridges between science and academic medicine, and in the mid 1940s he left the New York Psychoanalytic Institute to become first director of the Columbia Psychoanalytic Institute, a university-affiliated institute, in contrast to the free-standing New York Psychoanalytic Institute (Hale 1995:250).

Rado believed that psychoanalysis was a science of human behavior. Its cumulative insights about the mind were, to him, analogous to the observations of neuroscientists about the structure and function of the brain (Rado 1949). Rado was a formidable, charismatic teacher whose students included Irving Bieber, Lionel Ovesey, and Charles Socarides, all of whom disseminated and elaborated his ideas about homosexuality. He was probably the most influential psychoanalyst to conclude that homosexuality is inherently pathological. Rejecting Freud's theory of constitutional bisexuality, Rado concluded that all people were primarily heterosexual. Those who were erotically attracted to others of the same sex were seen by him as unconsciously attracted to those of the opposite sex. Their primary heteroerotic wishes were irrationally experienced as dangerous. Unconscious fears led to repression of heterosexual wishes and to the replacement in the conscious mind of the heterosexual erotic object by one of the same sex (Rado 1940).

The Psychoanalytic Treatment of Homosexual Patients
Prior to the APA Referendum in 1973

Sandor Rado's theory that homosexuality was due to an unconscious irrational fear of heterosexuality was accepted as valid by most American psychoanalysts (Bayer 1981). It fostered the widespread conviction that the sex of the consciously perceived object of desire could usually be altered with psychoanalysis. Pathological defenses could be undone—the argument went—resulting in the emergence into awareness of previously repressed heterosexual desires (Rado 1940; Ovesey, Gaylin, Hendin 1963; Ovesey and Gaylin 1965; Ovesey 1969).

Complications of treatment undertaken to convert homosexual individuals to heterosexual were more the rule than the exception during this phase of the history of psychoanalysis, however. Such complications included loss of self-esteem resulting from the many instances of what was then considered treatment failure as well as the wasting of financial resources on treatment that was deemed unsuccessful because the replacement of homosexual by heterosexual fantasies was never accomplished. A sense of betrayal and mistrust was experienced by many in the homosexual community toward organized psychoanalysis (Duberman 1991; Isay 1996; Goldman 1995).

A vivid description of psychoanalytic treatment during the postwar years has been provided by historian Martin Duberman (1991), presently director of the Center for Lesbian and Gay Studies of the City University in New York. The title of Duberman's book, *Cures*, belied his experiences as a patient. Here he describes his experience with Dr. Albert Igen (a pseudonym), professor of psychiatry at the Yale Medical School.

> I liked him immediately. Low-keyed and compassionate, he refrained from pompous pronouncements and optimistic predictions alike, telling me that for the sake of "sounder adjustment" we should indeed work to change my sexual orientation, but that there was no guarantee of success. "It will largely depend" he solemnly told me "on your wish to change." The ultimate rewards will be great, but since the process of change is fraught with frustration and difficulty, you must greatly want that change in order for it to happen. *(Duberman 1991:44)*

The analysis proceeded at three sessions per week. Dr. Igen interpreted his patient's homosexual activities as "acting out" a need for immediate gratification. When Duberman complained of feeling that his professional life was unfulfilling, Dr. Igen commented, "The cure for feelings of professional sterility was not a half-baked leap into emotional turmoil. My current concentration should be on therapy; until I resolved my conflicts, I could not hope to improve either my professional or my personal life" (50).

Dr. Igen subtly encouraged his patient to give up homosexual relationships and take up heterosexual ones in their place.

> After nearly a year and a half of therapy he said it was time for me to take hold. The failure of the affair with Billy should have conclusively demonstrated to me, Igen said, the futility of investing my hopes for sustained intimacy in a homosexual relationship. It was time to look elsewhere, time to close the "escape hatch," confront my underlying anxiety, move toward a heterosexual adjustment. *(Duberman 1991:52)*

The patient obediently courted a young woman for whom he felt no sexual desire.

> Dr. Igen kept the focus steady. He encouraged me to speculate about the source of my "unconscious resistance" to physical love with a woman. Though rarely theoretical he made reference to a possible "breast complex" and asked me if I had reacted violently to being weaned. When I laughed and said I couldn't remember as far back as yesterday's movie, let alone my experiences in the crib, he replied, with a pained expression that that too was part of the resistance! . . . "Is it any wonder you have had difficulty ever since in entrusting yourself to a female? You're chronically angry, angry at women and refuse to get it up for them. To enter a vagina is for you to risk being swallowed alive." *(Duberman 1991:58–59)*

About one and one-half years later Duberman broke off the treatment because his work took him to another city. His analyst assured him he seemed "on the verge of a cure." His sexual orientation, however, had not changed.

Later in his life Duberman, having moved to another city and again desirous of becoming heterosexual, tried psychodynamically oriented individual and group therapy with "Karl," who commented to his patient:

> What would cause you to defend your mother so vigorously as "a good woman" other than guilt?—which in turn is a mask for incestuous wish-

es you never worked through as a child. You and your mother are not separate people and that is why your gender identity remains faulty. Until you pass through a separation phase, you will never be your own person—and none of your relationships can become adult ones, which is to say post-familial.

(Duberman 1991:104)

Karl remarked about Duberman's persistent homosexual orientation:

There's a deep refusal to change yourself, a nihilistic insistence that you can't change. . . . Way down beneath the rhetoric of struggle, you think change is one of two things—easy or impossible. What it all adds up to is that you don't want to do the hard work: you don't want to control your artificial appetites in the name of allowing a deeper self to emerge.

(Duberman 1991:190)

The goal of sexual orientation change as a result of psychoanalysis was generally unattainable. The conviction that this end point was even possible to reach was unsupported by research. How do we understand this? Was the grandiosity of prediction limited to homosexuality, or were psychoanalysts generally promising behavioral change beyond anything that could reasonably be accepted?

There was a belief in the field that psychoanalysis could lead to total personality reorganization and repair damaged mental structures, thus minimizing the likelihood of future psychopathology (Knight 1941; Rado 1956). Karl Menninger put it this way: "Psychoanalysis remains . . . the supreme paradigm of psychotherapy . . . the most thoroughgoing, the most penetrative, the most intensive and persistent" (1963).

Numerous instances of prolonged treatment, assurances of progress, and failure to improve occurred in the psychoanalyses of patients who were *not* homosexual. In a well-known book about his own disappointing psychoanalysis, the author Dan Wakefield reported that after five years he still suffered from agonizing symptoms. According to Wakefield, he was assured that psychoanalysis was a medically effective treatment, as certain to work as setting a broken leg (Hale 1995). Wakefield terminated analysis in dismay, ultimately achieving help through other means (Wakefield 1988). Thorough discussion of the reasons for the trend toward excessive therapeutic optimism is beyond the scope of this book. Complications and inadequate results are only *part* of the story, however.

There is no question that for many patients psychoanalysis was invaluable. Many found the way to meaningful lives because of it, and some credit psychoanalysis with saving them from suicide. Physicians are constantly placed in the situation of having the responsibility to care for suffering patients despite the fact that scientific knowledge of illness and therapeutics is sparse or even absent. Surgery prior to the discovery of anesthesia, the treatment of bacterial infections prior to the discovery of antibiotics illustrate this. Patients *needed* surgery long before modern surgical techniques existed. Patients with pneumonia were admitted to hospitals before the introduction of penicillin.

It is understandable that well-intentioned practitioners, given what appeared to be a powerful new technique, tried to apply it whenever possible to diminish suffering. In the instance of psychoanalysis, results often *were* positive. Most experienced psychoanalysts had reason to believe that their methods often helped people.

We suspect that this occurred because most patients did not manifest a type of behavior whose origins were misunderstood, and whose treatment plan was invalid because of systematic errors built into the basic structure of psychoanalytic organization. Thus many patients who suffered from depression were no doubt greatly helped by psychoanalysis. This is because (later progress in psychopharmacology notwithstanding) the generally accepted psychoanalytic model of the mind *informed* their treatment. That was not the case with regard to change from homosexual to heterosexual orientation.

Psychoanalytic Training of Homosexual Analysts

During the postwar years, otherwise well-qualified applicants to psychoanalytic training institutes were routinely rejected solely because of their homosexual orientation. Ralph Roughton, a prominent contemporary psychoanalytic educator, recently observed:

> Applicants were told they were unanalyzable, or to "reapply when you're cured." Several gay psychiatrists have told me their stories of being advised not to apply for analytic training or of being rejected when they did. One respected leader in psychiatry, now retired, was rejected by two institutes when he acknowledged his homosexual orientation but was accepted by a third when he did not reveal it to interviewers. However,

after telling his training analyst in the first session, the analyst reported it and he was immediately dropped from the institute. *(Roughton 1995:15–16)*

Some homosexual psychiatrists, determined to become psychoanalysts, completed psychoanalytic training, despite its hazards. Usually they assumed a heterosexual lifestyle during this phase of their lives and often married (Isay 1996). By systematically rejecting for psychoanalytic training candidates who were gay or lesbian, the psychoanalytic institutes eliminated a potential source of clinical data that could cast doubt on the prevailing theory of homosexuality.

We have suggested that one reason for the acceptance of the model of homosexuality as psychopathology during the post–World War II years was an antiscientific attitude that dominated psychoanalysis, both in the United States and abroad. Although the specific problem psychoanalytic thinking had with homosexuality appears to have been largely corrected, difficulties remain in the larger task of integrating psychoanalysis and science. One window into this difficulty is an examination of the content of current psychoanalytic education.

Critiques of Modern Psychoanalytic Education

Otto Kernberg, an academic psychiatrist and psychoanalyst and now president of the International Psychoanalytic Association, published a searching critique of international psychoanalytic education (Kernberg 2000). He observed the widespread resistance of psychoanalytic institutes toward introduction of extrapsychoanalytic data into seminars and discussion groups. The examples he used (presently largely ignored) included the neurobiology of depression, reformulation of drive theory in the light of modern neurobiology, and the neuropsychology of affects. Even data garnered from observational studies of infants are often avoided. Kernberg also criticized psychoanalytic institutes for neglecting to develop research training and a research attitude, "reflecting a dangerous lack of concern for the scientific standing of psychoanalysis in the world that surrounds us" (109). He observed that "in many psychoanalytic institutes throughout the world there is a distrust of the university and clinical psychiatry and psychology; psychiatrists and psychologists who spend significant time in academic endeavours are suspected of not being true psychoanalysts" (109).

Absence of a generally positive attitude toward research and science has also been associated with lack of cross fertilization of analytic ideas across national boundaries." French Candidates frequently ignore significant contributions from Anglo-Saxon psychoanalysis; English-speaking psychoanalytic candidates systematically ignore key contributions from French psychoanalysis; both French and Anglo-Saxon candidates ignore significant contributions from Spanish, Italian or Portuguese languages. The mutual ignorance of French and German-speaking institutions is proverbial. *(108)*

Creating a number of research initiatives at the International Psychoanalytic Association, Kernberg (and others) have been working to foster a more accepting attitude toward science.

Similar criticisms to those of Kernberg were recently put forth by an American Psychoanalytic Association task force chaired by Dr. Allan Compton and charged with the mission of reassessing the current status of psychoanalytic science and making specific and concrete recommendations to the association "for its development in the future" (Compton 2000). The committee reported that science is presently not given high financial priority by the American Psychoanalytic Association and "receive[s] scant attention" on the agenda of meetings as well. "No one can recall, at least for the last two decades, any meeting of Council at which science, in the sense of research, was affording anything resembling a prominent position at a meeting." This curious situation existed despite the fact that many members of the American Psychoanalytic Association have positive attitudes about research or are themselves scholars and researchers. "To this point, however, the Association has tended to marginalize all of these people, their talents and their interests" (Compton 2000:8). The authors of this important report emphasized the enormous need for psychotherapy research:

> It can readily be argued that the decline in the prestige and practice of psychoanalysis over the last 20 to 30 years may be ascribed in significant part to our failure to attend to the principles of normative science, in particular, a demonstration of outcome results of the treatment and the dissemination of the outcome results that we do have.

Psychoanalysis and Literature

Kernberg's observations about the national boundary/language problem afflicting psychoanalysis suggests that the field is presently organized in a way similar to literature. French and German literature are, after all, distinct disciplines, and students of one do not necessarily have to be students of the other; one does not have to be a Cervantes scholar in order to teach German literature at a university. We have puzzled over the curious fact—noted by Kernberg and others—that despite the aspirations of psychoanalysis to be a therapeutic endeavor, much of its intellectual/educational effort emphasizes textual analysis, as if the field were a branch of literary theory. This blurs the distinction between fictional characters and living people who actually require the assistance of psychotherapists. Psychoanalytic writings that emphasize the textual analysis of narratives, each presenting a different "subjectivity" (as if it were a work of fiction), share a common perspective with literary criticism. There has always been a trend in organized psychoanalysis to regard the material verbalized by patients as the sole basis for understanding the aspects of psychology expressed in the psychoanalytic/psychotherapeutic situation. Those who believe this have argued that extrapsychoanalytic knowledge is irrelevant to psychoanalysis, since it is concerned only with superficial matters, not unconscious motivations. This argument has been vigorously challenged as out of date by many critics of psychoanalysis, including the neuroscientist and psychiatrist Eric Kandel (1999), who observed:

> During the first half of the twentieth century, psychoanalysis revolutionized our understanding of mental life. It provided a remarkable set of new insights about unconscious mental processes, psychic determinism, infantile sexuality, and perhaps most important of all, about the irrationality of human motivation. In contrast to these advances, the achievements of psychoanalysis during the second half of this century have been less impressive. *(Kandel 1999:505)*

> One hundred years after its introduction there is little new in the way of theory that can be learned by merely listening carefully to individual patients. We must, at last, acknowledge that at this point in the modern study of mind, clinical observation of individual patients, in a context like the psychoanalytic situation that is so susceptible to observer bias, is not a sufficient basis for a science of mind. *(Kandel 1999:506)*

We agree that it is particularly important for psychoanalysts to employ knowledge from other disciplines when considering etiology of specific forms of behavior. These include psychopathology such as depression or obsessive-compulsive behavior as well as normative phenomena such as the development of gender identity and sexual orientation. This conclusion, debatable and, indeed, debated fiercely by psychoanalysts during the twentieth century, seems beyond debate in the twenty-first.

The requirement of multidisciplinary knowledge for adequate understanding of normal and abnormal psychological functioning has posed special problems for organized psychoanalysis, because psychoanalysts and dynamic psychotherapists tend to be much more comfortable in the culture of the humanities than the culture of the sciences—in the world of meaning to a much greater extent than the world of knowledge. This has led psychoanalysis to be dependent on extrapsychoanalytic scientific advances in order to change its own models of the mind in keeping with modern knowledge—a point we made earlier in this chapter. In fact, the basic advances in information about human sexuality discussed throughout this book, those that have resulted in the most far-reaching and profound revisions in psychoanalytically oriented thinking about human behavior, have occurred almost entirely because of extra-analytic research. We doubt that any other field with clinical applications has been so dependent for modification of its paradigms on progress made independently in other fields. The way in which Masters and Johnson's direct observational studies of human sexual activity led psychoanalysis to change its paradigm of female psychosexual functioning and development, for example, has no parallel in other fields of clinical science.

The impediments to bridging the gap between the two disciplines of psychoanalysis and science are substantial. C. P. Snow observed in 1959 that in the Western European community two distinct and noncommunicating intellectual "cultures" had emerged, one of scientists, the other of humanists. Mistrust of individuals who studied the natural world was already well-established by the nineteenth century. Investigators from Galileo to Darwin had been roundly condemned by theologians who viewed the study of the natural world as the devil's work. In the nineteenth century, however, the term *scientist* first appeared, professional associations of "scientists" soon followed, and the fundamental aspects of the scientific method became widely disseminated. Intellectuals, particularly literary critics and scholars, expressed concern that science imposed a narrow, reductionistic worldview on those who practiced its methods (Snow 1959).

The "two-culture" idea seems useful in thinking about psychoanalytic education. Contemporary psychoanalytic thought is much more heavily weighted toward the culture of the humanities than the sciences. This is true despite recent attention paid to the topic of neuropsychoanalysis. For example, at psychoanalytic clinical conferences studies and other extrapsychoanalytic knowledge that might validate or invalidate ideas under consideration are rarely alluded to. The exclusive focus of discussion is almost always psychotherapeutic "process," e.g., textual analysis.

Most psychoanalysts are trained at psychoanalytic institutes, free-standing centers of learning and professional practice that are usually not associated with universities. Even though psychodynamic psychotherapists are not required to study at such institutes, and many never have, this is not the case for most of their teachers and supervisors. Thus standards of professional excellence, knowledge, attitude, and skill as a dynamic psychotherapist are probably more determined by psychoanalytic training institutes than they are by departments of psychology, psychiatry, or social work. The requirements for admission to psychoanalytic institutes vary. To the best of our knowledge there is no minimum science requirement that is accepted internationally.

Postmodernism and Psychoanalysis

In the 1960s and 1970s new social movements were born, and older ones found amplified voice in an increasingly receptive America. The gay rights movement was but one of these and took its place alongside the anti-Vietnamese War movement, black liberation, radical feminism, and other movements. Associated with this, a trend developed at universities that was critical of certain Western European intellectual traditions, including the idea that scientific advances inevitably led to social progress. The term *postmodernism* refers to a movement, present in many disciplines, that is critical of the intellectual perspectives of the Enlightenment. Sokal and Bricmont have described it as follows:

> Vast sectors of the humanities and the social sciences seem to have adopted a philosophy that we call for want of a better term "postmodernism," an intellectual current characterized by the more-or-less explicit rejection of the rationalist tradition of the Enlightenment, by theoretical discourses disconnected from any empirical test, and by a cognitive and cultural relativism that regards science as nothing more than a narration," a "myth" or a "social construction among others." (1998:1)

Associated with the abandonment of its authoritarian posture in the 1980s, organized psychoanalysis became increasingly permeable to intellectual trends generated in academia, including postmodernism.

In psychoanalytic psychology, for example, an idea that is basically postmodernist is that every single person is only knowable in terms of her or his unique subjectivity. The biographical narratives of each and every person are unique constructions whose complexity can be elucidated through analytic exploration. Although meanings can be elucidated for that person, objectification and categorization should be resisted. We feel that this view, admittedly not the dominant one among therapists, but sometimes expressed nonetheless, is incompatible with the therapeutic mission of psychoanalysts and psychotherapists. Our own perspective is compatible with that put forth by Charles Hanley in a recent discussion of subjectivity and objectivity in analysis.

Critical Realism

Charles Hanley criticized a trend in recent psychoanalytic thought that he termed "necessary interactionism," the idea that patient and analyst influence each other during the analytic process in a way that makes objective assessment of either by the other impossible. Analytic process in this view consists of the joint creation of narratives by analyst and patient: so-called reality is actually "intersubjective."

> If it turns out that psychoanalysts must instead take it for granted that psychoanalytic knowledge is subjective, then psychoanalysis will have to accept its status as one among a number of fundamentally untestable ways of thinking about the human psyche. Psychoanalysis would be obliged to find its place among the humanistic psychologies akin to those of Plato, Spinoza, Hobbes, Kank, Marx and the various religions.
>
> *(Hanley 1999)*

Hanley pointed out that extensive discussions have occurred throughout the history of philosophy about the existence of a universe independent of our senses. He argued that it is helpful to assume that there is indeed a reality independent of our persons. Despite the fact that we might have great difficulty sensing it, and are prone to make erroneous conclusions about it, "it" is nonetheless there, waiting to be observed and studied. He noted that

Freud clearly advocated this view, which he termed critical realism. "Critical realism is the implicit epistemology of common sense and of science" (Hanley 1999:441). This approach is relevant not only to the physical universe but also to the analytic and psychotherapeutic situation. Whereas aspects of analytic work are possibly unknowable and indescribable, Hanley believes, as do we and others, that its most important components are in fact accessible to scientific study (Bucci 1997; Dahl, Kaechele, and Thomae 1988; Luborsky et al. 1994).

Freud was a neurologist by training who based many of his theories on observation and intuition because the discipline of neurobiology of behavior was in its infancy and tools to test his ideas had not yet been developed. Always open to scientific discoveries about the mind and brain but sometimes incorrect in his hypotheses, he left us a psychoanalytic theory filled with leaps of brilliant insight—and errors as well. It is the task of modern psychoanalytic thinkers to integrate psychoanalytic theory with knowledge from the behavioral and neurosciences so that psychoanalysis acquires self-correcting mechanisms and retains its vitality. This process is associated with anxiety as old ideas abandoned and new ones raise more questions than they answer.

The experience of psychoanalysis with homosexuality was, in our view, a special instance of a general problem. The particular issue—misunderstanding gay/lesbian people—seems to have been largely corrected, although it is still apparent that, as of the writing of this book, traditional beliefs about homosexuality are still retained by psychoanalysis in various locations throughout the world. It is unclear what the field as a whole has learned from its struggles with the homosexuality issue, however. It seems to us that the reason psychoanalysis changed its ideas about homosexuality was because of a confluence of influences and pressures—mostly from outside the field itself. A crucial question that must be grappled with today is whether other instances of similarly dramatic misunderstandings of behavior exist in psychoanalytic psychology, because of the type of systematic bias that misled the field about homosexuality for so long.

References

Abel, G. G., C. Osborn, D. Anthony, and P. Gardos. 1992. Current treatments of paraphiliacs. *Annual Review of Sex Research* 2:255–291.

Acton, W. 1995 [1875]. The functions and disorders of the reproductive organs. In R. Barreca, ed., *Desire and the Imagination: Classic Essays in Sexuality*, p. 273. New York: Meridian.

Adams, H. E., L. W. Wright Jr., and B. A. Lohr. 1996. Is homophobia associated with homosexual arousal? *Journal of Abnormal Psychology* 105:440–445.

Alexander, F., and T. French. 1946. *Psychoanalytic Therapy.* New York: Ronald.

Allen, L. S., M. Hines, J. E. Shryne, and R. A. Gorski. 1989. Two sexually dimorphic cell groups in the human brain. *Journal of Neuroscience* 9:497–506.

Allen, L. S., and R. A. Gorski. 1992. Sexual orientation and the size of the anterior commissure in the human brain. *Proceedings of the National Academy of Sciences USA* 89:7199–7202.

American Academy of Pediatrics Committee on Adolescence. 1993. Homosexuality and adolescence. *Pediatrics* 92:631–634.

American Psychiatric Association. 1968. *Diagnostic and Statistical Manual of Mental Disorders (DSM-II).* 2d ed. Washington, D.C.: American Psychiatric.

—— 1980. *Diagnostic and Statistical Manual of Mental Disorders (DSM-III).* 3d ed. Washington, D.C.: American Psychiatric.

—— 1987. *Diagnostic and Statistical Manual of Mental Disorders (DSM-III-R).* Rev. 3d ed. Washington, D.C.: American Psychiatric.

—— 1994. *Diagnostic and Statistical Manual of Mental Disorders (DSM-IV).* 4th ed. Washington, D.C.: American Psychiatric.

—— 2000. Position statement on therapies focused on attempts to change sexual orientation (reparative or conversion therapies). *American Journal of Psychiatry* 157:1719–1721.

American Psychoanalyst. 2000. 34(1):2–5.

American Psychoanalytic Newsletter. 1962.

Ames, L. B. 1966. Children's stories. *Genetic Psychology Monographs* 73:337–396.

Arlow J. A. 1963. Conflict, regression, and symptom formation. *International Journal of Psycho-Analysis* 44:12–22.

—— 1969a. Fantasy, memory, and reality testing. *Psychoanalytic Quarterly* 38:28–51.

—— 1969b. Unconscious fantasy and disturbances of conscious experience. *Psychoanalytic Quarterly* 38:1–27.

—— 1984. On the nature and organization of the repressed. *Psychoanalytic Inquiry* 4:107–124.

Arnold, A. P., and R. A. Gorski. 1984. Gonadal steroid induction of structural sex differences in the central nervous system. *Annual Review of Neuroscience* 7:412–442.

Asch, S. 1988. The analytic concepts of masochism: A reevaluation. In R. A. Glick and D. I. Meyers, eds., *Masochism: Current Psychoanalytic Perspectives,* pp. 93–117. Hillsdale, N.J.: Analytic.

Atkinson, L., and K. J. Zucker, eds. 1997. *Attachment and Psychopathology.* New York: Guilford.

Al-Attia, H. M. 1996. Gender identity and role in a pedigree of Arabs with intersex due to 5 alpha-reductase-2 deficiency. *Psychoneuroendocrinology* 21:651–657.

Bacon, C. L. 1956. A developmental theory of female homosexuality. In S. Lorand and S. Balint, eds., *Perversions: Psychodynamics and Therapy,* pp. 131–160. New York: Random House.

Bailey, J. M., and D. Benishay. 1993. Familial aggregations of female sexual orientation. *American Journal of Psychiatry* 150:272–277.

Bailey, J. M., and K. J. Zucker. 1995. Childhood sex-typed behavior and sexual orientation: A conceptual analysis and quantitative review. *Developmental Psychology* 31:43–55.

Bailey, J. M., K. M. Kirk, G. Zhu, M. P. Dunne, and N. G. Martin. 2000. Do individual differences in sociosexuality represent genetic or environmentally contingent strategies? Evidence from the Australian twin registry. *Journal of Personality and Social Psychology* 78:537–545.

Bailey, J. M., M. P. Dunne, and N. G. Martin. 2000. Genetic and environmental influences on sexual orientation and its correlates in an Australian twin sample. *Journal of Personality and Social Psychology* 78:524–536.

Bailey, J. M., and R. C. Pillard. 1991. A genetic study of male sexual orientation. *Archives of General Psychiatry* 48:1089–1097.

Bailey, J. M., R. C. Pillard, K. Dawood, M. B. Miller, L. A. Farrer, S. Trivedi, and R. L. Murphy. 1999. A family history study of male sexual orientation using three independent samples. *Behavioral Genetics* 29:79–86.

Bailey, J. M., R. C. Pillard, M. C. Neale, and Y. Argei. 1993. Heritable factors influence sexual orientation in women. *Archives of General Psychiatry* 50:217–223.

Bailey, M. 1999. Homosexuality and mental illness. *Archives of General Psychiatry* 56:883–884.

Baker, L. A., I. L. Cesa, M. Gats, and C. Mellins. 1992. Genetic and environmental influences on positive and negative affect: Support for a two-factor theory. *Psychology and Aging* 7:158–163.

Baldwin, J. D., and J. I. Baldwin. 1997. Gender differences in sexual interest. *Archives of Sexual Behavior* 26:181–211.

Bardwick, J. M. 1971. *Psychology of Women*. New York: Harper and Row.

Baum, A., M. O'Keefe, and L. Davidson. 1990. Acute stressors and chronic response: The case of traumatic stress. *Journal of Applied Social Psychology* 20:1643–1654.

Baumeister, R. F. 2000. Gender differences in erotic plasticity: The female sex drive as socially flexible and responsive. *Psychological Bulletin* 126(3):375–380.

Bayer, R. V. 1981. *Homosexuality and American Psychiatry: The Politics of Diagnosis*. New York: Basic.

Beatty, W. W., A. M. Dodge, A. L. Traylor, and M. J. Meaney. 1981. Temporal boundary for the organization of social play in juvenile rats. *Physiology and Behavior* 26: 241–243.

Bekoff, M., and Byers, J. A., eds. 1988. *Animal Play*. Cambridge: Cambridge University Press.

Bell, A. P., M. S. Weinberg, and S. K. Hammersmith, 1981. *Sexual Preference: Its Development in Men and Women*. Bloomington: Indiana University Press.

Bell, B. R., and P. L. Bell. 1972. Sexual satisfaction among married women. *Medical Aspects of Human Sexuality* 6:136–144.

Bem, D. J. 1996. Exotic becomes erotic: A developmental theory of sexual orientation. *Psychological Review* 103:320–335

—— 2000. Exotic becomes erotic: Interpreting the biological correlates of sexual orientation. *Archives of Sexual Behavior* 29:531–548.

Bem, S. L. 1989. Genital knowledge and gender constancy in preschool children. *Child Development* 60:649–662.

Benedek, T. 1973. *Psychoanalytic Investigations: Selected Papers*. New York: Quandrangle.

Benedek, T., and B. B. Rubenstein. 1942. *The Sexual Cycle in Women: Psychosomatic Medicine*. Medicine Monographs 3, nos. 1 and 2. Washington, D.C.: National Research Council.

Benjamin, J. 1988. *The Bonds of Love: Psychoanalysis, Feminism, and the Problem of Domination*. New York: Pantheon.

Berenbaum, S. A. 1990. Congenital adrenal hyperplasia: Intellectual and psychosexual functioning. In C. Holmes, ed., *Psychoneuroendocrinology: Brain, Behavior and Hormonal Interactions*, pp. 227–260. New York: Springer-Verlag.

—— 1999. Effects of early androgens on sex-typed activities and interests in adolescents with congenital adrenal hyperplasia. *Hormonal Behavior* 35:102–10.

Berenbaum, S. A., and E. Snyder. 1995. Early hormonal influences on childhood sex-typed activity and playmate preferences: Implications for the development of sexual orientation. *Developmental Psychology* 3:31–42.

Berger, R. M., and J. J. Kelly. 1996. Gay men and lesbians grown older. In R. P. Cabaj and T. S. Stein, eds., *Textbook of Homosexuality and Mental Health*, pp. 305–316. Washington, D.C.: American Psychiatric.

Bergler, E. 1944. Eight prerequisites for psychoanalytic treatment of homosexuality. *Psychoanalytic Review* 31:253–286.

—— 1951. *Counterfeit Sex*. New York: Grune and Stratton.

—— 1952. *The Superego*. New York: Grune and Stratton.

—— 1956. *Homosexuality: Disease or Way of Life?* New York: Hill and Wang.

—— 1959. *One Thousand Homosexuals*. Patterson, N.J.: Pageant.

Berkovic, S. F., R. A. Howell, D. A. Hay, and J. L. Hopper, 1998. Epilepsies in twins: Genetics of the major epilepsy syndromes. *Annals of Neurology* 43:435–445.

Berthhold, K. A., and J. H. Hoover. 2000. Correlates of bullying and victimization among intermediate students in the midwestern USA. *School Psychology International* 21:65–78.

Bialer, Philip A. 2001. "Clinical issues and ethical concerns regarding attempts to change sexual orientation: An update." Symposium of the annual meeting of the American Psychiatric Association, New Orleans, Louisiana, May 9, 2001.

Bieber, I., H. J. Dain, and P. R. Dince, M. Drellich, H. Grand, R. Grundlach, M. Kremer, A. Rifkin, C. Wilbur, and T. Bieber. 1962. *Homosexuality: A Psychoanalytic Study of Male Homosexuals.* New York: Basic.

Birke, L. I. A., and G. Vines. 1987. Beyond nature versus nurture: Process and biology in the development of gender. *Woman's Studies International Forum* 10:555–570.

Blanchard, R., and A. F. Bogaert. 1996a. Homosexuality in men and number of older brothers. *American Journal of Psychiatry* 153:27–31.

—— 1996b. Biodemographic comparisons of homosexual and heterosexual men in the Kinsey interview data. *Archives of Sexual Behavior* 25:545–573.

Blanchard, R., and K. J. Zucker. 1994. Reanalysis of Bell, Weinberg, and Hammersmith's data on birth order, sibling sex ratio, and parental age in homosexual men. *American Journal of Psychiatry* 151:1375–1376.

Blanchard, R., K. J. Zucker, P. T. Cohen-Kettenis, L. J. G. Gooren, and J. M. Bailey. 1996. Birth order and sibling sex ration in two samples of Dutch gender-dysphoric homosexual males. *Archives of Sexual Behavior* 25:489–508.

Blanchard, R., K. J. Zucker, S. J. Bradley, and C. S. Hume. 1995. Birth order and sibling sex ratio in homosexual male adolescents and probably prehomosexual feminine boys. *Developmental Psychology* 31:22–30.

Blanchard, R., and P. M. Sheridan. 1992. Sibship size, sibling sex ratio, birth order, and parental age in homosexual and nonhomosexual gender dysphorics. *Journal of Nervous and Mental Disease* 180:40–47.

Blos, P. 1967. The second individuation process of adolescence. *Psychoanalytic Study of the Child* 22:162–186.

—— 1968. Character formation in adolescence. *Psychoanalytic Study of the Child* 23:245–263.

Blum, H. 1980. Paranoid and beating fantasies: An inquiry into the psychoanalytic theory of paranoia. *Journal of the American Psychoanalytic Association* 28:331–361.

Bornstein, M. H. 1989. Sensitive periods in development: Structural characteristics and causal interpretations. *Psychological Bulletin* 105:179–198.

Boston Lesbian Collective. 1987. *Lesbian Psychologies.* Urbana: University of Illinois Press.

Boswell, J. 1980. *Christianity, Social Tolerance, and Homosexuality.* Chicago: University of Chicago Press.

Bouchard, T. J. Jr. 1998. Genetic and environmental influences on adult intelligence and special mental abilities. *Human Biology* 70:253–275.

Bouchard, T. J. Jr., D. T. Lykken, M. McGue, N. L. Segal, and A. Tellegen. 1990. Sources of human psychological differences: The Minnesota Study of Twins Reared Apart. *Science* 250:223–228.

Bowlby, J. 1980. *Loss.* New York: Basic.

Bradford, J. M. W., and D. M. Greenberg. 1996. Pharmacological treatment of deviant sexual behavior. In *Annual Review of Sex Research* 7:283–306.

Bradford, S. M. W. 1995. Pharmacological Treatment of the Paraphilias. In J. M. Oldham and R. Bams, eds., *Annual Review of Psychiatry* 14:755–779. Washington, D.C.: American Psychiatric.

Bradley, S. J., G. D. Oliver, A. B. Chernick, and K. J. Zucker. 1998. Experiment of nurture: Ablatio penis at 2 months, sex reassignment at 7 months, and a psychosexual follow-up in young adulthood. *Pediatrics* 102:E91–E95.

Breedlove, M. S. 1994. Sexual differentiation of the human nervous system. *Annul Review of Psychology* 45:389–418.

Broido, E. M. 2000. Constructing identity: The nature and meaning of lesbian, gay, and bisexual identities. In R. M. Perez, K. A. DeBord, and K. J. Bieschke, eds., *Handbook of Counseling and Psychotherapy with Lesbian, Gay and Bisexual Clients,* pp. 13–33. Washington, D.C.: American Psychological Association.

Brown, L. S. 1995. Lesbian identities: Concepts and issues. In A. R. D'Augelli and C. J. Patterson, eds., *Lesbian, Gay, and Bisexual Identities Over the Lifespan,* pp. 3–23. New York: Oxford University Press.

Brown, T. R., P. A. Scherer, Y. Chang, C. J. Migeon, P. Ghirri, K. Murono, and Z. Zhou. 1993. Molecular genetics of human androgen insensitivity. *European Journal of Pediatrics* 152:S62–S69.

Bucci, W. 1997. *Psychoanalysis and Cognitive Science: A Multiple Code Theory.* New York: Guilford.

Bullough, V. 1976. *Sexual Variance in Society and History.* New York: Wiley.

Burgress, A., and L. Holmstrom. 1974. Rape trauma syndrome. *American Journal of Psychiatry* 131:981–986.

Buss, D. M., and D. R. Schmitt. 1993. Sexual strategies theory: An evolutionary perspective in human mating. *Psychological Review* 100:204–232.

Byne, W. B., and B. Parsons. 1993. Human sexual orientation: The biologic theories reappraised. *Archives of General Psychiatry* 50:228–239.

Byne, W., M. S. Lasco, E. Kemether, A. Shinwari, M. A. Edgar, S. Morgello, L. B. Jones, and S. Tobet. 2000a. The interstitial nuclei of the human anterior hypothalamus: An investigation of sexual variation in volume and cell size, number and density. *Brain Research* 856:254–258.

Byne, W., S. Tobet, L. A. Mattiace, M. S. Lasco, E. Kemether, M. A. Edgar, S. Mogello, M. S. Buchsbaum, and S. B. Jones. 2000b. The interstitial nuclei of the human anterior hypothalamus: An investigation of variation with sex, sexual orientation, and HIV status. Presented at the joint meeting of the Sixth International Conference on Hormones, Brain, and Behavior and the Society for Behavioral Neuroendocrinology, Madrid, 2000. *Hormones and Behavior* in press.

Cabaj, R. P., and T. S. Stein, eds. 1996. *Homosexuality and Mental Health: A Comprehensive Textbook.* Washington, D.C.: American Psychiatric.

Cameron, N. 1959. The paranoid pseudo-community revisited. *American Journal of Sociology* 55:52.

Cantarella, E. 1992. *Bisexuality in the Ancient World.* New Haven: Yale University Press.

Carr, B. R. 1998. Disorders of the ovaries and female reproductive tract. In R. H. Williams and J. D. Wilson, eds., *Williams Textbook of Endocrinology*, pp. 751–817. 9th ed. Philadelphia: Saunders.

Carter, C. S., I. I. Lederhendler, and B. Kirkpatrick, eds. 1997. *The Integrative Neurobiology of Affiliation.* New York: New York Academy of Sciences.

Cass, V. C. 1989. Homosexual identity formation: A theoretical model. *Journal of Homosexuality* 4:219–235.

—— 1996. Sexual orientation identity formation: A Western phenomenon. In R. P. Cabaj and T. S. Stein, eds., *Textbook of Homosexuality and Mental Health,* pp. 227–251. Washington, D.C.: American Psychiatric.

Chasseguet-Smirgel, J. 1986. *Sexuality and Mind: The Role of the Father and the Mother in the Psyche.* New York: New York University Press.

Chodoff, P. 1966. A critique of Freud's theory of infantile sexuality. *American Journal of Psychiatry* 123:507–518.

Chodorow, N. 1989. *Feminism and Psychoanalytic Theory.* New Haven/London: Yale University Press.

—— 1994. *Femininities, Masculinities, Sexualities: Freud and Beyond.* Lexington: University of Kentucky Press.

Chused, J. 1991. The evocative power of enactments. *Journal of the American Psychoanalytic Association* 39:615–639.

Coates, S. 1992. Gender identity disorder in boys: An integrative model. In J. W. Barron, M. N. Eagle, and D. L. Wolitzky, eds., *The Interface of Psychoanalysis and Psychology,* pp. 245–265. Washington, D.C.: American Psychological Association.

Cochran, S. D., and V. M. Mays. 2000a. Lifetime prevalence of suicide symptoms and affective disorders among men reporting same-sex sexual partners: Results from NHANES III. *American Journal of Public Health* 90:573–578.

—— 2000b. Relation between psychiatric syndromes and behavioral defined sexual orientation in a sample of the U.S. population. *American Journal of Epidemiology* 151:516–523.

Cohler, B. J., and R. M. Galatzer-Levy. 2000. *The Course of Gay and Lesbian Lives.* Chicago: University of Chicago Press.

Colapinto, J. 2000. *As Nature Made Him.* New York: Harper/Collins.

Coleman, E. 1982. Developmental stages of the coming out process. *Journal of Homosexuality* 7:2–3.

Coleman, E., and B. R. Simon-Rosser. 1996. Gay and bisexual male sexuality. 1996. In R. P. Cabaj and T. S. Stein, eds., *Textbook of Homosexuality and Mental Health,* pp. 707–721. Washington, D.C.: American Psychiatric.

Collaer, M. L. and M. Hines. M. 1995. Human behavioral sex differences: A role for gonadal hormones during early development. *Psychological Bulletin* 118:55–107.

Compton, A. 2000. Ad Hoc Strategic Task Force on Psychoanalytic Science. Report to Executive Council, American Psychoanalytic Association.

Costa, E. M. F., B. B. Mendonca, M. Inacio, I. J. P. Arnhold, F. A. Q. Silva, and O. Lodovici. 1997. Management of ambiguous genitalia in pseudohermaphrodites: New perspectives on vaginal dilation. *Fertility and Sterility* 67:229–232.

D'Augelli, A. R., and S. L. Hershberger. 1993. Lesbian, gay, and bisexual youth in community settings: Personal challenges and mental health problems. *American Journal of Community Psychology* 21:421–448.

Dahl, H., H. Kaechele, and H. Thomae, eds. 1988. *Psychoanalytic Process: Research Strategies.* New York: Springer-Verlag.

DeBrulin, G. 1982. From masturbation to orgasm with a partner: How some women bridge the gap—and why others don't. *Journal of Sex and Marital Therapy* 8:151–167.

DeFries, Z. 1979. A comparison of political and apolitical lesbians. *Journal of the American Academy of Psychoanalysis* 7:57–66.

Dekker, J., and W. Everaerd. 1988. Attentional effects on sexual arousal. *Psychophysiology* 25:45–54.

Diamond, M. 1982. Sexual identity, monozygotic twins reared in discordant sex roles and a BBC follow-up. *Archives of Sexual Behavior* 11:181–186.

—— 1993. Homosexuality and bisexuality in different populations. *Archives of Sexual Behavior* 22:291–310.

—— 1997. Sexual identity and sexual orientation in children with traumatized or ambiguous genitalia. *Journal of Sex Research* 34:199–211.

Diamond, M., and H. K. Sigmundson. 1997. Sex reassignment at birth: Long-term review and clinical implications. *Archives of Pediatrics and Adolescent Medicine* 151:298–304.

Dittmann, R. W., M. E. Kappes, and M. H. Kappes. 1992. Sexual behavior in adolescent and adult females with congenital adrenal hyperplasia. *Psychoneuroendocrinology* 17:153–170.

Domenici, T., and R. C. Lesser. 1995. *Disorienting Sexuality: Psychoanalytic Reappraisals of Sexuality Identities.* New York: Routledge.

Donohoe, P. K., and J. J. Schnitzer. 1996. Evaluation of the infant who has ambiguous genitalia and principles of operative management. *Seminars in Pediatric Surgery* 5:30–40.

Dover, K. J. 1989. *Greek Homosexuality.* Cambridge: Harvard University Press.

Downey, J. and R. C. Friedman. 1995. Internalized homophobia in lesbian relationships. *Journal of the American Academy of Psychoanalysis* 23:435–447.

—— 1996. The negative therapeutic reaction and self-hatred in gay and lesbian patients. In R. Cabaj and T. Stein, eds., *Homosexuality and Mental Health: A Comprehensive Textbook*, pp. 471–484. Washington, D.C.: American Psychiatric.

—— 1998. Female homosexuality: Classical psychoanalytic theory reconsidered. *Journal of the American Psychoanalytic Association* 46:471–506.

Drescher, J. 1998. *Pychoanalytic Therapy and The Gay Man.* Hillsdale, N.J.: Analytic.

—— 2001. A response to Richard C. Friedman's review of *Psychoanalytic Therapy and the Gay Man. Journal of Nervous and Mental Disease* 189(2):129–130.

Duberman, M. 1991. *Cures: A Gay Man's Odyssey.* New York: Dutton.

—— 1993. *Stonewall.* New York: Dutton.

Eckert, E. D., J. Bouchard, J. Bohlen, and L. Heston. 1986. Homosexuality in monozygotic twins raised apart. *British Journal of Psychiatry* 148:421–425.

Edelman, D. A. 1986. *DES/Diethylstilbestrol-New Perspectives.* Boston: MTP.

Edelson, M. 1984. *Hypothesis and Evidence in Psychoanalysis.* Chicago: University of Chicago Press.

Edmunds, L. 1985. *Oedipus: The Ancient Legend and Its Later Analogues*. Baltimore: Johns Hopkins University Press.

Ehrhardt, A. A., G. C. Grisanti, and H. F. L. Meyer-Bahlburg. 1977. Prenatal exposure to medroxyprogesterone acetate (MPA) in girls. *Psychoneuroendocrinology* 2:391–398.

Ehrhardt, A. A., and H. F. L. Meyer-Bahlburg. 1981. Effects of prenatal sex hormones on gender-related behavior. *Science* 211:1312–1318.

Ehrhardt, A. A., H. F. L. Meyer-Bahlburg, L. R. Rosen, J. F. Feldman, N. P. Veridiano, E. J. Elkin, and B. S. McEwen. 1989. The development of gender-related behavior in females following prenatal exposure to diethylstilbestrol (DES). *Hormones and Behavior* 23:526–541.

Ehrhardt, A. A., H. F. L. Meyer-Bahlburg, L. R. Rosen, J. F. Feldman, N. P. Veridiano, I. Zimmerman, and B. S. McEwen. 1985. Sexual orientation after prenatal exposure to exogenous estrogen. *Archives of Sexual Behavior* 14:57–77.

Ehrhardt, A. A., and J. Money. 1967. Progestin-induced hermaphroditism: IQ and psychosexual identity in a study of ten girls. *Journal of Sex Research* 3:83–100.

Ehrhardt, A. A., K. Evers, and J. Money. 1968. Influence of androgen and some aspects of sexually dimorphic behavior in women with the late-treated adrenogenital syndrome. *Johns Hopkins Medical Journal* 123:115–122.

Ehrhardt, A. A., R. Epstein, and J. Money. 1968. Fetal androgens and female gender identity in the early treated adrenogenital syndrome. *Johns Hopkins Medical Journal* 122:160–167.

Ehrhardt, A. A., and S. W. Baker, 1974. Fetal androgens, human CNS differentiation, and behavior sex differences. In R. C. Friedman, R. M. Richart, and R. L. Vande Wiele, eds., *Sex Differences in Behavior*, pp. 53–76. New York: Wiley.

Elbert, P., C. Pantev, C. Wienbruch, B. Rockstroh, and E. Taub. 1995. Increased cortical representation of the fingers of the left hand in string players. *Science* 270:305–307.

Ellis, H. 1897. *Sexual Inversion*. London: Wilson and Macmillan. Repr. 1975. New York: Arno.

—— 1938. *Psychology of Sex*. New York: Emerson.

—— 1942 [1896–1928]. *Studies in the Psychology of Sex*. 7 vols. New York: Random House.

Elsayed, S. M., M. Al-Maghraby, H. B. Hafeiz, and S. A. Taha. 1988. Psychological aspects of intersex in Saudi patients. *Acta Psychiatrica Scandinavica* 77:297–300.

Engel, G. 1962. *Psychological Development in Health and Disease*. Philadelphia: Saunders.

—— 1977. The need for a new medical model: A challenge for biomedicine. *Science* 196:129.

Erickson, M. T. 1993. Rethinking Oedipus: An evolutionary perspective of incest avoidance. *American Journal of Psychiatry* 150:411–416.

Erikson, E. H. 1959. The problem of ego identity. In *Identity and the Life Cycle*. Psychological Issues 1(1):101–164. New York: International Universities Press.

Everaerd, W., and E. Laan. 1994. Cognitive aspects of sexual functioning and dysfuntioning. *Sexual and Marital Therapy* 9:225–230.

Fabes, R. A. 1994. Physiological, emotional, and behavioral correlates of gender segregation. In C. Leaper, ed., *Childhood Gender Segregation: Causes and Consequences*, pp. 19–34. San Francisco: Jossey-Bass.

Fagen, R. 1981. *Animal Play Behavior*. Oxford: Oxford University Press.

Fagot, B. I. 1985. Changes in thinking about early sex role development. *Developmental Review* 5:83–98.

—— 1994. Peer relations and the development of competence in boys and girls. In C. Leaper, ed., *Childhood Gender Segregation: Causes and Consequences*, pp. 53–65. San Francisco: Jossey-Bass.

—— 1995. Psychosocial and cognitive determinants of early gender-role development. In R. C. Rosen, C. M. Davis, H. J. Ruppel Jr., and K. Heffernan, and S. L. Davis, eds., *Annual Review of Sex Research* 6:1–32. Mason City, Iowa: Society for the Scientific Study of Sexuality.

Fagot, B. I., B. Leinbach, and R. Hagan. 1986. Gender labeling and the adoption of sex-typed behaviors. *Developmental Psychology* 22:440–443.

Fairbairn, W. R. D. 1952. *Psycho-Analytic Studies of the Personality*. London: Routledge and Kegan Paul.

Faulkner, A. H. and K. Cranston. 1998. Correlates of same-sex sexual behavior in a random sample of Massachusetts high school students. *American Journal of Public Health* 88:262–266.

Fay, R. E., C. F. Turner, A. D. Klassen, and J. H. Gagnon. 1989. Prevalence and patterns of same-gender sexual contact among men. *Science* 243:338–348.

Fenichel, O. 1945. *The Psychoanalytic Theory of Neurosis*. New York: Norton.

Fergusson, D. M., L. J. Horwood, and A. L. Beautrais. 1999. Is sexual orientation related to mental health problems and suicidality in young people? *Archives of General Psychiatry* 56:876–880.

Fine, G. A. 1987. *With the Boys: Little League Baseball and Preadolescent Culture*. Chicago: University of Chicago Press.

Fisher, H. 1999. *The First Sex*. New York: Random House.

Fisher, S. 1973. *The Female Orgasm*. New York: Basic.

Fisher, S., and R. P. Greenberg. 1977. *The Scientific Credibility of Freud's Theories and Therapy*. New York: Basic. Repr. 1985. New York: Columbia University Press.

Flannery, R. 1990. Social support and psychological trauma: A methodological review. *Journal of Trauma and Stress* 3:593–610.

Ford, C. S., and F. A. Beach. 1951. *Patterns of Sexual Behavior*. New York: Ace.

Fox, T. O., S. A. Tobet, and M. J. Baum. 1999. Sex differences in human brain and behavior. In G. Adelman and B. Smith, eds., *Encyclopedia of Neuroscience*, pp. 1845–1849. 2d ed. Amsterdam: Elsevier Science.

Freud, A. 1937. *The Ego and the Mechanisms of Defense*. London: Hogarth.

—— 1965. *Normality and Pathology in Childhood: Assessments of Development*. Vol. 6. New York: International Universities Press.

Freud, S. 1900. *The Interpretation of Dreams*. In J. Strachey, ed. and trans., *The Standard Edition of the Complete Psychological Works of Sigmund Freud*, vols. 4, 5. London: Hogarth, 1953.

—— 1905. *Three Essays on the Theory of Sexuality*. In J. Strachey, ed. and trans., *The Standard Edition of the Complete Psychological Works of Sigmund Freud* 7:125–243. London: Hogarth, 1953.

—— 1907. Creative writers and daydreaming. In P. Gay, ed., *The Freud Reader*, pp. 436–443. New York: Norton, 1989.

—— 1910. Leonardo da Vinci and a memory of his childhood. In J. Strachey, ed. and trans., *The Standard Edition of the Complete Psychological Works of Sigmund Freud* 11:59–138. London: Hogarth, 1957.

—— 1911. Psychoanalytic notes on an autobiographical account of a case of paranoia (*Dementia Paranoides*). In J. Strachey, ed. and trans., *The Standard Edition of the Complete Psychological Works of Sigmund Freud* 12:3–82. London: Hogarth, 1958.

—— 1913. *Totem and Taboo.* In J. Strachey, ed. and trans., *The Standard Edition of the Complete Psychological Works of Sigmund Freud* 13:1–162. London: Hogarth, 1955.

—— 1915 [1905]. *Addendum to Three Essays on Sexuality.* London: Hogarth, 1953.

—— 1915–1916. *Introductory Lectures on Psychoanalysis,* parts 1 and 2. In J. Strachey, ed. and trans., *The Standard Edition of the Complete Psychological Works of Sigmund Freud,* vol. 15. London: Hogarth, 1963.

—— 1916–1917. *Introductory Lectures on Psychoanalysis,* part 3. In J. Strachey, ed. and trans., *The Standard Edition of the Complete Psychological Works of Sigmund Freud,* vol. 16. London: Hogarth, 1963.

—— 1916. Some character types met with in psychoanalytic work. In J. Strachey, ed. and trans., *The Standard Edition of the Complete Psychological Works of Sigmund Freud* 14:309–333. London: Hogarth, 1957.

—— 1917. Mourning and melancholia. In J. Strachey, ed. and trans., *The Standard Edition of the Complete Psychological Works of Sigmund Freud* 14:237–258. London: Hogarth, 1957.

—— 1918. From the history of an infantile neurosis. In J. Strachey, ed. and trans., *The Standard Edition of the Complete Psychological Works of Sigmund Freud* 17:3–122. London: Hogarth, 1955.

—— 1920. The psychogenesis of a case of homosexuality in a woman. In J. Strachey, ed. and trans., *The Standard Edition of the Complete Psychological Works of Sigmund Freud* 18:145–172. London: Hogarth, 1955.

—— 1921. Circular letter, with Otto Rank. In J. Marmor, ed., *Homosexual Behavior,* p. 395. New York: Basic, 1980.

—— 1922. Some neurotic mechanisms in jealousy, paranoia, and homosexuality. In J. Strachey, ed. and trans., *The Standard Edition of the Complete Psychological Works of Sigmund Freud* 18:221–232. London: Hogarth, 1955.

—— 1923. *The Ego and the Id.* In J. Strachey, ed. and trans., *The Standard Edition of the Complete Psychological Works of Sigmund Freud* 19:3–66. London: Hogarth, 1961.

—— 1924. The economic problem of masochism. In J. Strachey, ed. and trans., *The Standard Edition of the Complete Psychological Works of Sigmund Freud* 19:159–170. London: Hogarth, 1961.

—— 1930. *Civilization and Its Discontents.* In J. Strachey, ed. and trans., *The Standard Edition of the Complete Psychological Works of Sigmund Freud* 21:59–145. London: Hogarth, 1961.

—— 1931. Female sexuality. In J. Strachey, ed. and trans., *The Standard Edition of the Complete Psychological Works of Sigmund Freud* 21:223–243.

—— 1933. *New Introductory Lectures on Psycho-Analysis.* In J. Strachey, ed. and trans., *The Standard Edition of the Complete Psychological Works of Sigmund Freud* 22:3–182. London: Hogarth, 1964.

—— 1935. Letter to an American mother. In R. Bayer, ed., *Homosexuality and American Psychiatry: The Politics of Diagnosis*, p. 27. New York: Basic, 1981.

—— 1937. Analysis terminable and interminable. In J. Strachey, ed. and trans., *The Standard Edition of the Complete Psychological Works of Sigmund Freud* 22:209–253. London: Hogarth, 1964.

—— 1940. *An Outline of Psycho-Analysis.* In J. Strachey, ed. and trans., *The Standard Edition of the Complete Psychological Works of Sigmund Freud* 23:144–208. London: Hogarth, 1964.

Freund, K. 1963. A laboratory method of diagnosing predominance of homo- or heteroerotic interest in the male. *Behavior Research and Therapy* 12:355–359.

—— 1971. A note on the use of the phallometric method of measuring mild sexual arousal in the male. *Behavioral Therapy* 2:223–228.

Freund, K., R. Langevin, and D. H. Barlow. 1974. Comparison of two penile measures of erotic arousal. *Behavior Research and Therapy* 17:451–457.

Freund, K., R. Langevin, R. Chamberlayne, A. Deosoran, and Y. Zajac. 1974. The phobic theory of male homosexuality. *Archives of General Psychiatry* 31:495–499.

Friedman, R. C. 1983. Book Review: *Homosexuality* by Charles W. Socarides, M.D. *Journal of the American Psychoanalytic Association* 31:316–323.

—— 1988. *Male Homosexuality: A Contemporary Psychoanalytic Perspective.* New Haven: Yale University Press.

—— 1993a. Book review: *The Homosexualities: Reality, Fantasy and the Arts,* ed. C. Socarides and V. Volkan. *Journal of the American Psychoanalytic Association* 21:155–160.

—— 1993b. Book review: *The Homosexualities and the Therapeutic Process,* ed. C. Socarides and V. Volkan. *Journal of the American Psychoanalytic Association* 53:180–181.

—— 1997. Book review: *Reparative Therapy of Male Homosexuality: A New Clinical Approach,* by Joseph Nicolosi. *Archives of Sexual Behavior* 26:225–227.

—— 1998. Gender identity. *Psychiatric News* 33(2):10–31.

—— 1999. Homosexuality, psychopathology, and suicidality. *Archives of General Psychiatry* 56:887–888.

—— 2000. Book review of *Psychoanalytic Therapy and the Gay Man. Journal of Nervous and Mental Disease* 188:470–472.

—— 2001. A reply to Jack Drescher. *Journal of Nervous and Mental Disease* 189(2):130–131.

Friedman, R. C., and A. A. Lilling. 1996. An empirical study of the beliefs of psychoanalysts about scientific and clinical dimensions of homosexuality. *Journal of Homosexuality* 32:79–89.

Friedman, R. C., and J. Downey. 1993a. Neurobiology and sexual orientation: Current relationships. *Journal of Neuropsychiatric and Clinical Neurosciences* 5:131–153.

—— 1993b. Psychoanalysis, psychobiology, and homosexuality. *Journal of the American Psychoanalytic Association* 41:1159–1198.

—— 1993c. The psychoanalytic concept of bisexuality. Lecture of the Association for Psychoanalytic Medicine. New York, New York, February 2.

—— 1994. Special article: Homosexuality. *New England Journal of Medicine* 331:923–930.

—— 1995a. Biology and the Oedipus complex. *Psychoanalytic Quarterly* 64:234–264.

—— 1995b. Internalized homophobia and the negative therapeutic reaction in homosexual men. *Journal of the American Academy of Psychoanalysis* 23:99–113.

—— 1995c. Letter to the editor: MacIntosh Study Faulted. *Journal of the American Psychoanalytic Association* 43:304–305.

Friedman, R. C., and J. I. Downey, eds. 1999. *Masculinity and Sexuality: Selected Topics in the Psychology of Men.* Washington, D.C.: American Psychiatric.

Friedman, R. C., R. M. Richard, and R. L. Vande Wiele, eds. 1974. *Sex Differences in Behavior.* New York: Wiley.

Friedman, R. C., S. W. Hurt, M. S. Aronoff, and J. F. Clarkin. 1980. Behavior and the menstrual cycle. *Signs: Journal of Women in Culture and Society* 5:719–738. Repr. C. R. Stimpson and E. Spector Person, eds., *Women, Sex, and Sexuality,* pp. 192–212. Chicago: University of Chicago Press, 1980.

Friedman, T. 1999. *The Lexus and the Olive Tree.* New York: Random House.

Gabriel, M. A. 1996. *Aids Trauma and Support Group Therapy.* New York: Free.

Galenson, E. 1993. Sexuality in infancy and preschool-aged children. In A. Yates, ed., *Sexual and Gender Identity Disorders: Child and Adolescent Psychiatric Clinics of North America,* pp. 385–391. Philadelphia: Saunders.

Galenson, E., and Roiphe, H. 1971. The impact of early sexual discovery on mood, defensive organization, and symbolization. *Psychoanalytic Study of the Child* 26:195–216.

—— 1976. Some suggested revisions concerning early female development. *Journal of the American Psychoanalytic Association* 24:29–57.

—— 1980. The preoedipal development of the boy. *Journal of the American Psychoanalytic Association* 28:805–826.

—— 1981. *Infantile Origins of Sexual Activity.* New York: International Universities Press.

Gardner, R. A. 1969. Sexual fantasies in childhood. *Medical Aspects of Human Sexuality* 3:121–134.

Garofalo, R., R. C. Wolf, L. S. Wissow, E. R. Woods, and E. Goodman. 1999. Sexual orientation and risk of suicide attempts among a representative sample of youth. *Archives of Pediatric and Adolescent Medicine* 153:487–493.

Garofalo, R., R. C. Wolf, S. Kessel, J. Palfrey, and R. H. Durant. 1998. The association between health risk behaviors and sexual orientation among a school-based sample of adolescents. *Pediatrics* 101:895–902.

Gatz, M., N. L. Pedersen, S. Berg, B. Johansson, K. Johansson, J. A. Mortimer, S. F. Posner, M. Viitanen, B. Winblad, and A. Ahlbom. 1997. Heritability for Alzheimer's disease: The study of dementia in Swedish twins. *Journal of Gerontology* 52A:M117–M125.

Gay, P. 1988. *Freud: A Life for Our Time.* New York: Norton.

Geer, J. H., and G. M. Manguono-Mire. 1996. Gender differences in cognitive processes in sexuality. In R. C. Rosen, C. M. Davis, and H. J. Ruppel Jr., eds., *Annual Review of Sex Research* 6:90–124.

Gerson, B. P., and I. V. Carlier. 1992. Post-traumatic stress disorder: The history of the recent concept. *British Journal of Psychiatry* 16:742–744.

Geschwind, N., and A. M. Galaburda. 1985a. Cerebral lateralization: Biological mechanisms, associations and pathology. I: A hypothesis and a program for research. *Archives of Neurology* 42:428–459.

—— 1985b. Cerebral lateralization: Biological mechanisms, associations, and pathology. II: A hypothesis and a program for research. *Archives of Neurology* 42:521–552.

Gibbs, I., and I. Sinclair. 2000. Bullying, sexual harassment, and happiness in residential children's homes. *Child Abuse Review* 9:247–256.

Gilligan, C. 1982. *In a Different Voice.* Cambridge: Harvard University Press.

Gilligan, C., N. Lyons, and T. J. Hamner. 1989. *Making Connections.* Cambridge: Harvard University Press.

Gilligan, C., J. V. Ward, J. M. Taylor, and B. Bardige, eds. 1988. *Mapping the Moral Domain: A Contribution of Women's Thinking to Psychological Theory and Education.* Cambridge: Harvard University Press.

Gilmore, D. D. 1990. *Manhood in the Making.* New York: Yale University Press.

Glick, R., and D. I. Meyers. 1988. *Masochism: Current Psychoanalytic Perspectives,* pp. 93–117. Hillsdale, N.J.: Analytic.

Glick, R., and S. Roose, eds. 1993. *Rage, Power, and Aggression.* New Haven: Yale University Press.

Goffman, E. 1963. *Stigma: Notes on the Management of Spoiled Identity.* Englewood Cliffs, N.J.: Prentice-Hall.

Gold, S. R., and R. G. Gold. 1991. Gender differences in first sexual fantasies. *Journal of Sex Education and Therapy* 17:207–216.

Goldberg, J. S., R. Muir, and J. Kerr, eds. 1995. *Attachment Theory: Social, Developmental, and Clinical Perspectives.* Hillsdale, N.J.: Analytic.

Golden, C. 1987. Diversity and variability in women's sexual identities. In Boston Lesbian Psychologies Collective, ed., *Lesbian Psychologies: Aspirations and Challenges,* pp. 19–34. Urbana: University Illinois Press.

Goldman, S. B. 1995. An interview with Dr. Bertram Schaffner. In T. Domenici and R. C. Lesser, eds., *Disorienting Sexuality,* pp. 227–243. New York/London: Routledge.

Gonsiorek, J. C. 1995. Gay male identities: Concepts and issues. In A. R. D'Augelli and C.J. Patterson, eds., *Lesbian, Gay, and Bisexual Identities Over the Lifespan,* pp. 24–47. New York: Oxford University Press.

Goodman, L. A., M. P. Koss, L. F. Fitzgerald, N. F. Russo, and G. Puryear Keita. 1993. Male violence against women: Current research and future directions. *American Psychologist* 48:1054–1058.

Gooren, L., E. Fliers, and K. Courtney. 1990. Biological determinants of sexual orientation. *Annual Review of Sex Research* 1:175–196.

Gorski, R. A. 1991. Sexual differentiation of the endocrine brain and its control. In M. Motta, ed., *Brain Endocrinology,* pp. 71–103. 2d ed. New York: Raven.

Gorski, R. A., R. E. Harlan, C. D. Jacobson, J. E. Shryne, and A. M. Southam. 1980. Evidence for a morphological sex difference within the medial preoptic area of the rat brain. *Journal of Comparative Neurology* 193:529–539.

Goy, R. W., and B. S. McEwen, eds. 1980. *Sexual Differentiation of the Brain.* Cambridge: MIT Press.

Goy, R. W., and D. A. Goldfoot. 1974. Experimental and hormonal factors influencing development of sexual behavior in the male rhesus monkey. In F. O. Schmitt and F. G. Warden, eds., *The Neurosciences: Third Study Program,* pp. 571–581. Cambridge: MIT Press.

Green, B. 1990. Defining trauma: Terminology and generic stressor dimensions. *Journal of Applied Social Psychology* 20:1632–1642.

Green, B., J. Wilson, and J. Lindy. 1985. Conceptualizing post-traumatic stress disorder: A psychosocial framework. In C. R. Figley, ed., *Trauma and Its Wake.* New York: Brunner/Mazel.

Green, R. 1985. Gender identity in childhood and later sexual orientation: Follow-up of seventy-eight males. *American Journal of Psychiatry* 142:339–441.

—— 1987. *The "Sissy Boy Syndrome" and the Development of Homosexuality.* New Haven: Yale University Press.

Greenberg, D. F. 1988. *The Construction of Homosexuality.* Chicago: University of Chicago Press.

Greenberg, J. 1991. *Oedipus and Beyond: A Clinical Theory.* Cambridge: Harvard University Press.

Greenberg, J., and S. Mitchell. 1983. *Object Relations in Psychoanalytic Theory.* Cambridge: Harvard University Press.

Greenson, R. R. 1968. Disidentifying from mother. *International Journal of Psychoanalysis* 49:370–374.

Griffin, J. E. 1992. Androgen resistance: The clinical and molecular spectrum. *New England Journal of Medicine* 326:611–618.

Grinker, R., and J. Spiegel. 1945. *War Neuroses.* Philadelphia: Blakiston.

Grob, G. 1980. Psychiatry and social activism: The politics of a specialty in postwar America. *Bulletin of the History of Medicine* 60:477–501.

Groos, K. 1896. *Die Spiele der Tiere.* Jena: Fischer.

Gross, D. J., H. Landau, G. Kohn, A. Farkas, E. Elrayyes, R. el-Shawwa, E. E. Lasch, and A. Rosler. 1986. Male pseudohermaphroditism due to 17alpha-hydroxysteroid dehydrogenase deficiency: Gender reassignment in early infancy. *Acta Endocrinologica* 112:238–246.

Groth, A. N., and H. J. Birnbaum. 1978. Adult sexual orientation and attraction to underage persons. *Archives of Sexual Behavior* 7:175–181.

Group for the Advancement of Psychiatry (GAP). 1962. *Training in Psychiatry: The Preclinical Teaching of Psychiatry.* GAP Report no. 54. Washington, D.C.: American Psychiatric.

—— 2000. *Homosexuality and the Mental Health Professions: The Impact of Bias.* Hillsdale, N.J.: Analytic.

Grunbaum, A. 1984. *The Foundation of Psychoanalysis: A Philosophical Critique.* Berkeley: University of California Press.

—— 1998. A century of psychoanalysis: Critical retrospect and prospect. In M. Roth, ed., *Freud: Conflict and Culture,* pp. 1–16. New York: Knopf.

Habel, H. 1950. Zwillingsuntersuchungen an homosexuellen. *Zeitschr. Sexual Forsch.* 1:161–180.

Haldeman, D. C. 1991. Conversion therapy for gay men and lesbians: A scientific examination. In J. C. Gonsiorek and J. D. Weinrich, eds., *Homosexuality: Research Implications for Public Policy,* pp. 149–161. Newbury Park, Cal.: Sage.

—— 1994. The practice and ethics of sexual orientation conversion therapy. *Journal of Consulting and Clinical Psychology* 62:221–227.

Hale, N. C. 1995. *The Rise and Crisis of Psychoanalysis in the United States.* New York: Oxford University Press.

Hamer, D. H. 1999. Genetics and male sexual orientation. *Science* 285:803.

Hamer, D. H., S. Hu, V. L. Magnuson, N. Hu, and A. M. L. Pattatucci. 1993. A linkage between DNA markers on the X chromosome and male sexual orientation. *Science* 261:321–327.

Hampson, J. L., J. G. Hampson, and J. Money. 1955. The syndrome of gonadal agenesis (ovarian agenesis) and male chromosomal pattern in girls and women: Psychological studies. *Bulletin of the Johns Hopkins Hospital* 97:207–226.

Hanley, C. 1999. Subjectivity and objectivity in analysis. *Journal of the American Psychoanalytic Association* 47:427–445.

Hanson, A., and L. Hartmann. 1996. Latency development in prehomosexual boys. In R. P. Cabaj and T. S. Stein, eds., *Textbook of Homosexuality and Mental Health*, pp. 253–267. Washington, D.C.: American Psychiatric Press.

Harlow, H. F. 1986. *From Learning to Love: The Selected Papers of H. F. Harlow*. Ed. C. M. Harlow. New York: Praeger.

Harlow, H. F., and M. K. Harlow. 1965. The effect of rearing conditions on behavior. In J. Money, ed., *Sex Research: New Developments*, pp. 161–176. Baltimore: Johns Hopkins University Press.

Harry, J. 1983. Parasuicide, gender and gender deviance. *Journal of Health and Social Behavior* 24:350–361.

Hartmann, H. 1964. *Ego Psychology and the Problem of Adaptation*. New York: International Universities Press.

Hatfield, E., and R. L. Rapson. 1993. Historical and cross-cultural perspectives on passionate love and sexual desire. *Annual Review of Sex Research* 4:67–99.

Hays, R. B., J. Paul, M. Ekstrand, S. M. Kegeles, R. Stall, and T. J. Coates. 1997. Actual versus perceived HIV status, sexual behaviors and predictors of unprotected sex among gay and bisexual men who identify as HIV-negative, HIV-positive and untested. *AIDS* 11:1495–1502.

Heath, A. C., K. K. Bucholz, P. A. Madden, S. H. Dinwiddie, W. S. Slutske, L. J. Bierut, D. J. Statham, M. P. Dunne, J. B. Whitfield, and N. G. Martin. 1997. Genetic and environmental contributions to alcohol dependence risk in a national twin sample: Consistency of findings in women and men. *Psychological Medicine* 27:1381–1396.

Hedricks, C. A. 1994. Sexual behavior across the menstrual cycle: A biopsychosocial approach. *Annual Review of Sex Research* 5:122–173.

Heiman, J. 1977. A psychophysiological exploration of sexual arousal patterns in females and males. *Psychophysiology* 14:266–274.

—— 1980. Female sexual response patterns: Interactions of physiological, affective, and contextual cues. *Archives of General Psychiatry* 37:1311–1316.

Herbert, J. 1996. Sexuality, stress, and the chemical architecture of the brain. In R. C. Rosen, C. M. D. Davis, H. J. Ruppel Jr., S. L. Davis, and K. Johnson, eds., *Annual Review of Sex Research* 7:1–44. Mason City, Iowa: Society for the Scientific Study of Sexuality.

Herbert, S. E. 1996. Lesbian sexuality. In R. P. Cabaj and T. S. Stein, eds., *Textbook of Homosexuality and Mental Health*, pp. 723–742. Washington, D.C.: American Psychiatric.

Herdt, G., and M. McClintock. 2000. The magical age of ten. *Archives of Sexual Behavior* 29(6):587–606.

Herdt, G., ed. 1989. *Gay and Lesbian Youth*. New York: Harrington Park.

Herek, G. 1984. Beyond "homophobia": A social psychological perspective on attitudes toward lesbians and gay men. *Journal of Homosexuality* 10:1–21.

—— 1985. Beyond homophobia: A social psychological perspective on the attitudes toward lesbians and gay men. In J. DeCecco, ed., *Bashers, Baiters, and Bigots: Homophobia in American Society,* pp. 1–21. New York: Harrington Park.

—— 1991. Stigma, prejudice, and violence against lesbians and gay men. In J. Gonsiorek and J. Weinrich, eds., *Homosexuality: Research Implications for Public Policy,* pp. 60–80. Newbury Park, Cal.: Sage.

—— 1995. Psychological heterosexism in the United States. In A. R. D'Augelli and C. J. Patterson, eds., *Lesbian, Gay, and Bisexual Identities Over the Lifespan,* p. 321. Oxford: Oxford University Press.

—— 1996. Heterosexism and hompohobia. In R. P. Cabaj and T. Stein, eds., *Textbook of Homosexuality and Mental Health,* pp. 101–113. Washington, D.C.: American Psychiatric.

Herek, G. M., and K. T. Berrill, eds. 1992. *Hate Crimes: Confronting Violence Against Lesbians and Gay Men.* Newbury Park, Cal.: Sage.

Herrel, R., J. Goldberg, W. R. True, V. Ramarkrishnam, M. Lyons, S. Eisen, and M. T. Tsuang. 1999. Sexual orientation and suicidality: A co-twin controlled study in adult men. *Archives of General Psychiatry* 56:867–874.

Hertzberg, H. 1998. The Narcissus survey. *New Yorker,* January 5, 1998, pp. 27–30.

Hines, M. 1998. Abnormal sexual development and psychosexual issues. *Baillieres Clinical Endocrinology and Metabolism* 12(1):173–189.

Hines, M., and F. R. Kaufman. 1994. Androgen and the development of human sex-typical behavior: Rough and tumble play and sex of preferred playmates in children with Congenital Adrenal Hyperplasia (CAH). *Child Development* 65:1042–1053.

Hirschfeld, M. 1914. *Die Homosexualitaet des Mannes und des Weibes. Handbuck der Gesamtem Sexualwissenschaft in Einzeldarstellungen,* vol. 3. Berlin: Louis Marcus.

Hite, S. 1976. *The Hite Report.* New York: Macmillan.

Hochberg, Z., R. Chayen, N. Reiss, Z. Falik, A. Makler, M. Munichor, A. Farkas, H. Goldfarb, N. Ohana, and O. Hiort. 1996. Clinical, biochemical, and genetic findings in a large pedigree of male and female patients with 5alpha-reductase 2 deficiency. *Journal of Clinical Endocrinology and Metabolism* 81:2821–2827.

Holden, C. 1997. A gene is linked to autism. *Science* 276:905.

Holt, R. R. 1989. *Freud Reappraised.* New York: Guilford.

Holzman, P. S. 1976. The future of psychoanalysis and its institutes. *Psychoanalytic Quarterly* 65:250–273.

Hooker, E. 1957. The adjustment of the male overt homosexual. *J. Proj. Tech.* 21:18–31.

Horney, K. 1924. On the genesis of the castration complex in women. *International Journal of Psycho-Analysis* 5:50–65.

—— 1926. The flight from womanhood: The masculinity-complex in women as viewed by men and women. *International Journal of Psycho-Analysis* 7:324–339.

—— 1937. *The Neurotic Personality of Our Time.* New York: Norton.

—— 1939. *New Ways in Psychoanalysis.* New York: Norton.

Horowitz, M. J. 1976. *Stress Response Syndromes.* New York: Jason Aronson.

Hu, S., A. M. Pattatucci, C. Patterson, L. Li, D. W. Fulker, S. S. Cherny, L. Kruglyak, and D. H. Hamer. 1995. Linkage between sexual orientation and chromosome Xq28 in males but not in females. *Nature Genetics* 11:248–256.

Imperato-McGinley, J., L. Guerrero, T. Gautier, and R. E. Peterson. 1974. Steroid 5alpha-reductase deficiency in man: An inherited form of male pseudohermaphroditism. *Science* 186:1213–1215.

Imperato-McGinley, J., M. Miller, J. D. Wilson, R. E. Peterson, C. Shackleton, and D. C. Gajdusek. 1991. A cluster of male pseudohermaphrodites with 5alpha-reductase deficiency in Papua New Guinea. *Clinical Endocrinology* 34:293–298.

Imperato-McGinley, J., R. E. Peterson, T. Gautier, and E. Sturla. 1979. Androgens and the evolution of male-gender identity among male pseudohermaphrodites with 5alpha-reductase deficiency. *New England Journal of Medicine* 30:1233–1237.

Imperato-McGinley, J., T. Gautier, R. E. Peterson, and C. Shackleton. 1986. The prevalence of 5alpha-reductase deficiency in children with ambiguous genitalia in the Dominican Republic. *Journal of Urology* 136:867–873.

Inderbetzin, L. B., and S. T. Levy. 1990. Unconscious fantasy: A reconsideration of the concept. *Journal of the American Psychoanalytic Association* 38:113–130.

Isay, R. 1989. *Being Homosexual: Gay Men and Their Development.* New York: Farrar, Straus and Giroux.

—— 1991a. The development of sexual identity in homosexual men. In S. I. Greenspan and G. H. Pollock, eds., *The Course of Life*, vol. 4: *Adolescence*, pp. 453–467. Madison, Conn.: International Universities Press.

—— 1991b. The homosexual analyst: Clinical considerations. *Psychoanalytic Study of the Child* 46:199–216.

—— 1993. The homosexual analyst: Clinical considerations. In C. Cornett, *Affirmative Dynamic Psychotherapy with Gay Men*, pp. 177–198. Northvale, N.J.: Jason Aronson.

—— 1996. *Becoming Gay: The Journey to Self-Acceptance.* New York: Pantheon.

—— 1997. Remove gender identity disorder in DSM. *Psychiatric News* 32(2):9–13.

—— 1998. Heterosexually married homosexual men: Clinical and developmental issues. *American Journal of Orthopsychiatry* 68:424–432.

Jacobson, E. 1964. *The Self and the Object World.* New York: International Universities Press.

Johnson, A. M., J. Wadsworth, K. Wellings, J. Field, and S. Bradshaw. 1994. *Sexual Attitudes and Lifestyles.* Oxford: Blackwell Scientific.

Jones, E. 1927. The early development of female sexuality. *International Journal of Psycho-Analysis* 8:459–472.

Kagan, J. 1984. *The Nature of the Child.* New York: Basic.

Kahn, M. 1962. The role of infantile sexuality in early object relations in female homosexuality. In I. Rosen, ed., *The Pathology and Treatment of Sexual Perversions*, pp. 221–292. Oxford: Oxford University Press.

Kallman, F. J. 1952a. *Heredity in Health and Mental Disorder: Principles of Psychiatric Genetics in the Light of Comparative Twin Studies.* New York: Norton.

Kandel, E. R. 1999. Biology and the future of psychoanalysis: A new intellectual framework for psychiatry revisited. *American Journal of Psychiatry* 156:505–524.

Kaplan, H. S. 1979. *Disorders of Sexual Desire.* New York: Simon and Schuster.

Kaprio, J., M. Koskenvuo, and R. J. Rose. 1990. Change in cohabitation and intrapair similarity of monozygotic (MZ) twins for alcohol use, extraversion, and neuroticism. *Behavior Genetics* 20:265–276.

Kardiner, A., A. Karush, and L. Ovesey. 1959. A methodological study of Freudian theory. *Journal of Nervous and Mental Diseases 129:1. Repr. 1999. International Journal of Psychiatry* 2(5):489–542.

Kardiner, A., and H. Spiegel. 1947. *War Stress and Neurotic Illness.* New York: International Universities Press.

Katchadourian, H. A., and O. T. Lunde. 1972. *Fundamentals of Human Sexuality.* New York: Holt, Rinehart, and Winston.

Keegan, J. 1994. *A History of Warfare.* New York: Vintage.

Kendler, K. S., C. MacLean, M. Neale, R. Kessler, A. Heath, and L. Eaves. 1991. The genetic epidemiology of bulimia nervosa. *American Journal of Psychiatry* 148:1627–1637.

Kendler, K. S., L. M. Thornton, and C. O. Gardner. 2000. Stressful life events and previous episodes in the etiology of major depression in women: An evaluation of the "kindling" hypothesis. *American Journal of Psychiatry* 157:1243–1251.

Kendler, K. S., L. M. Thornton, S. E. Gilman, and R. C. Kessler. 2000. Sexual orientation in a U.S. national sample of twin and nontwin sibling pairs. *American Journal of Psychiatry* 157:1843–1846.

Kendler, K. S., M. C. Neale, R. C. Kessler, A. C. Heath, and L. J. Eaves. 1993. Panic disorder in women: A population-based twin study. *Psychological Medicine* 23:397–406.

Kennedy, H. 1980–1981. The third sex theory of Karl Heinrich Ulrichs. *Journal of Homosexuality* 6:103–111.

Kernberg, O. 1975. *Borderline Conditions and Pathological Narcissism.* New York: Jason Aronson.

—— 1976. *Object Relations Theory and Clinical Psychoanalysis.* New York: Jason Aronson.

—— 1980. *Internal World and External Reality.* New York: Jason Aronson.

—— 1988. Clinical dimensions of masochism. In R. A. Glick and D. I. Meyers, eds., *Masochism: Current Psychoanalytic Perspectives,* pp. 61–81. Hillsdale, N.J.: Analytic.

—— 1995. *Love Relations: Normality and Pathology.* New Haven: Yale University Press.

—— 2000. A concerned critique of psychoanalytic education. *International Journal of Psycho-Analysis* 81:97–121.

Kernberg, O., E. Burstein, L. Coyne, A. Applebaum, L. Horowitz, and H. Voth. 1972. Psychotherapy and psychoanalysis: Final report of the Menninger Foundation's Psychotherapy Research Project. *Bulletin of the Menninger Clinic* 36:1–275.

Kimura, O. 1999. *Sex and Cognition.* Cambridge: MIT Press.

Kinsey, A. C., W. B. Pomeroy, C. E. Martin. 1948. *Sexual Behavior in the Human Male.* Philadelphia: Saunders.

—— 1953. *Sexual Behavior in the Human Female.* Philadelphia: Saunders.

Kipnis, K., and M. Diamond. 1998. Pediatric ethics and the surgical assignment of sex. *Journal of Clinical Ethics* 9(4):398–408.

Kirkpatrick, M. 1984. Female homosexuality. Annual Meeting of American Psychoanalytic Association, San Diego, May 4.

—— 1987. Clinical implications of lesbian mother studies. *Journal of Homosexuality* 13:201–211.

—— 1989. Women in love in the 1980s. *Journal of the American Academy of Psychoanalysis* 17:535–542.

Klein, M. 1937. *The Psychoanalysis of Children.* 2d ed. London: Hogarth.

Klinger, R. L. 1996. Lesbian couples. In R. P. Cabaj and T. S. Stein, eds., *Textbook of Homosexuality and Mental Health,* pp. 339–352. Washington, D.C.: American Psychiatric.

Knight, R. P. 1941. Evaluation of the results of psychoanalytic therapy. *American Journal of Psychiatry* 11:434–446.

Kohlberg, L. 1976. *Moral Developmental and Behavior: Theory, Research, and Social Issues,* pp. 31–53. Ed. T. Lickona. New York: Holt, Rinehart and Winston.

—— 1981. *The Philosophy of Moral Development, Moral States, and the Idea of Justice: Essays on Moral Development.* New York: Harper and Row.

Kohut, H. 1971. *The Analysis of the Self.* New York: International Universities Press.

—— 1977. *The Restoration of the Self.* New York: International Universities Press.

Kolodny, R. C., W. H. Masters, J. H. Hendryx, and G. Toro. 1971. Plasma testosterone and semen analysis in male homosexuals. *New England Journal of Medicine* 285: 1170–1174.

Krafft-Ebing, R. 1965 [1886]. *Psychopathia Sexualis: A Medico-Forensic Study.* Trans. H. E. Wedeck. New York: Putnam.

Krystal, H. 1968. *Massive Trauma.* New York: International Universities Press.

—— 1978. Trauma and affects. *Psychoanalytic Study of the Child* 33:81–116.

Kwar, J. 1980. Transference and countertransference in homosexuality: Changing psychoanalytic views. *American Journal of Psychotherapy* 34:72–80.

Laan, E., and W. Everaerd. 1995. Determinants of female sexual arousal: Psychophysiological theory and data. *Annual Review of Sex Research* 6:32–77.

Lalumiere, M. L., R. Blanchard, and K. L. Zucker. 2000. Sexual orientation and handedness in men and women: A meta-analysis. *Psychological Bulletin* 126:1–18.

Langfeldt, T. 1981. Sexual development in children. In M. Cook and K. Howells, eds., *Adult Sexual Interest in Children,* pp. 99–120. New York: Academic.

Lasenza, S., P. L. Colucci, and B. Rothberg. 1996. Coming out and the mother-daughter bond. In J. Laird and R. J. Green, eds., *Lesbians and Gays in Couples and Families: A Handbook for Therapists,* pp. 123–136. San Francisco: Jossey-Bass.

Laumann, E. O., J. H. Gagnon, R. T. Michael, and S. Michaels. 1994. *The Social Organization of Sexuality: Sexual Practices in the United States.* Chicago: University of Chicago Press.

Leaper, C., ed. 1994. *Childhood Gender Segregation.* San Francisco: Jossey-Bass.

Leitenberg, H., and K. Henning. 1995. Sexual fantasy. *Psychological Bulletin* 117:469–496.

Leitenberg, H., M. J. Detzer, and D. Srebnik. 1993. Gender differences in masturbation and the relation of masturbation experiences in pre-adolescence and/or early adolescence to sexual behavior and sexual adjustment in young adulthood. *Archives of Sexual Behavior* 22:87–98.

LeVay, S. 1991. A difference in hypothalamic structure between heterosexual and homosexual men. *Science* 253:1034–1037.

—— 1993. *The Sexual Brain.* Cambridge: MIT Press.

—— 1996. *Queer Science.* Cambridge: MIT Press.

Lewes, K. 1988. *The Psychoanalytic Theory of Male Homosexuality.* New York: Simon and Schuster.

Lewis, D. O. 1989 [1967]. Adult antisocial behavior and criminality. In H. I. Kaplan and B. J. Sadock, eds., *Comprehensive Textbook of Psychiatry* 2:1400–1405. 5th ed. Baltimore: Williams and Wilkins.

Lewis, M. 1992. *Shame: The Exposed Self.* New York: Free.

Lidz, T., and R. W. Lidz. 1989. *Oedipus in the Stone Age: A Psychoanalytic Study of Masculinization in Papua, New Guinea.* Madison, Conn.: International University Press.

Lief, H. I., and H. S. Kaplan. 1986. Ego-dystonic homosexuality. *Journal of Sex and Marital Therapy* 12(14):259–266.

Lief, H. I., and P. Mayerson. 1965. Psychotherapy of homosexuals. In J. Marmor, ed., *Sexual Inversion,* pp. 302–344. New York: Basic.

Lifton, R. J. 1976. The human meaning of total disaster: The Buffalo Creek experience. *Psychiatry* 39:1–17.

Lilling, A. A., and R. C. Friedman. 1995. Bias toward gay patients by psychoanalytic clinicians: An empirical investigation. *Archives of Sexual Behavior* 24:563–570.

Lock, J., and H. Steiner. 1999. Gay, lesbian, and bisexual youth risks for emotional, physical, and social problems: Results from a community-based survey. *Journal of the American Academy of Child and Adolescent Psychiatry* 38:297–304.

Loewald, H. W. 1978. The Waning of the Oedipus complex. Plenary address, American Psychoanalytic Association, May 6. Repr. 1980. *Papers on Psychoanalysis,* pp. 384–404. New Haven: Yale University Press.

Losoya, S. H., S. Callor, D. C. Rowe, and H. H. Goldsmith. 1997. Origins of familial similarity in parenting: A study of twins and adoptive siblings. *Developmental Psychology* 33:1012–1023.

Lothane, Z. 1992. *In Defense of Schreber: Soul Murder and Psychiatry.* Hillsdale, N.J.: Analytic.

Luborsky, L., C. Popp, J. P. Barber, and D. Shapiro, eds. 1994. *Psychotherapy Research* 4(3/4):151–290 (special issue).

Lykken D. T., T. J. Bouchard Jr., M. McGue, and A. Tellegen. 1993. Heritability of interests: A twin study. *Journal of Applied Psychology* 78:649–661.

Lyons, M. J., W. R. True, S. A. Eisen, J. Goldberg, J. M. Meyer, S. V. Faraone, L. J. Eaves, and M. T. Tsuang. 1995. Differential heritability of adult and juvenile antisocial traits. *Archives of General Psychiatry* 52:906–915.

MacAlpine, I., and R. A. Hunter. 1953. The Schreber case: A contribution to schizophrenia, hypochondria, and psychosomatic symptom formation. *Psychoanalytic Quarterly* 11:328–371.

McClearn, G. E., B. Johansson, and S. Burg. 1997. Substantial genetic influence on cognitive abilities in twins eighty or more years old. *Science* 276:1560–1563.

McClintock, M., and G. Herdt. 1996. Rethinking puberty: The development of sexual attraction. *Current Directions in Psychological Science* 5:167–183.

Maccoby, E. E. 1990. Gender and relationships: A developmental account. *American Psychologist* 45:513–520.

—— 1998. *The Two Sexes: Growing Up Apart, Coming Together.* Cambridge: Harvard University Press.

Maccoby, E. E., and C. N. Jacklin. 1974. *The Psychology of Sex Differences.* Palo Alto: Stanford University Press.

McConaghy, N. 1993. *Sexual Behavior: Problems and Management.* New York: Plenum.

—— 1999. Unresolved issues in scientific sexology. *Archives of Sexual Behavior* 28:285–319.

McConaghy, N., and M. A. Blaszczynski. 1980. A pair of monozygotic twins discordant for homosexuality: Sex-dimorphic behavior and penile volume responses. *Archives of Sexual Behavior* 9:123–131.

McConigle, M. M., T. W. Smith, L. S. Benjamin, and C. W. Turner. 1993. Hostility and nonshared family environment: A study of monozygotic twins. *Journal of Research in Personality* 27:23–34.

McCormick, C. M., and S. F. Witelson. 1991. A cognitive profile of homosexual men compared to heterosexual men and women. *Psychoneuroendocrinology* 16:459–473.

McCormick, C. M., S. F. Witelson, and E. Kingstone. 1990. Left-handedness in homosexual men and women: Neuroendocrine implications. *Psychoneuroendocrinology* 15:69–76.

McDougall, J. 1980. *Plea for a Measure of Abnormality*. New York: International Universities Press.

McEwen, B. A. 1983. Gonadal steroid influences on brain development and sexual differentiation. In R. Greep, ed., *Reproductive Physiology* 4:99–145. Baltimore: University Park Press.

McGue, M., and T. J. Bouchard Jr. 1998. Genetic and environmental influences on human behavioral difference. *Annual Review of Neuroscience* 21:1–24.

McWhirter, D. P., and A. M. Mattison. 1984. *The Male Couple: How Relationships Develop*. New York: Prentice-Hall.

—— 1996. Male couples. In R. P. Cabaj and T. S. Stein, eds., *Textbook of Homosexuality and Mental Health,* pp. 329–337. Washington, D.C.: American Psychiatric.

Magee, M., and D. Miller. 1997. *Lesbian Lives: Psychoanalytic Narratives, Old and New*. Hillsdale, N.J.: Analytic.

Malyon, A. K. 1982. Psychotherapeutic implications of internalized homophobia in gay men. *Journal of Homosexuality* 7:59–69.

Mann, J., and D. Tarantola, eds. 1996. *AIDS in the World II*. New York: Oxford University Press.

Marmor, J. 1980. *Homosexual Behavior*. New York: Basic.

—— 1996. Nongay therapists working with gay men and lesbians: A personal reflection. In R. P. Cabaj and T. S. Stein, eds., *Textbook of Homosexuality and Mental Health,* pp. 539–545. Washington, D.C.: American Psychiatric.

Masica, D. N., J. Money, and A. A. Ehrhardt. 1971. Fetal feminization and female gender identity in the testicular feminizing syndrome of androgen insensitivity. *Archives of Sexual Behavior* 1:131–142.

Masson, J. M., ed. and trans. 1985. *The Complete Letters of Sigmund Freud to Wilhelm Fleiss, 1887–1904*. Cambridge: Harvard University Press.

Masters, W. H., and V. E. Johnson. 1966. *Human Sexual Response*. Boston: Little, Brown.

Mattison, A. M., and D. P. McWhirter. 1995. Lesbians, gay men, and their families. *Psychiatric Clinics of North America* 18:123–137.

Meaney, M. J. 1989. The sexual differentiation of social play. *Psychiatric Development* 3:247–261.

Meaney, M. J., A. M. Dodge, and W. W. Beatty. 1981. Sex dependent effects of amygdaloid lesions on the social play of prepubertal rats. *Physiological Behavior* 26:467–472.

Meaney, M. J., and B. S. McEwen. 1986. Testosterone implants into the amygdala during the neonatal period masculinize the social play of juvenile female rats. *Brain Research* 398:324–328.

Meaney, M. J., J. Stewart, and W. W. Beatty. 1985. Sex differences in social play: The socialization of sex roles. In J. S. Rosenblatt, C. Bear, C.M. Busnell, and P. Plater, eds., *Advances in the Study of Behavior* 15:33. San Diego: Academic.

Meissner, W. W. 1981. *Internalization in Psychoanalysis.* Psychological Issues Monograph no. 50. New York: International Universities Press.

Mendez, J. P, A. Ulloa-Aguirre, J. Imperato-McGinley, A. Brugmann, M. Delfin, B. Chavez, C. Shackleton, S. Kofman-Alfaro, and G. Perez-Palacios. 1995. Male pseudohermaphroditism due to primary 5alpha-reductase deficiency: Variation in gender identity reversal in seven Mexican patients from five different pedigrees. *Journal of Endocrinological Investigation* 18:205–213.

Mendonca, B. B., M. Inacio, E. M. F. Costa, I. J. P. Arnhold, F.A. Silva, W. Nicolau, W. Bloise, D. W. Russell, and J. D. Wilson. 1996. Male pseudohermaphroditism due to steroid 5alpha-reductase 2 deficiency: Diagnosis, psychological evaluation, and management. *Medicine* 75:64–76.

Mendonca, B. B., W. Bloise, I. J. P. Arnhold, M. C. Batista, S. P. de Almeida Toledo, M. C. F. Drummond, W. Nicolau, and E. Mattar. 1987. Male pseudohermaphroditism due to nonsalt-losing 3alpha-hydroxysteroid dehydrogenase deficiency: Gender role change and absence of gynecomastia at puberty. *Journal of Steroid Biochemistry* 28:669–675.

Menninger, K. 1963. *The Vital Balance.* New York: Viking.

Meston, C. M., and P. F. Frohlich. 2000. The neurobiology of sexual function. *Archives of General Psychiatry* 11:1012–1033.

Meyer, I. H. 1995. Minority stress and mental health in gay men. *Journal of Health and Social Behavior* 36:38–56.

Meyer-Bahlburg, H. F. L. 1993. Psychobiologic research on homosexuality. In A. Yates, ed., *Sexual and Gender Identity Disorders: Child and Adolescent Psychiatric Clinics of North America,* pp. 489–500. Philadelphia: Saunders.

—— 1998. Gender assignment in intersexuality. *Journal of Psychology and Human Sexuality* 10:1–21.

—— 1999. Variants of gender differentiation. In H.-C. Steinhausen and F. C. Verhulst, eds., *Risks and Outcomes in Developmental Psychopathology,* pp. 298–313. New York: Oxford University Press.

Meyer-Bahlburg, H. F. L., A. A. Ehrhardt, L. R. Rosen, R. S. Gruen, N. P. Veridiano, H. F. Neuwalder, and F. H. V. Neuwalder. 1995. Prenatal estrogens and the development of homosexual orientation. *Developmental Psychology* 31:12–21.

Meyer-Bahlburg, H. F. L., G. C. Grisanti, and A. A. Ehrhardt. 1977. Prenatal effect of sex hormones on human male behavior: Medroxyprogesterone acetate (MPA). *Psychoneuroendocrinology* 2:383–390.

Meyer-Bahlburg, H. F. L., J. F. Feldman, P. Cohen, P. Cohen, and A. A. Ehrhardt. 1988. Perinatal factors in the development of gender-related play behavior: Sex hormones versus pregnancy complications. *Psychiatry* 51:260–271.

Michaels, S. 1996. The prevalence of homosexuality in the United States. In R. P. Cabaj and T. S. Stein, eds., *Textbook of Homosexuality and Mental Health*, pp. 43–63. Washington, D.C.: American Psychiatric.

Mitchell, E. D., and B. S. Mason. 1935. *The Theory of Play*. New York: Barnes.

Mitchell, S. 1988. *Relational Concepts in Psychoanalysis: An Integration*. Cambridge: Harvard University Press.

Monette, P. 1992. *Becoming A Man*. New York: Harcourt Brace Jovanovich.

Money, J. 1955. Hermaphroditism, gender, and precocity in hyperadrenocorticism: Psychologic findings. *Bulletin of the Johns Hopkins Hospital* 96:253–264.

—— 1988. *Gay, Straight, and In-Between: The Sexology of Erotic Orientation*. New York: Oxford University Press.

—— 1994. *Sex Errors of the Body and Related Syndromes: A Guide to Counseling Children, Adolescents, and Their Families*. 2d ed. Baltimore: Brookes.

Money, J., and A. A. Ehrhardt. 1972. *Man and Woman, Boy and Girl: The Differentiation and Dimorphism of Gender Identity from Conception to Maturity*. Baltimore: Johns Hopkins University Press.

Money, J., A. A. Ehrhardt, and D. N. Masica. 1968. Fetal feminization induced by androgen insensitivity in the testicular feminizing syndrome: Effect on marriage and maternalism. *Johns Hopkins Medical Journal* 123:105–114.

Money, J., and D. Mathews. 1982. Prenatal exposure to virilizing progestins: An adult follow-up study of twelve women. *Archives of Sexual Behavior* 11:73–83.

Money, J., H. Devore, and B. F. Norman. 1986. Gender identity and gender transposition: Longitudinal outcome study of 32 male hermaphrodites assigned as girls. *Journal of Sex and Marital Therapy* 12:165–181.

Moore, B. E., and B. D. Fine. 1990. *Psychoanalytic Terms and Concepts*, pp. 86–87. New Haven: American Psychoanalytic Association and Yale University Press.

Moore, B. E., and B. D. Fine, eds. 1995. *Psychoanalysis: The Major Concepts*. New Haven: Yale University Press.

Morel, B. A. 1857. *Traite des Degenerescences Physiquales de L'Espece Humain*. Paris: Bailliere.

—— 1860. Traite des Maladies Mentales. Paris: Masson

Morris, J. M. 1953. The syndrome of testicular feminization in male pseudohermaphrodites. *American Journal of Obstetrics and Gynecology* 65:1192–1211.

Morris, J. M., and V. B. Mahesh. 1963. Further observations on the syndrome "testicular feminization." *American Journal of Obstetrics and Gynecology* 87:731–748.

Morrison, A. P. 1989. *Shame*. Hillsdale, N.J.: Analytic.

Moyer, K. E. 1974. Sex differences in aggression. In R. C. Friedman, R. M. Richard, and R. L. Vande Wiele, eds., *Sex Differences in Behavior*, pp. 335–372. New York: Wiley.

Moyer, K. E., ed. 1976. *Physiology of Aggression*. New York: Raven.

Muehrer, P. 1995. Suicide and sexual orientation: A critical summary of recent research and directions for future research. *Suicide and Life Threatening Behavior* 25(Suppl): 72–81.

Mynard, H., S. Joseph, and J. Alexander. 2000. Peer-victimisation and posttraumatic stress in adolescents. *Personality and Individual Differences* 29:815–821.

Nansel, T. R., M. Overpeck, R. S. Pilla, W. J. Ruan, B. Simons-Morton, and P. Scheidt. Bullying behaviors among U.S. youth: Prevalence and association with psychosocial adjustment. *Journal of the American Medical Association* 285:2131–2132.

Neubauer, P. B., and A. Neubauer. 1990. *Nature's Thumbprint: The New Genetics of Personality.* New York: Columbia University Press.

Nicolopoulou, A. 1997. Worldmaking and identity formation in children's narrative play-acting. In B. Cox and C. Lightfood, eds., *Sociogenic Perspectives in Internalization,* pp. 157–187. Hillsdale, N.J.: Erlbaum.

Nicolopoulou, A., B. Scales, and J. Weintraub. 1994. Gender differences and symbolic imagination in the stories of four year olds. In A. H. Dyson and C. Geneshi, eds., *The Need for Story: Cultural Diversity in Classroom and Community,* pp. 102–123. Urbana, Ill.: National Council of Teachers of English.

Nicolosi, J. 1991. *Reparative Therapy of Male Homosexuality.* Northvale, N.J.: Jason Aronson.

O'Connell, P., D. Pepler, and W. Craig. 1999. Peer involvement in bullying: Insights and challenges for intervention. *Journal of Adolescence* 22:437–452.

O'Connor, N., and J. Ryan. 1993. *Wild Desires and Mistaken Identities: Lesbianism and Psychoanalysis.* New York: Columbia University Press.

Oates, W. J., ed. 1948. *Basic Writings of St. Augustine.* New York: Random House.

Ochberg, F. M. 1995. *Post-Traumatic Therapy and Victims of Violence.* New York: Brunner/Mazel.

Offerdahl, J. 1993. *Sports Illustrated,* July, p. 48.

Olds, D. D. 1994. Connectionism and psychoanalysis. *Journal of the American Psychoanalytic Association* 42:581–613.

Oliner, S. P., and P. M. Oliner. 1988. *The Altruistic Personality.* New York: Free.

Oliver, M. B., and J. S. Hyde. 1993. Gender differences in sexuality: A meta analysis. *Psychological Bulletin* 14:29–51.

Oomura, Y., H. Yoshimatsu, and S. Aou. 1983. Medial preoptic and hypothalamic neuronal activity during sexual behavior of the male monkey. *Brain Research* 266:340–343.

Oomura, Y., S. Aou, Y. Koyama, and H. Yoshimatsu. 1988. Central control of sexual behavior. *Brain Research Bulletin* 20:863–870.

Ovesey, L. 1969. *Homosexuality and Pseudohomosexuality.* New York: Science House.

Ovesey, L., and W. Gaylin. 1965. Psychotherapy of male homosexuality: Prognosis, selection of patients, technique. *American Journal of Psycho-Therapy* 19:385–396.

Ovesey, L., W. Gaylin, and H. Hendin. 1963. Psychotherapy of male homosexuality. *Archives of General Psychiatry* 9:19–31.

Panel. 1983. Toward a further understanding of homosexual men. Presented at the American Psychoanalytic Association, New York. Summary by R. C. Friedman in *Journal of the American Psychoanalytic Association* 34(1986):193–206.

—— 1989. Enactments in psychoanalysis. Presented at the American Psychoanalytic Association, San Francisco.

—— 1998. Homophobia: Analysis of a "permissible" prejudice. Presented at the American Psychoanalytic Association, New York.

Paredes, R. G., and M. J. Baum. 1997. Role of the medial preoptic area/anterior hypothalamus in the control of masculine sexual behavior. In R. C. Rosen, C. M. D. Davis,

H. J. Ruppel Jr., S. L. Davis, and K. Johnson, eds., *Annual Review of Sex Research* 7:68–102. Mason City, Iowa: Society for the Scientific Study of Sexuality.

Patterson, C. 1995. Lesbian mothers, gay fathers and their children. In A. R. D'Augelli and C. J. Patterson, eds., *Lesbian, Gay, and Bisexual Identities Over the Lifespan,* pp. 262–290. Oxford: Oxford University Press.

—— 1996. Lesbian mothers and their children: Findings from the Bay Area Families Study. In J. Laird and R. J. Green, eds., *Lesbians and Gays in Couples and Families: A Handbook for Therapists,* pp. 420–437. San Francisco: Jossey-Bass.

Pelligrini, A. D., and P. I. Smith. 1998. Physical activity play: The nature and functions of a neglected aspect of play. *Child Development* 69:577–598.

Peplau, L. A., L. D. Garnets, L. R. Spalding, T. D. Conley, and R. C. Veniegas. 1998. A critique of Bem's "Exotic Becomes Erotic" theory of sexual orientation. *Psychological Review* 105(2):387–394.

Perachio, A. A., L. D. Marr, and M. Alexander. 1979. Sexual behavior in male rhesus monkeys elicited by electrical stimulation of preoptic and hypothalamic areas. *Brain Research* 177:127–144.

Perez-Palacios, G., A. Brügmann, J. Imperato-McGinley, S. Bassol, E. Valdes, J. P. Mendez, and A. Ulloa-Aguirre. 1984. Variability on the gender identity in the syndrome of 5alpha-steroid reductase deficiency. *Prostate* 5:355.

Perez-Palacios, G., B. Chavez, J. P. Mendez, J. Imperato-McGinley, and A. Ulloa-Aguirre. 1987. The syndromes of androgen resistance revisited. *Journal of Steroid Biochemistry* 27:1101–1108.

Persky, H., H. I. Lief, D. Strauss, W. R. Miller, and C. P. O'Brien. 1978. Plasma testosterone level and sexual behavior of couples. *Archives of Sexual Behavior* 7:157–173.

Persky, H., L. Dresbach, W. R. Miller, C. P. O'Brien, M. A. Khan, H. I. Lief, N. Charney, and D. Strauss. 1982. The relation of plasma androgen levels to sexual behaviors and attitudes of women. *Psychosomatic Medicine* 44(4):305–319.

Person, E. 1980. Sexuality as the mainstay of identity. In C. R. Stimpson and E. Person, eds., *Women, Sex, Sexuality.* Chicago: University of Chicago Press.

—— 1995. *By Force of Fantasy.* New York: Basic.

Person, E., N. Terestman, W. Myers, E. Goldberg, and C. Salvadori. 1989. Gender differences in sexual behaviors and fantasies in a college population. *Journal of Sex and Marital Therapy* 15:187–198.

Pfaff, D. W. 1999. *Drive: Neurobiological and Molecular Mechanisms of Sexual Motivation.* Cambridge: MIT Press.

Phoenix, C. H., R. W. Goy, A. A. Gerall, and W. C. Young. 1959. Organizing action of prenatally administered testosterone propionate on the tissues mediating mating behavior in the female guinea pig. *Endocrinology* 65:369–382.

Pitcher, E. G., and E. Prelinger. 1963. *Children Tell Stories: An Analysis of Fantasies.* New York: International Universities Press.

Plomin, R., and D. Daniels. 1987. Why are children in the same family so different from one another? *Behavioral and Brain Sciences* 10:1–16.

Ploog, D. W., and P. D. MacLean. 1963. Penile display in the squirrel monkey. *Animal Behavior* 11:32–39.

Pollack, W. P. 1998. *Real Boys.* New York: Holt.

Ponse, B. 1978. *Identities in the Lesbian World.* Westport: Greenwood.

Posner, R. A. 1992. *Sex and Reason.* Cambridge: Harvard University Press.

Prentky, R. A., and V. L. Quinsey, eds. 1988. Human sexual aggression: Current perspectives. *Annals of the New York Academy of Sciences,* vol. 528.

Price, J. H., D. D. Allensworth, and K. Hilman. 1985. Comparison of sexual fantasies of homosexuals and heterosexuals. *Psychological Reports* 57:871–877.

Price, R. A., K. K. Kidd, D. J. Cohen, D. L. Pauls, and J. F. Leckman. 1985. A twin study of Tourette syndrome. *Archives of General Psychiatry* 42:815–820.

Quigley, C. A., A. De Bellis, K. B. Marschke, M. K. El-Awady, E. M. Wilson, and F. S. French. 1995. Androgen receptor defects: Historical, clinical, and molecular perspectives. *Endocrine Reviews* 16:271–321.

Quinn, S. 1987. *A Mind of Her Own: The Life of Karen Horney.* New York: Summit.

Quinodez, J. M. 1989. Female homosexual patients in psychoanalysis. *International Journal of Psycho-Analysis* 70:55–63.

Racker, H. 1968. *Transference and Countertransference.* New York: International Universities Press.

Radmayr, C., Z. Culig, J. Glatzl, F. Neuschmid-Kaspar, G. Bartsch, and H. Klocker. 1997. Androgen receptor point mutations as the underlying molecular defect in 2 patients with androgen insensitivity syndrome. *Journal of Urology* 158:1553–1556.

Rado, S. 1940. A critical examination of the concept of bisexuality. *Psychosomatic Medicine* 2:459–467.

—— 1949. An adaptational view of sexual behavior. In P. Hoch and J. Zubin, eds., *Psychosexual Development in Health and Disease,* pp. 167–172. New York: Grune and Stratton.

—— 1956. *Psychoanalysis of Behavior: Collected Papers of Sandor Rado.* New York: Grune and Stratton.

Ramafedi, G. 1999. Suicide and sexual orientation: Nearing the end of controversy? *Archives of General Psychiatry* 56:885–886.

Rangell, L. 1991. Castration. *Journal of the American Psychoanalytic Association* 39:3–23.

Raphael, S. M., and M. K. Robinson. 1980. The older lesbian: Love relationships and friendship patterns. *Alternative Lifestyles* 3:207–229.

Redlich, F. C., and D. X. Freedman. 1966. *The Theory and Practice of Psychiatry.* New York: Basic.

Reiss, D., E. M. Hetherington, R. Plomin, G. W. Howe, S. J. Simmens, S. H. Henderson, T. J. O'Connor, D. A. Bussell, E. R. Anderson, and T. Law. 1995. Genetic questions for environmental studies: Differential parenting and psychopathology in adolescence. *Archives of General Psychiatry* 52:925–936.

Remafedi, G., J. A. Farrow, and R. W. Deisher. 1991. Risk factors for attempted suicide in gay and bisexual youth. *Pediatrics* 87:8679–875.

Remafedi, G., S. French, M. Story, M. D. Resnick, and R. Blum. 1998. The relationship between suicide risk and sexual orientation: Results of a population-based study. *American Journal of Public Health* 88:57–60.

Reynolds, A. L., and W. F. Hanjorgiris. 2000. Coming out: Lesbian, gay, and bisexual identity development. In R. M. Perez, K. A. DeBoard, and K. J. Bieschke, eds., *Handbook of Counseling and Psychotherapy with Lesbian, Gay, and Bisexual Clients,* pp. 35–55. Washington, D.C.: American Psychological Association.

Rice, G. 1999. Response to Hamer's Genetics and Sexual Orientation. *Science* 285:803.

Rice, G., C. Anderson, N. Risch, and G. Ebers. 1995. Male homosexuality: Absence of linkage to micro satellite markers on the X-chromosome in a Canadian study. Paper presented at the annual meeting of the International Academy of Sex Research, Provincetown, Massachusetts.

Rich, C. L., R. C. Fowler, D. Young, and M. Blenkush. 1986. San Diego suicide study: Comparison of gay to straight males. *Suicide and Life Threatening Behavior* 16:448–457.

Richardson, J. 1996. Setting limits on gender health. *Harvard Review of Psychiatry* 4:49–53.

Robinson, J. L., J. Kagan, J. S. Reznick, and R. Corley. 1992. The heritability of inhibited and uninhibited behavior: A twin study. *Developmental Psychology* 28:1030–1037.

Robinson, P., ed. 1989. Havelock Ellis. In Havelock Ellis, *The Modernization of Sex*, pp. 1–42. Ithaca: Cornell University Press.

Roiphe, H., and E. Galenson. 1972. Early genital activity and the castration complex. *Psychoanalytic Quarterly* 41:334–347.

—— 1973. Object loss and early sexual development. *Psychoanalytic Quarterly* 42:73–90.

—— 1981. *Infantile Origins of Sexual Identity*. New York: International Universities Press.

Rose, R. 1985. Psychoendocrinology. In J. D. Wilson and D. W. Foster, eds., *Williams Textbook of Endocrinology*, pp. 653–682. Philadelphia: Saunders.

Rosen, R. C., and J. G. Beck. 1988. *Patterns of Sexual Arousal: Psychophysiological Processes and Clinical Applications*. New York: Guilford.

Rosenstein, L. D., and E. D. Bigler. 1987. No relationship between handedness and sexual preference. *Psychological Reports* 60:704–706.

Rosler, A., and G. Kohn. 1983. Male pseudohermaphroditism due to 17-hydroxysteroid dehydrogenase deficiency: Studies on the natural history of the defect and effect of androgens on gender role. *Journal of Steroid Biochemistry* 19:663–674.

Rotheram-Borus, M. J., and J. Hunter. 1994. Suicidal behavior and gay related stress among gay and bisexual male adolescents. *Journal of Adolescent Research* 9:498–508.

Roudinesco, E. 1990. *Jacques Lacan and Co.* Chicago: University of Chicago Press.

Roughton, R. 1995a. *American Psychoanalyst* 29(4):15–16.

—— 1995b. Action and acting out. In B. E. Moore and B. D. Fine, eds., *Psychoanalysis: The Basic Concepts*, pp. 130–145. New Haven: Yale University Press.

Roy, A., G. Rylander, and M. Sarchiapone. 1997. Genetic studies of suicidal behavior. *Psychiatric Clinics of North America* 20:595–611.

Roy, A., N. L. Segal, B. S. Centerwall, and C. D. Robinette. 1991. Suicide in twins. *Archives of General Psychiatry* 48:29–32.

Royce, R. A., A. Sena, W. Cates Jr., and M. S. Cohen. 1997. Current concepts: Sexual transmission of HIV. *New England Journal of Medicine* 336:1072–1079.

Rudnytsky, P. L. 1987. *Freud and Oedipus*. New York: Columbia University Press.

Ruse, M. 1981. Are there gay genes? Sociobiology and homosexuality. *Journal of Homosexuality* 6:5–34.

Rutgers, J. L., and R. E. Scully. 1991. The androgen insensitivity syndrome (testicular feminization): A clinicopathologic study of 43 cases. *International Journal of Gynecological Pathology* 10:126–144.

Saghir, M. T., and E. Robins, E. 1973. *Male and Female Homosexuality: A Comprehensive Investigation*. Baltimore: Williams and Wilkins.

Salmon, G., A. James, E. L. Cassidy, M. Javaloyes, and J. Auxiliadora. 2000. Bullying a review: Presentations to an adolescent psychiatric service and within a school for emotionally and behaviorally disturbed children. *Clinical Child Psychology and Psychiatry* 5:563–579.

Sanders, A. R. 1998. Poster presentation, 149th annual meeting of American Psychiatric Association, Toronto.

Sanders, G., and L. Ross-Field. 1987. Neuropsychological development of cognitive abilities: A new research strategy and some preliminary evidence for a sexual orientation model. *International Journal of Neuroscience* 36:1–16.

Sanders, J. 1934. Homosexueele tweelingen nederl genesk. *Nederl. Genesk.* 78:3346–3352.

Sandfort, T. G., R. de Graaf, R. V. Bijl, and P. Schnabel. 1999. Sexual orientation and psychiatric disorders: Findings from the Netherlands Mental Health Survey and Incidence Study. NEMESIS. Poster presented at the Thirty-Fifth Annual Meeting of the International Academy of Sex Research, June 23–27.

—— 2001. Same-sex sexual behavior and psychiatric disorders: findings from the Netherlands Mental Health Survey and Incidence Study (NEMESIS). *Archives of General Psychiatry* 58:85–91.

Sandler, J. 1986. Reality and the stabilizing function of unconscious fantasy. *Bulletin of the Anna Freud Centre* 9:177–194.

Sandler, J., and A. Sandler. 1983. The "second censorship," the "three-box model," and some technical implications. *International Journal of Psycho-Analysis* 64:413–433.

Saudino, K. J., and R. Plomin. 1996. Personality and behavioral genetics: Where have we been and where are we going? *Journal of Research in Personality* 30:335–347.

Savin-Williams, R. C. 1994. Verbal and physical abuse as stressors in the lives of lesbian, gay male, and bisexual youths: Associations with school problems, running away, prostitution and suicide. *Journal of Consulting and Clinical Psychology* 62:261–269.

—— 1996. Self-labeling and self-disclosure among gay, lesbian, and bisexual youths. In J. Laird and R. J. Green, eds., *Lesbians and Gays in Couples and Families: A Handbook for Therapists,* pp. 153–183. San Francisco: Jossey-Bass.

Schacter, S., and J. Singer. 1962. Cognitive, social, and physiological determinants of emotional state. *Psychological Review* 69:379–399.

Schafer, R. 1968. *Aspects of Internalization.* New York: International Universities Press.

—— 1974. Problems in Freud's psychology of women. *Journal of the American Psychoanalytic Association* 22:459–485.

Schmidt, C. 1984. Allies and persecutors: Science and medicine in the homosexuality issue. *Journal of Homosexuality* 10:127–140.

Schrut, A. 1993. Is Castration anxiety and the Oedipus complex a viable concept? Presented at the meeting of The American Academy of Psychoanalysis, San Francisco, May 22, 1993.

—— 1994. The Oedipus complex: Some observations and questions regarding its validity and universal existence. *Journal of the American Academy of Psychoanalysis* 22:727–751.

Schwaber, E. A. 1985. *The Transference in Psychotherapy: Clinical Management.* New York: International Universities Press.

Science 2001. The human genome. 291:1145–1434.

Searles, H. F. 1965. *Collected Papers on Schizophrenia and Related Subjects*. New York: International Universities Press.

Segal, N. L. 1999. *Entwined Lives: Twins and What They Tell Us About Human Behavior*. New York: Plume.

Segal, N. L., M. W. Dysken, T. J. Bouchard Jr., N. L. Pedersen, E. D. Eckert, and L. L. Heston. 1990. Tourette's disorder in a set of reared-apart triplets: Genetic and environmental influences. *American Journal of Psychiatry* 147:196–199.

Seidman, S. N., and R. O. Rieder. 1994. A review of sexual behavior in the United States. *American Journal of Psychiatry* 151:330–341.

Sell, R. L., J. A. Wells, and D. Wypij. 1995. The prevalence of homosexual behavior and attraction in the United States, the United Kingdom, and France: Results of national population-based samples. *Archives of Sexual Behavior* 24:235–248.

Severino, S. K., and M. L. Moline. 1989. *Premenstrual Syndrome: A Clinician's Guide*. New York: Guilford.

Shaffer, D., P. Fisher, R. H. Hicks, M. Parides, and M. Gould. 1995. Sexual orientation in adolescents who commit suicide. *Suicide and Life Threatening Behavior* 25(Suppl): 64–71.

Shapiro, D. 1981. *Autonomy and Rigid Character*. New York: Basic.

Sheldon, A., and L. Rohleder. 1995. Sharing the same world, telling different stories: Gender differences in co-constructed pretend narratives. In D. Slobin, J. Gerhardt, A. Kyratzis, and G. Jiansheng, eds., *Social Interaction, Social Context and Language*, pp. 613–632. New York: Erlbaum.

Sherman, D. K., M. K. McGue, and W. G. Iacono. 1997. Twin concordance for attention deficit hyperactivity disorder: A comparison of teachers' and mothers' reports. *American Journal of Psychiatry* 154:532–535.

Sherwin, B. 1991. The psychoendocrinology of aging and female sexuality. *Annual Review of Sex Research* 2:181–199.

Siegel, E. 1988. *Female Homosexuality: Choice Without Volition*. Hillsdale, N.J.: Analytic.

Siegelman, M. 1974. Parental backgrounds of male homosexuals and heterosexuals. *Archives of Sexual Behavior* 3:3–19.

Slap, J. W. 1986. Some problems with the structural model and a remedy. *Psychoanalysis and Psychology* 3:47–58.

Slap, J. W., and A. J. Saykin. 1983. The schema: basic concept in a nonmetapsychological model of the mind. *Psychoanalysis and Contemporary Thought* 6:305–325.

Slijper, F. M. E., S. L. S. Drop, J. C. Molenaar, and S. M. P. F. de Muinck Keizer-Schrama. 1998. Long-term psychological evaluation of intersex children. *Archives of Sexual Behavior* 27:125–144.

Slimp, J. C., B. L. Hart, and R. W. Goy, 1978. Heterosexual, autosexual, and social behavior of adult male rhesus monkeys with medial preoptic-anterior hypothalamic lesions. *Brain Research* 142:105–122.

Slob, A. K., J. J. van der Werfften Bosch, E. V. van Hall, F. H. de Jong, W. C. Weijmar Schultz, and F. A. Eikelboom. 1993. Psychosexual functioning in women with complete testicular feminization: Is androgen replacement therapy preferable to estrogen? *Journal of Sex and Marital Therapy* 19:201–209.

Snow, C. P. 1959. *The Two Cultures*. Cambridge: Cambridge University Press.

Socarides, C. 1963. The historical development of theoretical and clinical concepts of overt female homosexuality. *Journal of the American Psychoanalytic Association* 11: 386–414.

—— 1968. A provisional theory of etiology in male homosexuality: A case of pre-oedipal origin. *International Journal of Psycho-Analysis* 49:27–37.

—— 1978. *Homosexuality*. New York: Jason Aronson.

Sokal, A., and J. Bricmont. 1998. *Fashionable Nonsense: Postmodern Intellectuals' Abuse of Science*. New York: Picador.

Sophocles. 1947. *The Theban Plays: King Oedipus, Oedipus at Colonus, Antigone*. Trans. E. F. Watling. London: Penguin.

Stein, T. S. 1993. Overview of new developments in understanding homosexuality. *Review of Psychiatry* 12:9–40.

Stein, T. S., and C. J. Cohen. 1986. *Contemporary Perspectives on Psychotherapy with Lesbians and Gay Men*. New York: Plenum.

Stern, J. M. 1989. Maternal behavior: Sensory, hormonal and neural determinants. In F. R. Brush and S. Levine, eds., *Psychoendocrinology*, p. 149. San Diego: Academic.

Stoleru, S., M. C. Gregoire, D. Gerard, J. Decety, E. Lafarge, L. Cinotti, F. Lavenne, D. Lebars, E. Vernet-Maury, H. Rada, C. Collet, B. Mazoyer, M. G. Forest, F. Magnin, A. Spira, and D. Comar. 1999. Neuroanatomical correlates of visually evoked sexual arousal in human males. *Archives of Sexual Behavior* 28:1–23.

Stoller, R. 1968. *Sex and Gender: On the Development of Masculinity and Femininity*. Vol. I. New York: Science House.

—— 1975a. *Perversion: The Erotic Form of Hatred*. London: Karnac.

—— 1975b. Pornography and perversion. In R. Stoller, *Perversion: The Erotic Form of Hatred*, pp. 63–92. London: Karnac.

—— 1979. *Sexual Excitement: Dynamics of Erotic Life*. New York: Pantheon.

—— 1985. Gender identity disorders in children and adults. In H. I. Kaplan and B. J. Sadock, eds., *Comprehensive Textbook of Psychiatry* 1:1034–1041. 4th ed. Baltimore: Williams and Wilkins.

Stone, L. 1995. Transference. In B. E. Moore and B. D. Fine, eds., *Psychoanalysis: The Major Concepts*, pp. 110–120. New Haven: Yale University Press.

Stone, M. 1980. *The Borderline Syndromes*. New York: McGraw-Hill.

—— 1986. *Essential Papers on Borderline Disorders: One Hundred Years at the Border*. New York: New York University Press.

Sullivan, H. S. 1953. *The Interpersonal Theory of Psychiatry*. New York: Norton.

Sulloway, F. J. 1979. *Freud, Biologist of the Mind: Beyond the Psychoanalytic Legend*. New York: Basic.

Swaab, D. F., and M. A. Hofman. 1990. An enlarged suprachiasmatic nucleus in homosexual men. *Brain Research* 537:141–148.

Swan, G. E., D. Carmelli, and L. R. Cardon. 1997. Heavy consumption of cigarettes, alcohol, and coffee in male twins. *Journal of Studies on Alcohol* 58:182–190.

Taha, S. A. 1994. Male pseudohermaphroditism: Factors determining the gender of rearing in Saudi Arabia. *Urology* 43:370–374.

Thorne, B. 1993. *Gender Play: Girls and Boys in School*. New Brunswick, N.J.: Rutgers University Press.

Troiden, R. 1979. Becoming homosexual: A model of gay identity acquisition. *Psychiatry* 42:362–373.

Tyson, P. 1982. A developmental line of gender identity, gender role, and choice of love object. *Journal of the American Psychoanalytic Association* 30:59–84.

—— 1994. Theories of female psychology. *Journal of the American Psychoanalytic Association* 42:447–469.

Tyson, P., and R. L. Tyson. 1990. *Psychoanalytic Theories of Development: An Integration.* New Haven: Yale University Press.

Ursano, R. J., S. M. Sonnenberg, and S. G. Lazar. 1998. *Concise Guide to Psychodynamic Psychotherapy.* Washington, D.C.: American Psychiatric.

Valzelli, L. 1981. *Psychobiology of Aggression and Violence.* New York: Raven.

Wakefield, C. 1988. *Returning: A Spiritual Journey.* New York: Doubleday.

Walker, L. E. 1991. Post-traumatic stress disorder in women: Diagnosis and treatment of battered women's syndrome. Special Issue: Psychotherapy with victims. *Psychotherapy* 28:21–29.

Wallen, K., and J. E. Schneider, eds. 2000. *Reproduction in Context.* Cambridge: MIT Press.

Waller, N. G., B. A. Kojetin, T. J. Bouchard Jr., D. T. Lykken, and A. Tellegen. 1990. Genetic and environmental influences on religious interests, attitudes, and values: A study of twins reared apart and together. *Psychological Science* 1:138–142.

Wallerstein, R. S. 1986. *Forty-Two Lives in Treatment.* New York: Guilford.

Walsh, M. R., ed. 1987. *The Psychology of Women: Ongoing Debates.* New Haven: Yale University Press.

Warmington, E. H., and P. G. Rouse, eds. 1984. *Great Dialogues of Plato,* pp. 86–88. Trans. W. H. D. Rouse. New York: Mentor.

Weinberg, G. H. 1972. *Society and the Healthy Homosexual.* New York: St. Martin's.

Whitam, F. L., M. Diamond, and J. Martin. 1993. Homosexual orientation in twins: a report on sixty-one pairs and three triplet sets. *Archives of Sexual Behavior* 22:187–206.

Whitam, F. L., and M. Zent. 1984. A cross-cultural assessment of early cross-gender behavior and familial factors in male homosexuality. *Archives of Sexual Behavior* 13:427–439.

Whitam, F. L., and R. M. Mathy. 1991. Childhood cross-gender behavior of homosexual females in Brazil, Peru, the Philippines, and the United States. *Archives of Sexual Behavior* 20:151–170.

Wiedeman, G. H. 1962. Survey of psychoanalytic literature on overt male homosexuality. *Journal of the American Psychoanalytic Association* 10:386–409.

—— 1974. Homosexuality: A survey. *Journal of the American Psychoanalytic Association* 22:651–696.

—— 1995. Sexuality. In B. E. Moore and B. D. Fine, eds., *Psychoanalysis: The Major Concepts,* pp. 334–345. New Haven: Yale University Press.

Wilson, E. O. 1978. *On Human Nature.* Cambridge: Harvard University Press.

Winnicott, D. W. 1967. *Playing and Reality.* Harmondsworth: Penguin.

Wolf, M. E., and A. D. Mosnaims, eds. 1990. *Post-Traumatic Stress Disorder: Etiology, Phenomenology, and Treatment.* Washington, D.C.: American Psychiatric.

Wolfson, A. 1984. Toward the further understanding of homosexual women. Annual Meeting of the American Psychoanalytic Association, San Diego, May 4.

Wolmann, B. 1975. Principles of interactional psychotherapy. *Psychotherapy: Theory, Research and Practice* 12:149–159.

Wright, L. 1997. *Twins—and What They Tell Us About Who We Are.* New York: Wiley.

Wright, R. 1994. *The Moral Animal.* New York: Vintage.

Wurmser, L. 1981. *The Mask of Shame.* Baltimore: Johns Hopkins University Press.

Yates, A. ed. 1993. *Sexual and Gender Identity Disorders: Child and Adolescent Psychiatric Clinics of North America.* Philadelphia: Saunders.

Young-Bruehl, E. 1996. *The Anatomy of Prejudice.* Cambridge: Harvard University Press.

Zucker, K. J. 1991. Gender identity disorder. In S. R. Hooper, G. W. Hybnd, and R. E. Mattison, eds., *Child Psychopathology: Diagnostic Criteria and Clinical Assessment,* pp. 305–342. Hillsdale, N.J.: Erlbaum.

—— 1996. Commentary on Diamond's "Prenatal predisposition and the clinical management of some pediatric conditions." *Journal of Sex and Marital Therapy* 22:148–160.

—— 1999a. Intersexuality and gender identity differentiation. In R. C. Rosen, C. J. Davis, H. J. Ruppel Jr., and S. L. Davis. *Annual Review of Sex Research* 10:1–69. Mason City, Iowa: Society for the Scientific Study of Sexuality.

—— 1999b. Commentary on Richardson's 1996 Setting limits on gender health. *Harvard Review of Psychiatry* 7:347–42.

Zucker, K. J., and R. Green. 1991. Gender identity disorders. In M. Lewis, ed., *Child and Adolescent Psychiatry: A Comprehensive Textbook,* pp. 604–613. Baltimore: Williams and Wilkins.

Zucker, K. J., and S. J. Bradley. 1995. *Gender Identity Disorder and Psychosexual Problems in Children and Adolescents.* New York: Guilford.

Zucker, K. J., S. J. Bradley, G. Oliver, J. Blake, S. Fleming, and J. Hood. 1996. Psychosexual development of women with congenital adrenal hyperplasia. *Hormones and Behavior* 30:300–318.